Basic Child Psychiatry

Basic Child Psychiatry

FOURTH EDITION

Philip Barker

MB, BS, FRCP(Ed), FRCPsych., FRCP(C), DPM, DCH

*Professor of Psychiatry and Paediatrics, University of Calgary
Psychiatrist, Alberta Children's Hospital*

University Park Press
Baltimore

Fourth edition published in the USA and Canada by
University Park Press
300 North Charles St.
Baltimore, MD 21201

First published in Great Britain 1971 by
Crosby Lockwood Staples
Second and third editions published in
Great Britain by Granada Publishing Limited
in Crosby Lockwood Staples, 1976 and 1979
Fourth edition published in Great Britain
by Granada Publishing Ltd, 1983

Library of Congress Cataloging in Publication Data

Barker, Philip Alan.
  Basic child psychiatry.

  Includes bibliographies and index.
  1. Child psychiatry. I. Title.
[DNLM: 1. Child psychiatry. WS350 B255b]
RJ499.B27   1979   618.9'28'9   82–73567
ISBN 0–8391–1820–1

Printed in Great Britain

To Heather, Edmund, Elsa, Lorna, Brenda and Alice

Contents

Foreword   xi

Introduction   xiii

1   **Normal Development**   1
    The first year of life – The second year – The pre-school period –
    Middle childhood – Adolescence – Family Development

2   **Causes, Classification and Prevalence of Child**
    Psychiatric Disorders   20
    Causes – Constitutional factors – Physical disease and injury –
    Temperamental factors – Environmental factors – Classification
    of psychiatric disorders in children and adolescents – Prevalence
    of child psychiatric disorders

3   **Assessing Children and their Families**   39
    Taking the history – Examining the child – The family – Family
    interviews – The choice of assessment procedure – The
    formulation

4   **Conduct Disorders**   58
    Definition – Prevalence – Causes – Description – Juvenile
    delinquency – Treatment – Outcome

5   **Neurotic Disorders**   73
    Definition – Prevalence – Causes – Description – Anxiety
    neuroses – Phobic states – Obsessive-compulsive neuroses –
    Hysteria – Neurotic-depressive conditions – School refusal –
    Other neurotic syndromes – Treatment – Outcome

6   **Psychotic Disorders**   94
Infantile autism and other infantile psychoses — Disintegrative
psychoses — Schizophrenic psychoses — Affective disorders —
Suicide in children — Acute and subacute confusional states

7   **Enuresis, Encopresis and the Hyperkinetic Syndrome**   121
Enureses — Encopresis — Hyperkinetic syndrome of childhood

8   **Other Clinical Syndromes**   139
Adjustment reactions — Personality disorders — Tics and Gilles de
la Tourette's syndrome — Stuttering — Elective mutism — Epilepsy

9   **Specific Delays in Development**   161
Specific reading retardation — Specific arithmetical disorders —
Language disorders — Articulation disorders — Specific motor
retardation — Mixed developmental disorders

10   **Psychosomatic Disorders**   173
Causes — Description — Treatment — Outcome — Anorexia
nervosa

11   **The Psychiatry of Infants and Young Children**   184
Prevalence of disorders — Assessment of infants and young
children — Common problems — Sleep problems — Feeding
problems — Breath-holding spells — Thumb-sucking and
nail-biting — Treatment

12   **Emotional Disorders in Mentally Handicapped
Children**   193
Mental handicap — Prevalence of emotional disorders —
Causes and clinical associations — Treatment

13   **Disorders in Adolescence**   200
Prevalence — Unresolved childhood disorders — Disturbances
related to stresses of puberty and adolescence — Adolescent
drug taking — Adult-type mental disorders arising in
adolescence — Suicidal behaviour in adolescence — Treatment
of Adolescents

14   **Psychological Tests**   217
Intelligence tests — Tests of educational attainment —
Personality tests — Projective tests — Tests of specific psycholo-
gical functions — General points

15   Legal Aspects of Child Psychiatry and Problems of Child Abuse   227
Writing reports for courts — Child abuse — Sexual abuse and incest — Custody and access disputes

16   Treatment of Child Psychiatric Disorders   241
Individual psychotherapy — Help for the parents — Family therapy — Group therapy — Behaviour therapy — Drug treatment — Inpatient treatment — Day treatment — Alternative families — Educational measures — Speech and language therapy — Removal from parental care

17   Prevention of Child Psychiatric Disorders   268
Types of prevention — Primary prevention — Risk factors in primary prevention — Protective factors — Preventive measures — Secondary prevention — Tertiary prevention — Other points concerning prevention

References   279

Glossary   299

Index   308

Foreword

It is a pleasure to be asked once again, to write the Foreword to the fourth edition of Dr Philip Barker's book. In writing the Foreword for the third, I remarked on the speed of succession of new editions as pointing to the book's continuing usefulness and popularity. Once again this has obviously been maintained.

What are the changes incorporated in this new edition? As Dr Barker states in his Introduction, classification has been modified in order to incorporate that of DSM-III of the American Psychiatric Association and ICD-9, the more commonly used classification outside the North American Continent. This, which has obviously been a not altogether easy task, seems, however, to have been successfully accomplished.

As for the rest, the other new changes together with fresh topics included are again listed in the Introduction. Some, such as sleep apnoea and the use of lithium carbonate in adolescence, are subjects of considerable interest and along with other fresh developments reflect current changes in the practice of child and adolescent psychiatry. As in the case of previous editions, the text is highly readable and easy to assimilate. The avoidance so far as possible of technical jargon is commendable.

There are as yet few good books of moderate size on child psychiatry. This is surely one of them.

Sir William H. Trethowan
Professor of Psychiatry,
University of Birmingham.

Introduction

Like the earlier ones, this edition of *Basic Child Psychiatry* is intended to give the newcomer to the field the basic facts of the subject and guidance as to where to obtain further information. Perhaps the citing of a larger number of references in this new edition will also make the book of value to more advanced students seeking to further their reading in particular areas of child psychiatry.

I hope the book will be of use to undergraduate and postgraduate medical students, as well as to students of social work, child care, psychology, education, nursing and related subjects. In order to make it comprehensible to those working in a wide range of disciplines, medical and psychological jargon have been avoided as far as possible; such terms as have proved necessary are explained either in the text or in the glossary.

The book has once again been extensively revised to incorporate advances in the field. An important change has been the use of the third *Diagnostic and Statistical Manual* (DSM-III) of the American Psychiatric Association. This has been used along with the ninth edition of the *International Classification of Diseases* (ICD-9), to make the book useful worldwide. The multiaxial modification of the latter scheme for use in children, by Professor Michael Rutter and his colleagues at the Institute of Psychiatry, London, is also explained. DSM-III, of course, is already a multiaxial scheme. While the arrangement of chapters, and sections of chapters, is similar to that in the third edition, I have throughout explained how the various disorders being discussed are categorised, using each of the two methods of classification.

The section on encopresis has been completely re-written, with the aim of making the aetiology, types and treatment of this sometimes very distressing symptom even clearer than in previous editions. Substantial changes have been made to the chapters on the psychiatry of infancy and young children and on disorders in adolescence. Subjects mentioned for the first time in this edition include sleep apnoea, neurolinguistic programming, incest and its relevance in child psychiatry and the use of lithium carbonate in adolescence. There is also a new section on the assessment of young children. On the other hand, the section on epilepsy has been shortened, and emphasis has been placed on this subject's psychiatric importance: information on epilepsy and its treatment, which has become very much more complex in recent years, is readily available in textbooks of paediatrics and neurology.

The case histories are all from my own practice, except for the case of Quentin, the boy with snake phobia mentioned in Chapter 16; he was treated by Mary Browning, then psychologist at the Charles Burns Clinic, Birmingham. Names and other data which might identify the children or their families have been changed.

During recent years increasing use has been made of family approaches to the understanding and treatment of children's disorders. This development led me to wonder whether more material about families and their treatment should be included in *Basic Child Psychiatry*. After much consideration, however, I came to the conclusion that it would be better to leave this book as an introductory textbook of child psychiatry and instead to write another text on family therapy. Consequently the companion volume *Basic Family Therapy* was published in 1981 and should be regarded as complementing *Basic Child Psychiatry*. Although I have made frequent reference to the family approach to children's disorders in this book, and have included a short section on family therapy in Chapter 16, readers wanting to know about the family approach should refer to *Basic Family Therapy*. I hope that the two books, taken together, will provide a comprehensive and easily understood introduction to the whole area of the assessment and treatment of children, adolescents and their families.

As in the development of previous editions of the book, I have received much help from many colleagues, who are now becoming too numerous to mention by name. I should however like to acknowledge my debt to Dr Philip Connell, who originally introduced me to child psychiatry and taught me the basics of the subject. In the preparation of this edition I am particularly grateful to my wife, Heather, who not only typed the book but struggled at the same time to master a less-than-perfect word processing programme. She worked exceedingly hard in order to meet the publisher's deadline, something which would not have been achieved without her assistance. Karen McMordie also helped by proofreading the text, and for this I am most grateful. Responsibility for the contents, and any errors that may remain, of course remains mine. Once again Richard Miles, of Granada Publishing, has been helpful, supportive and courteous during the preparation of this fourth edition. It is enormously helpful to an author to have such an efficient and pleasant colleague with whom to deal.

Philip Barker.

CHAPTER ONE

Normal Development

Psychiatric disorders in childhood and adolescence have to be looked at against the background of the normal process of development from helpless infant to independent adult. When emotional, social and intellectual functioning are assessed, the range of normal for the child's age and social setting must be taken into account. What is normal is best learnt by contact with developing children and their families.

There are many theories of child development. Among the more important are the psychoanalytic approach of Freud (1905), Erik Erikson's psychosocial approach (1965, 1968) and the work of Jean Piaget, which has been concisely summarised by Beard (1969) and described more fully by Flavell (1963). Important contributions to the study of children's development have also been made by Anna Freud (1966) and Melanie Klein (1948). More recently the importance of the process of 'bonding' between parents and children has become clear; John Bowlby has made a study of this and has published a good, concise account of the process (1977), as well as books on attachment and related processes (1969, 1979).

This chapter can only sketch out the main features of child and adolescent development. Readers without first-hand experience with children of various ages should seek such experience, in addition to consulting texts such as those recommended in this chapter.

It must also be remembered that the development of children has to be considered along with that of the family, for child and family are always a unit in constant interaction. Family development will be considered after child development has been briefly reviewed.

The First Year of Life

Following birth, infants are totally dependent on those caring for them. They may respond in various ways however. Their responses in turn influence the behaviour of those looking after them. Thomas and Chess (1977) have shown that newborn babies show different *behavioural styles*. They distinguished nine traits: activity level, rhythmicity of biological functions (sleeping, eating, etc.), adaptability, approach or withdrawal in new situations, intensity of emotional reaction (to both pleasant and unpleasant situations), reaction threshold (the ease with which the child copes with changed circumstances), quality of mood, distractibility and 'attention span-persistence'. The course of events during infancy depends in part on the 'fit' between the child's behavioural style and the parents' temperaments and ways of reacting.

The first year of life is called the 'oral' stage by psychoanalysts because the baby's main satisfactions seem to arise from feeding and sucking things. Erikson (1965) calls this period that of 'basic trust versus basic mistrust'. This is the first of his 'eight ages of man'. A healthy outcome occurs when the child experiences the world, during this period, as nurturing, reliable and trustworthy. The child who has this experience develops the capacity for intimate relationships. The child who lacks this warm, nurturing experience may show impaired capacity for intimacy.

There is a rapid development of motor functions in the first year, culminating in walking at about one year, though the range of normal is wide. There are also big developments in social behaviour. By three weeks the child smiles at people's faces. At first this is a reflex response, but by six months children learn to distinguish people and will selectively smile at their mothers and other familiar people. This leads, at about eight months, to signs of fear and anxiety in the presence of strangers. Soon afterwards *separation anxiety* appears. This is anxiety upon separation from mother, especially if in an unfamiliar place or with unfamiliar people. It is a sign that the child has developed a close relationship with the mother. For this to occur it is necessary for the child to have been cared for constantly by the same person (mother or mother-substitute), and for there to have been a reasonably good 'fit' between the child's behavioural style and the parent's temperament. The process is called *bonding*.

Bowlby (1977) has described the development of *attachment*

behaviour in early childhood. This behaviour is characterised by the subject attaining or keeping physical proximity to the object of attachment. Such a child is said to have bonded to that person. In infancy this is commonly the mother. The process is held to be a biological phenomenon, characteristic of many primate species. Attachment theory conceives of this behaviour as being a class of behaviour at least as important as feeding and sexual behaviour, but distinct and different. Features of it in the first year are crying, calling, stranger anxiety and separation anxiety, these all being behaviours which tend to bring about proximity to the mother-figure. The theory states that an infant's attachment results primarily from the availability of a familiar figure. The more social interaction there is with the figure, the more likely it is the subject will become attached to the person. The process does not depend on gratification of needs. Indeed in monkeys attachment can occur to a soft, cuddly dummy as well as to a live mother monkey (Harlow, 1958).

By the end of the first year the child should have a close, secure relationship with mother (or mother-substitute), and an ordered pattern of feeding and sleeping should have been established. Fixed, rigid feeding schedules are not nowadays usual in western countries, and semi-solid foods tend to be introduced earlier, often at two or three months. These factors seem to make weaning less of a problem than it once was. Nevertheless giving up breast or bottle is one of the first demands made on the infant. Its successful accomplishment is a good augury for the many other changes required later.

Intellectual development proceeds rapidly in the first year. Piaget (Beard, 1969) calls the first two years of life the *sensori-motor period*. During this period children learn certain basic things about their relationship to the environment. They discover that objects exist apart from themselves, and continue to exist when they do not perceive them. They also learn simple cause-and-effect relationships. They come to understand spatial relationships, and acquire some idea of how one thing can symbolise another. All these processes, however, involve action by the child and depend on current sensory input and motor activity.

The Second Year

Rapid development continues in the second year. Children start to walk and so become able actively to explore their environments.

They also start to talk. More demands are made of them, particularly over bowel and bladder training and limiting their exploratory behaviour.

Erikson (1965) considers the main issue of the second year to be that of 'autonomy versus shame and doubt'. The child should develop a feeling of being in control of his or her self, combined with pleasant, self-confident feelings. These features contrast with feelings of shame and doubt about oneself and one's body. The acquisition of bowel and bladder control is an important process. During this period children should obtain pleasure from gradually gaining control of their sphincters, and indeed of their bodies generally. Erikson's views differ from classical psychoanalytic theory in that he does not relate anal activity and defecation to sexual gratification, to which he gives a less central role.

The successful performance of the developmental tasks of the second year requires a warm, secure relationship between children and their parents. In such contexts children want to please their parents, and will be made anxious by parental disapproval. They learn to inhibit or release their behaviour accordingly. This applies not only to bowel and bladder training (which may not be started until the end of the second year or even the third year), but also to motor behaviour generally.

Attachment behaviour should be well established by the second year (Bowlby, 1977). It contrasts with exploratory behaviour, which becomes possible once the child can walk. From a secure base the child can move into the environment to explore it, returning to mother when frightened or tired. As the child grows, the time and distance he can be away from mother or family base steadily increase.

Nevertheless some exploratory behaviour has to be limited. Chidren must learn not to play with fire, run out into the roadway, drop crockery on the floor and so on. There is usually some resistance to such learning, often expressed as temper tantrums. These commonly start in the second year and are a normal reaction when a child's wishes are not gratified. They can, nevertheless, cause great concern to an inexperienced mother, as when a previously well-behaved child suddenly starts throwing himself or herself on the floor, screaming, kicking and waving arms around. Normally, however, tantrums are a transient feature of the toddler period, which die away as children learn to accept the constraints placed on their behaviour by their parents and others. This process is of course greatly helped by a secure loving relationship between children and parents.

The development of speech and its comprehension considerably refine the process of communication between child and parents. These important features of the second and subsequent years are discussed more fully in Chapter 9.

The second year sees the end of Piaget's period of sensori-motor intelligence and the beginning of the period of *concrete operations of classes, relations and numbers.* This begins with the start of the acquisition of language, which occurs about mid-way through the second year, and extends up to about eleven or twelve years of age. It has a number of sub-stages. It will be discussed further in the following section.

During the second year, children continue to see themselves as the centre of their world and remain closely dependent on their parents.

The Pre-school Period (ages two to five)

During this period there is further development of intellectual functions, especially a rapid increase in the complexity of language used and understood (see Chapter 9). A big advance in socialisation is made; the child learns to live as a member of the family group. Because of the importance of the development of sexual identity and feelings, psychoanalysts have called this the 'genital stage'. It is the period during which the child learns his or her sexual identity; Erikson considers this period to be that in which the issue of 'initiative versus guilt' must be resolved. A successful outcome is a child who feels able to do many exciting, even almost magical, things as opposed to being frightened and guilty about taking the initiative. Erikson believes that failure at this stage results in a child who feels that others will be angry with, or even destroy, him if he does what he wants. Ideally the child should emerge confident in his abilities but with his impulses under adequate control.

Other features of this period are identification with the parents, and the consequent development of the motivation to do certain things, or be a certain kind of person; the beginning of conscience formation; the establishment of methods of dealing with anxiety and guilt; and the development of patterns of behaviour towards individuals outside the family. The child still feels at the centre of the world, and tends to consider inanimate objects as having feelings and opinions.

The establishment of the sex role starts with the acquisition of a general idea that people are divided into male and female categories. This is fostered by the different appearance, clothing and behaviour of the sexes. The child then comes to feel a member of one or other group. This is brought about partly through the child becoming aware of the anatomical differences between the sexes, and partly because of the operation of inborn biological factors. The parents are normally the child's main models of the male and female roles. Sex play, often with undressing or sexual exploration, is common at this time (Newson and Newson, 1968). Interest in the genitals of siblings and playmates is common and normal. As sexual awareness develops, the boy or girl is faced with the problem of his or her position *vis-à-vis* the parents, and there is often for a time a feeling of rivalry with the parent of the same sex for the affection of the other parent, the 'oedipal' stage. Normally this problem is resolved by close identification with the parent of the same sex. Its persistence in severe form beyond about six years of age is abnormal.

While the appropriate sex role is being adopted most children go through a period of uncertainty and curiosity on the subject. Fear of loss of male characteristics ('castration fears') in the boy and concern about lack of male genitals in the girl, are frequent causes of transient anxiety at this stage. Masturbation is so common in this period as to be a normal phenomenon. If sensibly handled it usually lessens in frequency or ceases; if it continues the child normally learns to avoid it at socially unsuitable times.

The development of conscience is important. It arises through the adoption of parents' standards, which in turn results from identification with the parents. The child comes to feel that certain types of attitudes and actions are right and others wrong, and thus feels guilty about activities which are in the 'wrong' category. The child made anxious in this way will often be unaware, at the conscious level, of the cause of the anxiety. It is due of course to the standards of the parents which have been made the child's own (or 'internalised'). Obviously if the child lacks a stable relationship with parents or parent-substitutes the process of conscience formation will be impaired. Conscience, and the capacity to feel guilty, tend to be poorly developed in children brought up in large impersonal institutions, and in those who have been moved frequently from one home to another during their early years.

Defence mechanisms are means whereby the individual copes with feelings of anxiety which might otherwise not be tolerable. Anxiety is a normal, indeed an essential, experience. It may arise from an act or threat from outside (for example the 'stranger anxiety' mentioned above), from the lack of familiar or expected objects or experiences, or from the operation of conscience. It may also be communicated, as from an anxious parent with whom a child is closely identified.

At first anxiety is directly expressed, but then it comes to be dealt with more often through the operation of 'defences' (or defence mechanisms) appearing in the pre-school period. Normal anxieties. are dealt with this way as are the abnormal anxieties occurring in psychiatric disorders. The use of defence mechanisms (or mental mechanisms) is in itself a normal process. A basic one is *repression*, the consigning to the unconscious of ideas not acceptable (because too threatening, anxiety-producing or otherwise intolerable) at the conscious level. The ideas or feelings repressed may, however, continue to influence the individual's behaviour and emotional state. They may be expressed in dreams, during hypnosis or in the course of psychoanalysis.

The repressed ideas may be denied at the conscious level, and actions or attitudes arising from them may be *rationalised*, that is an alternative consciously acceptable explanation given. Thus the child asked to go to the shops may say he is too tired or is frightened of the shopkeeper, but his reluctance may arise from repressed (and so unconscious) anxiety about what will happen to his mother while he is away, or a fear that she may play with his brother towards whom he feels (again perhaps unconsciously) some jealousy. *Compensation* is an attempt to make up for unconsciously felt inferiority; *reaction formation* is a more extreme form of compensation, the individual developing character traits or behaviour the exact opposite of the 'true', unconscious ones. For example, the individual who unconsciously wishes someone dead may consciously feel and show special solicitide and concern for that person.

Displacement and *projection* involve the transfer of feelings from one to another, more acceptable, object. Thus the child who hates his father may repress this and consciously express much of the hate towards, for example, his teacher. 'Projection' is the attribution of one's disclaimed characteristics on to another person. So the individual tempted by the desire to steal (about which he feels guilty) may repress this and unjustly attribute the propensity to steal to others.

Obsessional ideas are apparently irrational but nevertheless intrude into the consciousness. They have their origin in unconscious anxiety or guilt, and represent a sort of 'magical' way of dealing with guilt. Though seen as illogical, and resisted by the subject, they nevertheless continue to intrude themselves into consciousness. *Compulsions* are actions arising from such thoughts. Examples of 'normal' compulsions in children are avoiding the cracks in paving stones and touching lamp-posts as they are passed. Such actions are usually means of dealing with the normal anxieties of this period. Indeed, anxiety resulting from any cause in everyday life may be dealt with by means of these mechanisms. So may guilt feelings arising from the newly developed conscience. All these mental processes are, in themselves, normal phenomena which can be found operating in all of us.

Fantasy is important to children. A rich and vivid fantasy life is normal in children in the two- to five-year-old range, and persists into later childhood. It is a means of temporarily substituting for the real world, one in which desires and wishes can be fulfilled regardless of reality. Young children especially have a complex fantasy life, often expressed in play with other children and with dolls and toys. Despite their apparent involvement in such play, they normally remain able to distinguish fantasy from reality. Persistent inability to do so is a sign of deviant development. Children lacking siblings or friends to play with may invent imaginary playmates with names and detailed descriptions. They may carry on long conversations with them. One boy, an only child, always insisted on a place at table being set for his 'friend'. This ceased however soon after he started attending a nursery school at age four.

Fantasy ideas and play help young children to understand the world of which they are gradually becoming aware. Relationships such as mother–child, father–child, sibling–sibling, teacher–pupil and patient–nurse can be enacted and explored. The knowledge that it is all fantasy makes this safe and less anxiety-provoking than in real life. Children develop their own inner lives, partly corresponding to reality, partly fantasy, and the world can be distorted to meet their current emotional needs. As development proceeds fantasy becomes less prominent, but most adults nevertheless resort to it sometimes.

The term *transitional object* was given by Winnicott (1965) to items to which children develop enduring attachments, which are not part of the child's body nor objects (such as pacifiers) provided by the parents for oral gratification, and which appear to provide comfort and reassurance in stressful situations (Busch *et al.*, 1973). The object may be a piece of blanket or other material, a teddy bear or a toy of some sort. It is treated by the child as of special value. It may be cuddled or sucked and the child may want to take it every-where but especially to bed at bedtime. It is sometimes known as a 'security blanket'; it is believed to take the place, temporarily, of the mother to whom the child has been attached and to be a substitute for her in stressful situations when she is absent. It appears that transi-tional objects are not used by institutionalised infants (Provence and Lipton, 1962).

Transitional objects are by no means universal and Litt (1981), in a valuable study, found that they were significantly more common in a group of private paediatric patients than in a group of black lower-middle and lower income patients attending a clinic in Cleve-land, Ohio. Their use seemed to bear some relationship to the nature of the child-rearing practices used in their families. They are encoun-tered chiefly in the age range 2 to 5.

'Transitional phenomena' such as rituals, songs, stories and parti-cular movements, have been described as serving a similar function to transitional objects (Hong, 1978).

The pre-school period is one of rapidly increasing socialisation. By the end of it the business of learning to live in a group of three (the other two being the parents) should have been mastered. Progress should also have been made in coming to terms with any siblings, though some degree of rivalry at this stage is normal.

Temper tantrums usually continue in the two- to five-year age range but lessen in intensity and should have largely died out by the time the child starts school.

In many countries children have an organised pre-school experi-ence (nursery school, playgroup or kindergarten), before starting primary school at age five or six. This is usually a useful and con-structive experience, especially for children who lack siblings or neighbourhood friends of similar age. It is a first, gentle step into the world outside the family. The child can spend a few hours each day in a sheltered but warm and stimulating environment, in the company of other children of similar age and of understanding adults. This experience is likely to make it easier for the child to enter school.

The child's awareness of and curiosity about the environment increase rapidly in the two- to five-year period. This is a concomitant of intellectual development and advance in the use of language. Healthy children of this age are naturally curious about their environments. They want to know why things are as they are, how things work and what is their own relation to everything. This often results in the constant asking of questions about the what, how and why of a vast range of matters. Irrational fears are common.

Attachment behaviour continues to be readily activated until about the end of the third year. In the normally developing child it then becomes less readily elicited. Bowlby (1977) believes, however, that it remains a feature of the behaviour of a healthy person of any age.

The pre-school period comprises the first part of Piaget's 'period of concrete operations'. This is subdivided, the first section (about 18 months to 7 years) being a *pre-operational period.* This is again subdivided into a *pre-conceptual stage* (up to about four) and an *intuitive stage.* In the pre-conceptual stage children become increasingly able to represent one thing by another, so that they can use language symbols and can represent things by drawing them but they cannot yet form true concepts nor properly understand that an item belongs to a class of objects. Between ages 4 and 5 this sub-stage gives way to the intuitive sub-stage which is dealt with in the next section.

Middle Childhood (ages five or six to ten)

By the start of this period the child should have a clear conception of his position in the family group as well as a clearly defined identity as boy or girl. Psychoanalysts refer to it as the *latency period,* because psychosexual development has been considered relatively quiescent. This view has been questioned by Rutter (1971b). In many non-western cultures sex play and lovemaking have been found to be common in this period, and recent research in the USA has yielded similar findings. In western society there may be greater concealment of sexual interests and activities but they are nevertheless present. Masturbation in boys gets common as middle childhood proceeds. It is less common in girls. Heterosexual play also increases and Broderick and Rowe (1968), in a study of 1029 boys and girls in the age range 10–12, found definite evidence of a set of stages which most pre-adolescents go through on their way to 'social heterosexual maturation'.

Erikson (1968) calls this period the stage of *industry versus inferiority*. A healthily developing child gains satisfaction from doing the things which are taught, in one way or another, to children in all cultures at this stage. Children learn the 'fundamentals of technology' and come to enjoy the personal satisfaction, recognition from others and chance to relate to other people which result. The main danger is that the child will develop instead a sense of inadequacy and inferiority. This happens when children despair of their skills and capabilities or of their status among partners. The development of self-esteem is thus a central issue.

In western society the main formal vehicle for teaching skills to children is school, but instruction is also carried out in the home and in activities like Cub Scouts, Brownies, religious teaching groups and more informal associations with neighbourhood groups. Children's adjustment to school, and any other social groups they may enter, is a crucial matter. They must learn to cope with a more complex and less supportive social environment than the family group, as well as mastering reading, writing and numerical concepts. The teacher becomes an important person. Children's attitudes towards learning depend largely on their relationships with their teachers, though parents' attitudes are important too. Ideally parents and teachers should co-operate in the information and values they present and should complement each other.

Gradually the children get an idea of their capacities and limitations, as well as working out patterns of social behaviour which may be in various degrees active or passive, leader or follower, outgoing or inturning. Temperamental characteristics continue to be important determinants of the child's behaviour. Garside and his colleagues (1975) studied 39 temperamental attitudes in a group of 209 school children aged 5 to 7. They found that among 30 of these attitudes there were four clusters representing four dimensions of temperamental style: (a) withdrawal, poor adaptation and dependence; (b) high activity, intensity and distractibility; (c) moodiness and sulkiness; and (d) irregularity. Each of these features may thus be present in any degree in a child at this age.

During this period there is further development of the use of defence mechanisms against anxiety and guilt. This parallels the continuing development of the conscience. Children come to have their own patterns of psychological defences, depending partly on constitutional and partly on environmental, especially family, factors. Standards of social behaviour are further refined and ideas of right and wrong elaborated. The personality and attitudes which a child has acquired by the end of this period tend to persist into adult life.

Piaget describes the period from about 4½ to 7 years as the *intuitive sub-stage*. Children can give reasons for their actions and beliefs, but their thinking remains 'pre-operational'. Such thinking depends on immediate perceptions, rather than on mental representation of the relevant concepts. This imposes great limitations, including the attribution of causation to something which just happens to occur at the same time, frequent changes of opinion and a continuance of the young child's egocentric attitude. Life and feelings are still attributed to inanimate objects, and relationships between classes are not well understood. This stage is followed at about age 7 by the *subperiod of concrete operations*. This in turn continues until the onset of adolescence which marks the start of the period of *formal operations*.

The main changes in the concrete operational period are that children can internalise the properties of objects and their thinking becomes less egocentric. The capacity to internalise properties means that children can put objects in order, or classify them by size, shape or colour, without physically comparing them with each other. They can, as it were, arrange them in their minds and thus come up with answers much more rapidly. The other principal change affects play and activities with others. Previously children have mainly played on their own or in the company of others; now we see the start of co-operative play. Piaget considers this to be related to their increased capacity to perceive relationships.

Beard (1969) warns that at this stage thinking is still largely intuitive, however, and that the development of individuals is often more piecemeal than Piaget suggested. Children's verbal fluency may conceal the fact that they have not yet grasped concepts such as weight or numerical relationships — as when they know their multiplication tables by rote, but do not understand what they signify.

Adolescence

Adolescence starts at puberty. While emotional and physical development do not always go hand in hand, the onset of menstruation in the girl and seminal emissions in the boy are usually taken as marking puberty's onset. The age of onset is most often between eleven and thirteen in girls and between thirteen and seventeen in boys but the range of normal is wider. The biological changes are spread over a longer period of time. The pattern of production of sex hormones starts to change, in both sexes, between the ages of eight and ten. The physical changes, including a marked growth spurt, the growth of the genitals and of hair in certain parts of the body, and breast development in girls, are spread over several years. The period tends to be longer in boys (four to five years) than in girls (usually three to four years).

Erikson (1965) considers that the main issue to be dealt with during the adolescent period is that of *identity versus role confusion.* With the end of childhood proper, the youth must now achieve a view of his or her own identity and individual characteristics. By the end of the adolescent period the young person should know who he or she is, and be confident in making this identity known to the world. This personal identity becomes the basis for the individual's relationships. Those who have failed to negotiate this period success-fully do not know who they are or where they want to go in life. Identity formation has of course started much earlier in childhood, but the process intensifies during adolescence and should have been largely completed by the end of the person's teens.

The Group for the Advancement of Psychiatry, in a helpful little book on normal adolescence (1968), has defined four main develop-mental tasks. These are changing from being nurtured and cared for to being able to nurture and care for others; learning to work and acquiring the skills to become materially self-supporting; accepting and becoming proficient in the adult sexual role and coping with heterosexual relationships; and finally moving out of the family of origin to form a new family of procreation.

Adolescence sees a marked increase in heterosexual interests and activity. The early adolescent usually first makes tentative and unself-confident approaches to the opposite sex. In time these approaches become more direct and self-assured. By late adolescence the individual should be able to enter into relationships involving tender affection as well as sexual feelings. In due course the person becomes able to enter into deeper and more lasting heterosexual relationships. These processes enable the third and fourth of the above development tasks to be accomplished.

The ways in which adolescents' developing sexual feelings are expressed depend greatly on sociocultural standards and on family rules and restrictions. Masturbation is almost universal in boys, though less common in girls. Heterosexual activities start earlier in girls than boys, but precise information is hard to obtain. A study of English teenagers in the early 1960s (Schofield, 1965), showed the onset of dating and kissing to be usually between 13 and 16, but the range was much wider. By age 18 about one-third of the boys studied and one-sixth of the girls had had sexual intercourse, and there seemed to be evidence of a small group of very promiscuous girls. It is unlikely however, that a similar survey in England today would yield the same results and behaviour in other sociocultural settings would certainly be different.

In the lives of most adolescents peer group relations are very important. Adolescents make friends easily and deep, sometimes lasting relationships commonly develop, especially among girls. As well as having individual friendships, adolescents often belong to groups. These provide support for the members in the sometimes anxiety-provoking task of moving out of the family group to become autonomous adults. With group support adolescents can do things they could not manage on their own. Groups may be as small as two or three, but membership may run to ten, twenty or even more. An adolescent may belong to more than one group, and the membership of larger groups may change quite often. The influence of the group is often beneficial but can be harmful, as in the case of delinquent gangs.

Relationships with parents gradually change in the adolescent period. The nature of these changes has been reviewed by Rutter and his colleagues (1976) using especially the results of an epidemiological study in the Isle of Wight. It is clear from this research, and other studies reviewed, that parent—child alienation is not common, certainly at age 14 (the age group studied in the Isle of Wight). It may be a little commoner in late adolescence, but most adolescents trust their parents, share many of their parents' values and accept the need for parents to set restrictions and controls on their behaviour. The process of moving out of the family group thus proceeds smoothly and gradually in most instances. Research in both Britain and North America suggests that alienation, breakdown and overt rebellion are more characteristic of that small segment of the teenage population that is referred for psychiatric care.

The same review (Rutter *et al.*, 1976) used the Isle of Wight findings to discover whether 'inner turmoil' is characteristic of adolescence, as sometimes alleged. There was some support for this notion in that more than one-fifth of these 14- and 15-year-olds reported feeling miserable and depressed in response to a questionnaire and a similar proportion reported sleep difficulties. In psychiatric interviews with a sample of adolescents from the general population studied, nearly one-half reported some misery or depression, though only one in eight actually looked sad to the psychiatrist. Self-depreciation was less common, occurring in about 20 per cent, than reported misery. Only about 7 per cent of either sex had entertained suicidal ideas. There is thus some evidence of what might be called emotional turmoil, but in some cases it was apparently quite mild and just over half the group showed none at all.

Piaget calls adolescence the period of *formal operations*. This is characterised by much more flexible thinking. The main features, as summarised by Beard (1969), are the ability to accept assumptions for the sake of argument and to make hypotheses and set up propositions to test them, and the ability to look for general properties and laws in symbolic (especially verbal) material and so to invent imaginary systems and conceive things beyond what is tangible, finite and familiar. Adolescents also become aware of their own thinking, using it to justify the judgements they make, and they become able to deal with such complex ideas as porportionality and correlation.

The Group for the Advancement of Psychiatry (1968) has summarised the resolution of adolescence as being characterised by:

1. The attainment of separation and independence from parents.
2. The establishment of sexual identity.
3. The commitment to work.
4. The development of a personal moral system.
5. The capacity for lasting relationships and for both tender and genital sexual love in heterosexual relationships.
6. A return to the parents in a new relationship based on a relative equality.

The ease with which these developmental challenges are met depends largely on the adolescent's relationships with his or her parents. Developments earlier in childhood are thus crucial. The more secure relationships have been, the easier the handing over of responsibility to the young person will be. Despite widely differing sociocultural norms, it seems that the handover of responsibility by parents to adolescents usually goes quite smoothly. Serious emotional turmoil or disturbance are the exception, not the rule.

Family Development

Development does not stop when adolescence is superseded by adulthood. Erikson (1965) describes three more 'ages of man'. The first is that of *intimacy versus isolation.* The young adult, having completed his or her search for identity, is now ready for intimacy with others, in close relationships including sexual union. Failure at this stage results in isolation. Instead of developing close relationships the individual may isolate, or even destroy, forces and people that appear threatening in some way.

The next stage is that of *generativity versus stagnation.* The essence of generativity is the establishing and guiding of the next generation, not only, nor even necessarily, by parenthood, though for many this is central. Failure to achieve generativity leads to a sense of stagnation and personal impoverishment. The final stage is that of *ego integrity versus despair.* Ego integrity is the mature integration of one's life's experiences, people and things taken care of, triumphs and disappointments accepted. It is the feeling of things accomplished, and life lived satisfactorily. Failure to achieve ego integrity results in despair, a characteristic of which is fear of death due to the feeling that time is now too short to live another live.

The above three stages are of interest to those who work with children, since they describe the developmental stages through which parents and grandparents go. The adults in the child's world are the basis from which the family is created, and it is important to look at the stages of development of the family as well as those of the child. The functions of families and their development are discussed more fully in *Basic Family Therapy* (Barker, 1981a), and in books by Duvall (1977) and by Carter and McGoldrick (1980).

The first stage in family development is the courtship of a man and a woman. Following successful courtship the young couple form a group whose task is to teach any children they have about how to live in a family and also about the customs and cultural values of society. Fleck (1976) summarises the evolutionary tasks of the family as being 'effecting a marital coalition capable of forming a triad of parents and infant, nurturing and weaning the infant to enable it to exist as a body apart from the mother, and imparting language and intrafamilial modes epitomised by the resolution of the oedipal phase. The family must introduce the child into society in school and through 'peer relationships'. The family goes on to help the child through the developmental tasks of adolescence and finally to emancipation from the family group.

In other words the family is a developing system, and it must progress in the right way for the child's development to be healthy. A 'system' is made up of a group of dynamically interrelated and interdependent parts (in the case of a family the family members). The behaviour of the parts cannot be understood in isolation from the whole, which itself is more than the sum of the parts. Family systems are 'open' in that there is interchange between them and the surrounding environment. Every system has a pattern of functioning with built-in feedback mechanisms and a set of rules which determine how it operates. Family members are not consciously aware of the rules that govern their system, but the professional studying a family and its level of development needs to discover what they are. Systems theory and the investigation and assessment of family systems will be discussed further in the following two chapters. In studying developing children, the important questions about the family are whether the family system has reached a state of development such as to help its children through the developmental tasks they are currently facing, and also to see how each child's temperament and other characteristics are themselves affecting the system.

Duvall describes the following eight stages in family development:

(a) Married couples – without children.
(b) Childbearing families – oldest child from birth to 30 months.
(c) Families with pre-school children – oldest child 2½ to 6 years.
(d) Families with school children – oldest 6 to 13 years.
(e) Families with teenagers – oldest child 13 to 20 years.
(f) Families launching young adults – from first to last child's leaving home.
(g) Middle-aged parents – 'empty nest' to retirement.
(h) Ageing family members – retirement to death of both spouses.

Families are considered to be 'expanding' until the first child leaves home. This event usually marks the start of the 'contracting' phase, though occasionally additional children are born after the first child leaves the home.

The move from one of the above stages to the next involves, in each case, a change in the implicit rules governing the family system. Marriage partners are usually at first greatly influenced by their families of origin (Minuchin, 1974). Various compromises and adjustments are necessary to enable the two people to live together satisfactorily, and in some marriages these are not made and the relationship either breaks down or continues in a state of unhappiness or tension. Further changes in the rules are necessary as one stage succeeds another.

The extended family situation may also dictate alteration of the family rules, as when a grandparent or other relative dies, moves away from the area or comes to live in the family. Changes in the parents' employment, periods of unemployment, moving to a different place of residence and many other factors have their effects, great or small, in the developing family system.

Barnhill and Longo (1978) define nine 'transition points', based on Duvall's stages of family development. These are:

0–I   Commitment of the couple to each other.
I–II   Developing new parent roles, as husband and wife become father and mother.
II–III   Accepting the new personality, as the child grows up.
III–IV   Introducing the child to institutions outside the family, such as school, church, scouts, sports and so on.
IV–V   Accepting adolescence, with the various changed roles associated with this and the parents' need to come to terms with the rapid social and sexual changes occurring in their son or daughter.
V–VI   Allowing the child to experiment with independence in late adolescence and early adulthood.
V–VII   Preparations to launch, the term used by Barnhill and Longo for the acceptance by the parents of their child's independent adult role, including starting his or her own family.
VI–VIII   Letting go – facing each other again, when child-rearing is finished and the couple face each other as husband and wife alone again.

VIII–IX   Accepting retirement and/or old age, with the changed life
            style involved.

   Barnhill and Longo believe that families are especially subject to
stress when a 'family life cycle transition' has not been successfully
managed.
   In short, the family is a changing, open system with the task of
facilitating the development of its members. In turn the changing
needs and behaviours of the members cause shifts in the family's
rules and pattern of functioning. A complete assessment needs to
look at the individuals concerned and also the family system as a
whole.

CHAPTER TWO

Causes, Classification and Prevalence of Child Psychiatric Disorders

Causes

It is unusual to find a single clear-cut cause for a childhood psychiatric disorder. For the most part, child psychiatric disorders are not 'disease entities' like appendicitis or measles, but complex reactions to a variety of factors in a developing personality. Four main groups of factors require to be considered in every case:

Constitutional factors
The effects of physical disease or injury
Temperamental factors
Environmental factors

Constitutional factors

Constitutional factors are those with which the child is born. These result from the child's genetic make-up and any damage or ill-effects the foetus may have suffered during pregnancy or birth.

Few of the psychiatric disorders of childhood are known to be caused by *specific genetic factors,* though such factors are responsible for some forms of mental handicap (Penrose, 1972). In these cases the genetic effect is to cause low intelligence rather than bring about emotional disturbance, though emotional disturbance may be present also. *Phenylpyruvic oligophrenia,* or *phenylketonuria,* is a form of mental handicap inherited as a recessive trait, and due to a specific inborn enzyme defect; and the commonest distinct form of handicap, *Down's syndrome* or *mongolism,* is associated with the presence of an additional chromosome. Many rarer forms of mental handicap are also genetically determined.

It is possible that specific genetic factors contribute to disturbed behaviour in other ways. Some boys have an extra Y chromosome, so that their sex chromosome pattern is XYY instead of the usual XY. As a group, men and boys with this abnormality are unusually tall, though the height of some is within the normal range. There is also an association between aggressive and antisocial behaviour and the presence of an extra Y chromosome (Nielson and Christenson, 1974). Yet the association is not marked and most boys with an extra Y chromosome do not show such behaviour, while most who do show it do not have an extra chromosome.

More important than specific genetic factors are *polygenic influences.* These are the outcome of the operation of a combination of genes which together affect the probability of some disorder or characteristic being manifest. Whether or not the disorder does occur depends on the unique combination of environmental and genetic factors in each individual. The best way of determining whether polygenic factors play a part in causing a disorder is by the study of twins. If they do, the disorder under consideration will be commoner in monozygotic (MZ) twins (who are genetically identical) than in dizygotic twins (who are genetically dissimilar) brought up in the same environment. Another approach is to study MZ twins who are separated early in life, as by adoption into different families, and see whether there is concordance for the feature under study as often as in MZ twins reared in the same family. This shows the effects of different environments on genetically similar children.

Shields (1976) has reviewed the results of twin studies and has concluded that polygenic factors are marked in the case of intelligence, where they may account for up to 80 per cent of the variance in a population. This explains why intelligence may vary widely in children brought up in the same family. In some cases, however, as with children brought up in very adverse circumstances, the contribution of the environment may be much greater. It appears that a person's maximum intellectual potential is limited by his or her genetic make-up and that the right environmental factors are needed for this potential to be realised.

It appears also that children of exceptionally high intelligence may have difficulties in adjustment. Robinson (1981), in an excellent review, suggests that the very bright children he has studied may not fare as well as children of more modest abilities. However, research studies of this issue are lacking: many reports are anecdotal accounts of particular children whose high intelligence happened to contribute to difficulties for them in their particular families, peer groups and schools. Whether this is a common problem in 'gifted' children generally is unclear.

Personality variation is more difficult to measure than intelligence but it seems that here again genetic factors are important, if rather less so than with intelligence (Shields, 1976). Present knowledge suggests that some basic features of personality are genetically determined. These leave room for development to take various lines. They are rather like foundations which permit a variety of types of house to be built on them, but which, by their size, shape and strength nevertheless place definite limits on the final result.

Temperamental attributes, evident in early childhood, also appear to be determined to an important degree by polygenic factors (Torgersen and Kringlen, 1978). Genetic influences seem to have only minor effects upon conduct disorders and delinquency but are rather more important in the case of neurotic disorders.

An *adverse intrauterine environment* can affect the foetus in ways which influence subsequent psychological development. A number of diseases (for example rubella, toxoplasmosis and syphilis) transferred from the mother may affect the nervous system of the developing foetus. So also may an insufficient supply of oxygen.

There is evidence that injury at birth, and also premature birth, are associated with abnormal development or behaviour disturbance in later life. For example, a follow-up study of a group of 561 Edinburgh children born in the period 1953—1960 has shown that in children with lower birth weights there is a higher incidence of mental and of physical handicap, as well as of disturbed behaviour (Drillien, 1969). Since then, however, the development of intensive care units for the newborn seems to have helped improve the outlook for babies of low birth weight. Hack and her colleagues (1979) found that 82 per cent of surviving babies weighing between 1000 and 1500 grams at birth were developing normally two years later. The remaining 18 per cent had serious neurological or intellectual impairment, or both. Driscoll and his colleagues (1982) studied infants weighing less than 1000 grams at birth. Of 54 such infants admitted to a neonatal intensive care nursery 26 survived, though two died later. Of 23 followed up, 19 (83 per cent) were neurologically normal, though the overall complication rate, including mental retardation, was 30 per cent. Thus small babies are still at risk even though their outlook is better than it used to be.

The *foetal alcohol syndrome* is due to alcohol abuse by pregnant women. It consists of growth deficiency, various physical abnormalities and mental retardation. The physical abnormalities include short palpebral fissure, a thin upper lip and abnormalities of nose, eyes, ears and heart. The syndrome is reviewed by Little and Streissgath (1981).

The British Child Development Study involved nearly 16 000 children from birth through into their teens. When these children were assessed at age seven (Davie *et al.*, 1972), significant associations were found between 'social adjustment' (as measured by the Bristol Social Adjustment Guide, see Chapter 14) and birth order (first-born children being better adjusted than those born later); smoking in pregnancy (the mothers who smoked heavily having children who were less well adjusted at seven); period of gestation (the most favourable being 38 to 42 weeks); and birth weight, those with very low birth weights being less well adjusted. While these associations do not prove that the factors mentioned are causal, they do suggest the possibility that the developing child may be affected adversely during pregnancy and birth in such ways, even though there is no gross, obvious evidence of damage.

Physical Disease and Injury

Physical disease or injury may contribute to the development of psychiatric disorder. Brain disease or damage may produce impairment of intelligence, loss of particular motor or sensory functions, epilepsy or (probably) specific forms of abnormal behaviour like motor overactivity. It can also have less specific effects; in the Isle of Wight epidemiological studies, children with definite evidence of brain damage were found to have psychiatric disorders five times as often as the general child population, and three times as commonly as children with chronic physical handicaps not involving the brain (Rutter *et al.*, 1970).

Brain damage may be caused by injury, infection, metabolic

abnormality or tumour, and by some degenerative disorders of unknown cause. Development of the brain can also be adversely affected by severe malnutrition in early life. Exactly what effect this has on behaviour and intelligence is uncertain and study of the matter is made difficult by the usual association of malnutrition with other adverse social circumstances. It is probable however that intelligence is impaired. This complex subject has been helpfully reviewed by Ricciuti (1981). 'Non-accidental injury', usually by parents, is an established cause of brain injury in children. It too may accompany undernutrition, psychological neglect, or both (Scott, 1977).

Infections which may cause injury to the brain include various virus and bacterial diseases causing infection of the brain as a whole (encephalitis) and localised infection, which for example, may spread from the ear or paranasal sinuses.

Many inborn errors of metabolism have been discovered in the past few decades. These frequently cause mental retardation and other handicapping conditions (Ellis, 1980). There is disordered synthesis of a particular protein, often an enzyme, with consequent disruption of cell function. Examples include the lipidoses, in which fatty substances accumulate in the brain and other tissues; galactosaemia, in which the carbohydrate galactose accumulates; and errors of amino acid metabolism, such as *phenylketonuria, homocysteinuria* and *histidinaemia.*

Physical diseases not directly affecting the brain can also have psychological repercussions. They may act through the physical handicap they impose or the anxiety, or guilt, they cause in child, parents or both. The possible effects on a child of a severe physical handicap such as may occur in cerebral palsy, or of blindness, are obvious. Much can be done to enable such children to lead a full life and to prevent them developing emotional problems as complications of their physical ones. It often requires skill and patience, however, and a standard of care greater than that needed by physically healthy children. Many other chronic conditions, for instance diabetes, asthma, congenital heart disease and the various forms of dwarfism may cause emotional problems, through their physically handicapping effects, their possible restricting effects on the child's social life, the anxiety and fears of death they may cause, and their effects on the attitudes of family and perhaps friends and teachers.

Injuries, especially serious ones such as severe burns, can have similar effects, causing guilt in parents and children — each of whom may think the injury their fault. Anger, withdrawal and depression may also occur in the children and their families. But many years ago Woodward and Jackson (1961), at Birmingham Accident Hospital, showed in studies of burnt children that much depends on the way child and family are handled during treatment.

Temperamental Factors

There is evidence that adverse temperamental characteristics contribute to the genesis of psychiatric disorders in children. Thomas and Chess (1977), identified a subgroup of 'difficult children'. These showed irregularity of biological function, a tendency to respond to new stimuli by withdrawal, slow adaptation to changes in the environment, unhappy and unpleasant mood states and 'intense reaction', that is a relatively large behavioural response to an environmental stimulus. These features were identifiable before the age of two and the children with this cluster of characteristics more often later developed behaviour disorders. By contrast a group of 'easy children' showed a happy, contented mood, high regularity of biological functions, rapid adaptability, reactions to stimuli that were of low or mild intensity and a positive approach to new situations. These children developed behaviour disorders less often.

Graham and colleagues (1973) studied a group of mainly working class children in London and found a significant association of three temperamental characteristics — low regularity, low malleability and low fastidiousness — with later behaviour problems in school, as rated independently by the teacher. They concluded that temperamental characteristics probably act by making the child more vulnerable to family stress or other adversity. Thus what might be a passing problem in one family could, as a result of the parental reaction it evokes, lead to a big problem in another.

Although temperament seems to be in part genetically determined, environment apparently affects it as well. Indeed it is probable that the temperamental attributes of all family members are gradually modified over time as they interact with each other. Cameron (1977), in another study using data from the New York longitudinal study, has found that there are associations between temperamental changes over time in children, and parental characteristics. Seventy items on which parents were rated using interviews given them when the children were aged 3 were subject to cluster analysis. One cluster of parental characteristics was described as 'parental disapproval, intolerance and rejection'. These parental features were associated, by the second year, with daughters who were less persistent and less active in their reactions than the majority, and also with change in their daughters' temperaments over a 2–3 year period towards less adaptability and less positive mood.

An interesting study by Torgersen (1981) compared monozygotic (MZ) and dizygotic (DZ) twins at different ages, on the various temperamental variables described by Thomas and Chess (1977), at 2 months, 9 months and 6 years of age. At the first two ages the MZ twins were more alike on all nine of Thomas and Chess characteristics, and at 9 months the difference was statistically significant for all nine variables. At 6 years the differences between the MZ and DZ twins were much less, suggesting that environmental factors had modified the original genetically determined differences — not a surprising finding. So in this respect, as in many other areas of development, genetics and environment combine to bring about the final result. More interesting is the fact that the three factors identified as showing the least evidence for a genetic factor at age 6 — regularity, adaptability and mood — were identified by Thomas, Chess and Birch (1968) as risk factors for the development of behaviour disorders. (Withdrawal and high intensity were the other two so identified.) This suggests that environmental factors may be the principal, though not the only ones influencing the development of behaviour disorders in early and middle childhood.

Environmental Factors

The family environment is very important to the developing child. The family should provide a sheltered training ground in which the individual learns to live as a member of a society. Families are miniature societies in which children make their first attempts at adapting to others and in which they learn patterns of social behaviour which tend to persist throughout life. The child's family should facilitate development from a state of complete dependence in infancy to one of independence of the family in adult life. Poor early adjustment in family life is likely to be followed by poor adjustment in society at large. Attitudes towards parents may later become generalised and applied to a much wider circle of people. At any particular age too much must not be asked of children in the way of self-control and responsibility for their actions, but at the same time too much must not be done for them. If too much is done the process of growing up and becoming independent may be retarded. If too little, a child's level of anxiety may become intolerably great and psychiatric disorder may develop.

Childhood should thus be a process of gradual transfer of responsibility from parents to child. This process requires, for a background, a secure and stable family setting, with reasonably consistent and constant parent figures. This does not mean there must never be disagreements or arguments, or that members of the family will not sometimes become angry with one another or with the child. On the contrary, it is essential that children be exposed to a range of emotions and situations as they will be in adult life. The repression by parents of all their emotions would in itself be harmful to their children.

So the whole family must be considered when a psychiatric assessment is made of a child. Children who are deprived of a normal family group in which to grow up suffer a serious handicap. How well they develop depends partly upon their own personality resources, but largely upon the substitute environment in which they live.

In looking at environmental, especially family factors, use is being increasingly made of *general systems theory*. This was originally conceived by von Bertalanffy (1948) and has been found useful as a theoretical basis by many family therapists (Barker, 1981a). General systems theory deals with interactions and the rules which govern them, rather than with individual phenomena. As applied to families it involves 'viewing the family unit as a biosocial sub-system within a larger cultural-social system' (Brown, 1972). The family is regarded as a system made up of parts (its members) which are dynamically interrelated and interdependent. The behaviour of the parts cannot be understood in isolation from the whole, which is itself more than the sum of the parts. The system is 'open' in that it is in constant interaction with forces outside itself, in the wider sociocultural setting. It is thus a part of, usually, several 'supra-systems', such as the extended family, the neighbourhood network, the village, the tribe and so on. Families usually also contain sub-systems, such as parental, marital and child subsystems. Individuals can, and usually do, belong to more than one system, for example to systems at school or at work as well as in the family.

Every system has a *boundary*. Certain materials, feelings and communications can pass through the boundary and others cannot. It is thus selectively permeable in both directions. Some system boundaries are rigid and well defined, others are flimsy and blurred. The more rigid the boundary, the harder communication across it is; the more flimsy, the easier communication becomes. Minuchin (1974) uses the term 'disengagement' for situations in which there is a very rigid boundary and 'enmeshment' for situations in which there is a weak boundary.

All systems are governed by rules. In family systems the members are not aware of most of the rules, which nevertheless operate powerfully to maintain the system. This process is often called 'homeostasis'. French (1977) has defined two processes, one of which is concerned with maintaining homeostasis, the other with changing the rules when necessary. Type I process involves all the mechanisms which maintain the steady state of the system, with its fixed reference points. Type II process involves a change in the reference points leading to a new and different homeostatic balance. The former is much easier to achieve than the latter and is always the preferred method that is tried in the face of stress. The latter is however sometimes essential, as when family circumstances change, and failure to achieve the necessary adjustments may precipitate symptoms in one or more family members.

Disturbed behaviour in a family member or members is often found to be associated with a 'dysfunctional' family system. That is to say the rules and way of functioning of the system depend on one or more members being symptomatic or disabled in some way. The family system is then not operating, as it should, to realise each member's potential for healthy development and constructive activities.

Haley (1976) has pointed out that central to many problems is a malfunctioning hierarchy. To take a simple example, consider a three-member family in which there is over-involvement of one parent and child, let us say mother and son, to the exclusion of the other parent. This can lead to various problems for the son who may become overdependent on the mother and in time get to be so immature and anxious that he develops school refusal (see Chapter 5). Instead of the parental couple helping the boy to grow up, one of them is keeping him a baby while the other is uninvolved in the family. That parent may instead have an intense involvement in his work or in some other relationship outside the family. Another possible outcome is obesity in the son, the focus of the close, involved relationship leading to the mother overfeeding the child whose weight problem then becomes another of her concerns: fruitless attempts at treatment and dieting can then perpetuate the dysfunctional over-involvement. In such cases a therapist's task would be to lessen the involvement of mother and son, and increase that of mother and father. The aim would be to change the subsystem pattern as follows:

Methods whereby this may be done will be discussed in Chapter 16.

Many other and more complex dysfunctional family patterns are possible. They may involve three generations, or even four; and extended family members, or even non-members of the family, may be important too. Dysfunctional systems can, and indeed often do, occur elsewhere, for example in schools, places of work and neighbourhood groups. The therapist wishing to understand a person's disturbed behaviour may have to look at systems such as these as well as at the family system, in order to do so.

The study of family systems has led to the identification of certain roles into which family members may be cast. A commonly used term is 'scapegoat', although it is not strictly accurate. The term has biblical origins, and the use of a scapegoat was one of the procedures laid down by Moses for use by the people of Israel. The priest was to lay his hands on the head of the goat and 'confess over it all the iniquities of the Israelites and all their acts of rebellion, that is all their sins' (New English Bible, 1970). Having laid the sins on the goat's head, the goat was to be sent into the wilderness to 'carry all their iniquities upon itself into some barren waste'. It is true that the 'scapegoated' family member (often a symptomatic child) appears to be the person upon whom all the family's problems and difficulties are projected, but that person is usually maintained in the family system, rather than being sent out into a barren waste. Some families depend on having a 'bad' child for their (often precarious) stability.

The 'acting-out', difficult child may be the only thing that keeps the parents, or the whole of the rest of the family, together. The symptomatic member may be the only subject the parents can be united about.

Another abnormal role is that of the 'parental' child. Some parental functions in relation to younger siblings may be appropriate for an older child, but if too much responsibility is given to the child — and especially if the delegation of authority is not explicit — the child may be unable to function as required and become symptomatic; or it may be that some other member presents as the identified parent. In extreme cases there is reversal of roles, the child taking care of the parent, while at the same time the inversion of roles is camouflaged (see Skynner, 1976, page 417).

While it can be helpful to regard the family as a system when trying to understand a child's current behaviour, it is clear also that past experiences can be very relevant. The quality of the parental care a child receives undoubtedly affects that child's development, and sometimes severe problems are seen in children who have been seriously deprived (Bowlby, 1961). Loss of a parent can also have serious effects. The effects vary and it is not only the actual loss, but also the circumstances preceding and following it that are important. The matter is discussed more fully in the book *Maternal Deprivation Reassessed* (Rutter, 1972).

Psychiatric disorder in a parent can adversely affect that parent's children. It seems that maternal depression increases the risk of pregnancy and birth complications (Zax *et al.*, 1977) and may also affect a mother's capacity to care for her child (Wolkind, 1981). Moreover depression is a common condition, especially in working class women (Brown *et al.*, 1975), and it seems to be associated with behaviour problems in the children (Wolkind, 1981).

A child's school environment is also important, as also is the wider social setting in which child and family live. The importance of the school environment was strikingly demonstrated in a study of secondary school children in London (Rutter *et al.*, 1979; Rutter, 1980a). After making careful allowance for the types of children admitted to different secondary schools, and the extent to which they were at risk, student outcome varied greatly according to the nature of the secondary school. Factors which favourably influenced behaviour and attainments were:

1. A reasonable balance between intellectually able and less able children.
2. The ample use of rewards, praise and appreciation by teachers.
3. A pleasant, comfortable and attractive school environment.
4. Plenty of opportunity for children to be responsible for and participate in the running of the school.
5. An appropriate emphasis on academic matters.
6. Good models of behaviour provided by teachers.
7. The use of appropriate group management skills in classrooms.
8. Firm leadership in the school, combined with a decision-making process involving all staff and leading to a cohesive approach in which staff members support each other.

This is an important study with major implications for the prevention of child psychiatric disorders.

The wider social environment is also important. The prevalence rates for psychiatric disorders − in adults as well as children − are much higher in inner city areas than in rural areas or small towns. Rutter (1981) has reviewed the relationship between city life and psychiatric disorder in his usual lucid and thorough way. He concludes that the reported differences in prevalence rates are real, though inner cities are not homogeneous; even within them prevalence rates vary a good deal.

The increased rates of psychiatric disorder apply to boys and girls, men and women and to crime, delinquency, depression and 'emotional disturbance' − that is neurotic disorders (see Chapter 5). It seems that various aspects of the ecology of cities, including the schools, contribute to the causation of these disorders. Although certain factors, notably those operative in the schools, affect children directly, many have their effect through the family. The greatest effect seems to be on 'early onset, chronic disorders in children which are associated with severe family pathology'. Rutter's (1981) article contains a fuller discussion of these issues and reference to the main relevant research findings.

In summary, children bring with them into their families, and later their schools and neighbourhood groups, certain genetic characteristics and temperamental styles. These are modified as a result of any organic brain damage or disease they may suffer, and also powerfully by their environments. Ideally, children's family, school and neighbourhood environments should be adaptively functioning systems into which they can fit to the mutual benefit of themselves and the other members of the systems. In that case the needs and assets of family members are mutually complementary. Sometimes they are not, however, and this is often due to a poor 'fit' between the temperaments and personalities of different family members, as well as to specific problems in individual members. But many severe individual handicaps are compatible with the absence of psychiatric disorder. Thus a boy with a severe learning disorder may do well if he is in a special class for learning-disordered children and belongs to a warm, accepting family which takes a constructive and helpful attitude towards his disability. Should either or both of these conditions not be met, psychiatric disorder may result. Indeed all the people in a child's environment — parents, siblings, other relatives, teachers, fellow-students at school, neighbourhood folk — contribute to that child's development as models for identification, people loved or feared and so on. At the same time each child has an effect, great or small, on the various systems of which he or she is a part.

It will be clear from the above that it is seldom possible to assign a single cause to a child psychiatric disorder. These problems are usually multifactorial in origin.

Classification of Psychiatric Disorders in Children and Adolescents

No entirely satisfactory classification of child psychiatric disorders exists, but recent years have seen the development of *multiaxial systems* which have already proved valuable. These systems provide a series of parameters, or axes, upon which every disorder must be classified. They avoid some of the problems of systems such as that proposed in 1966 by the Group for the Advancement of Psychiatry; this consisted of a list of conditions, some of which were defined on the basis of aeiology, others according to the psychopathology present, or on the subject's intellectual level or developmental course and so on. This approach is like classifying chalk along with cheese. By contrast, multiaxial schemes lay down the axes to be used, and each should have 'no abnormality' and 'information unavailable' codings. They can then separate out the clinical syndrome present from the aetiological factors and from level of intellectual functioning. This is important in dealing with disorders of multifactorial origin, as child psychiatric disorders usually are.

Two multiaxial systems are available. One (Rutter *et al.*, undated), devised at the Institute of Psychiatry, University of London, has the additional merit of being based, in four out of its five axes, on the ninth edition of the *International Classification of Diseases* (World Health Organisation, 1977a). The items in this classification have been subdivided so that those which cover clinical psychiatric syndromes form the first axis, those which cover 'specific delays in development' constitute the second, those dealing with intellectual level form the third and all the remaining codes in the ICD — that is all non-psychiatric disorders — make up the fourth axis. In addition, a fifth axis has been devised which deals with 'abnormal psychosocial situations'. This does not form part of the ninth edition of the ICD. Operational definitions are provided for all axes except the fourth. The main categories on the five axes are shown below.

Classification of the Main Categories (ICD–9)

Axis One (Clinical Psychiatric Syndrome)
Psychoses (290–299)

Code 290   Senile and Presenile Organic Psychotic Conditions
291   Alcoholic Psychoses
292   Drug Induced Psychoses
293   Transient Organic Psychotic Conditions
294   Other Organic Psychotic Conditions (Chronic)
295   Schizophrenic Psychoses
296   Affective Psychoses
297   Paranoid States
298   Other Non-organic Psychoses
299   **Psychoses Specific to Childhood**

Neurotic Disorders, Personality Disorders and Other Non-Psychotic Mental Disorders (300–316)

Code 300   **Neurotic Disorders**
301   Personality or Character Disorders
302   Sexual Deviations and Disorders
303   Alcohol Dependence
304   Drug Dependence
305   Non-Dependent Abuse of Drugs
306   Physical Conditions arising from Mental Factors
307   **Special Symptoms or Syndromes not Elsewhere Classified**
308   Acute Reaction to Stress
309   **Adjustment Reaction**
310   Specific Non-Psychotic Disorders following Brain Damage

311   Depressive Disorders not Elsewhere Classified
312   **Disturbances of Conduct not Elsewhere Classified**
313   **Disturbances of Emotions Specific to Childhood and Adolescence**
314   **Hyperkinetic Syndrome of Childhood**
316   Psychic Factors Associated with Diseases Classified Elsewhere

Axis Two (Specific Delays in Development)

No Specific Delay
Specific Reading Retardation
Specific Arithmetical Retardation
Other Specific Learning Difficulties
Developmental Speech/Language Disorder
Specific Motor Retardation
Mixed Developmental Disorder
Other Specified
Unspecified

Axis Three (Intellectual Level)

Normal variation
Mild Mental Retardation
Moderate Mental Retardation
Severe Mental Retardation
Profound Mental Retardation
Unspecified Mental Retardation
Intellectual Level Unknown

Axis Four (Medical Conditions) Includes all remaining codes in ICD.

Axis Five (Abnormal Psychosocial Situations)

No significant distortion or inadequacy of psychosocial environment
Mental disturbance in other family members
Discordant intra-familial relationships
Lack of warmth in intra-familial relationships
Familial over-involvement
Inadequate or inconsistent parental control
Inadequate social, linguistic or perceptual stimulation
Inadequate living conditions
Inadequate or distorted intra-familial communication
Anomalous family situation
Stresses or disturbance in school or work environment
Migration or social transplantation
Natural disaster

Other intra-familial psychosocial stress
Other extra-familial psychosocial stress
Persecution or adverse discrimination
Other psychosocial disturbance in society in general
Other (Specified)
Not known

In axis I, the items likely to be most used in childhood and adolescence are printed in heavy type, though any may be used.

The other multiaxial scheme is described in the third edition of the *Diagnostic and Statistical Manual* (DSM–III) of the American Psychiatric Association (1980). It is designed for use with psychiatric patients of all ages. It comprises five axes:

I   Mental disorders and 'conditions not attributable to a mental disorder that are a focus of attention or treatment'.

II Personality disorders (for adults and, in some cases, for children and adolescents); and specific developmental disorders (for children and adolescents and, in some cases, for adults).

III Physical disorders or conditions. These are to be classified according to a modification of the ICD–9 developed in the U.S.A. and known as the ICD–9–CM; this is similar to the ICD–9 but unfortunately just sufficiently different to cause confusion (Barker and Swinson, 1980).

IV Severity of psychosocial stressors. This is rated on a seven point scale, with also an 'unspecified' category. The seven grades of severity are:

Code Term	Examples (children and adolescents)
(1) None	No apparent psychosocial stressor
(2) Minimal	Vacation with family
(3) Mild	Change in school teacher; new school year
(4) Moderate	Chronic parental fighting; change to new school; illness of close relative; birth of sibling
(5) Severe	Death of peer; divorce of parents; arrest; admission to hospital; persistent, harsh parental discipline
(6) Extreme	Death of parent or sibling, repeated physical or sexual abuse
(7) Catastrophic	Multiple family deaths

V   Highest level of adaptive functioning in past year. This is coded
as in Table 1.

TABLE 1:   AXIS V OF DSM–III

Level	Examples (children and adolescents)
(1) Superior – Unusually effective functioning in social relations, occupational functioning, and use of leisure time.	A 12-year-old gets superior grades in school, is extremely popular among her peers, and excels in many sports. She does all of this with apparent ease and comfort.
(2) Very good – Better than average functioning in social relations, occupational functioning and use of leisure time.	An adolescent boy gets excellent grades, works part-time, has several close friends, and plays banjo in a jazz band. He admits to some distress in 'keeping up' with everything.
(3) Good – No more than slight impairment in either social or occupational functioning.	An 8-year-old boy does well in school, has several friends, but bullies younger children.
(4) Fair – Moderate impairment in either social relations or occupational functioning; or some impairment in both.	A 10-year-old girl does poorly in school, but has adequate peer and family relations.
(5) Poor – Marked impairment in either social relations or occupational functioning; or some impairment in both.	A 14-year-old boy almost fails in school and has trouble getting along with his peers.
(6) Very poor – Marked impairment in both social relations and occupational functioning.	A 6-year-old needs special help in all subjects and has virtually no peer relationships.
(7) Grossly impaired – gross impairment in virtually all areas of functioning.	A 4-year-old boy needs constant restraint to avoid hurting himself and is almost totally lacking in skills.
(8) Unspecified	No information

In axes I and II a very large number of conditions, many of them
symptoms rather than syndromes or specific disorders, is listed. The
conditions 'usually first evident in infancy, childhood or adolescence'
are divided as follows:

I   Mental retardation: various degrees of severity are listed.

II   Behaviour (overt)
　　　Attention deficit disorder
　　　Conduct disorder

III Emotional
　　　Anxiety disorders of childhood or adolescence
　　　Other disorders of infancy, childhood or adolescence; these
　　　include 'reactive attachment', 'schizoid', 'oppositional' and
　　　'identity' disorders and elective mutism.

IV   Physical
　　　Eating disorders
　　　Stereotyped movement disorders (various forms of 'tic'
　　　disorders)
　　　Other disorders of infancy, childhood or adolescence stutter-
　　　ing, enuresis, encopresis, sleep disorders.

V   Developmental
　　　Pervasive developmental disorders (see Chapter 6)
　　　Specific developmental disorders (these are classified under
　　　axis II (see Chapter 9).

Other categories which 'often will be appropriate for children and
adolescents' are:

Organic mental disorders   Somatoform disorders
Substance use disorders   Personality disorders
Schizophrenic disorders   Psychosexual disorders
Affective disorders   Adjustment disorders
Schizophreniform disorder   Psychological factors affecting
Anxiety disorders   physical condition

A strength of the DSM—III is that detailed operational definitions
are given for the various conditions named, with quite specific diagnostic criteria. Its categories, and the diagnostic criteria suggested,
will be discussed in later chapters when the various classes of child
psychiatric disorders are described.

The DSM—III has many limitations as a diagnostic system for
children (Rutter and Shaffer, 1980), not the least being the failure to
provide a separate axis for level of intellectual functioning. It also has
a tendency to elevate symptoms (pica, rumination and sleepwalking,
for instance) to the level of 'disorders'. It is nevertheless in widespread use in North America and has a number of helpful features.

Prevalence of Child Psychiatric Disorders

Several studies of the prevalence of psychiatric disorders in children have been carried out in Britain. The Isle of Wight study (Rutter *et al.*, 1970), was designed to cover all the 10- and 11-year-old children in the island in 1965. The researchers concluded that the prevalence of psychiatric disorders, as they defined them, in this island of small towns and rural areas was 6.8 per cent. Psychiatric disorder was considered present if 'abnormalities of behaviour, emotions or relationships were sufficiently marked and sufficiently prolonged to be causing persistent suffering or handicap in the child himself, or distress or disturbance in the family or community'. There were nearly twice as many boys with psychiatric disorder as there were girls.

A subsequent survey, by some of the same workers, in an inner London borough showed a rate of disturbance about double that in the Isle of Wight (Rutter, 1972). Prevalence rates thus vary considerably, and they probably vary also in different age groups. Leslie (1974) studied 13- to 14-year-olds in Blackburn, a British industrial town. Prevalence rates are given separately for each sex, the relevant percentages being:

	Boys	*Girls*
Moderate disorder	6.2	2.6
Severe disorder	14.6	11.0
Total	20.8	13.6

A study in an Australian town of about 2000 inhabitants suggested prevalence rates of 10 per cent in children and 16 per cent in adolescents (Krupinski *et al.*, 1967).

Psychiatric disorders in children and adolescents are thus a major problem affecting large numbers of individuals. The prevalence of particular types of disorder will be considered when the different syndromes are described, and the prevalence of disorders in young children is discussed in Chapter 11.

CHAPTER THREE

Assessing Children and their Families

A flexible approach is needed when assessing children and their families. Many psychiatrists prefer to interview child and parents separately, but some start by seeing the family as a whole. When child and parents are separated for the interview, the parents may be seen first. A disadvantage of this, however, is that the child may feel, often rightly, that the parents have been reporting unfavourably on him or her. This can make it harder to gain the child's confidence. On the other hand, if the parents have been seen first the interviewer is better aware of the nature of the problem and so can try to steer the course of the interview accordingly. With children the relative advantages of the two approaches are often evenly balanced. Adolescents, however, are usually best seen first and on their own.

Seeing the whole family together avoids the pitfalls inherent in seeing sections of it separately, though it can make it more difficult to obtain a comprehensive, factual history. Some psychiatrists believe that observing the family group together, and seeing how the members interact with each other, is more important than obtaining facts about the history and symptoms. Moreover facts can if necessary be ascertained by means of later interviews with family members. Increasing use is being made nowadays of family interview methods and allied to this is the increasing acceptance of the family, rather than the individual child, as the unit for treatment. Family interviews will be considered later after guidelines for assessing children and their parents in the more traditional way have been given.

Taking the History

If possible both parents should be seen, but sometimes only one, usually the mother, attends with the child. It is a good plan to state, when the appointment is made, that both parents should attend if possible. If only one can come on the first occasion, attempts should be made to see the other later. It is important that if at all possible both parents should be concerned with the study and treatment of the child from the start, even if one is a step-parent or they are unmarried.

It is best to let the parents start by talking freely about the problems which have led to the consultation. They should be allowed to explain the situation as they see it, in their own way and with a minimum of prompting. When they have finished speaking of one issue they can be asked if there are any others and if so, again allowed to explain in their own words. By thus allowing the parents to speak freely, information is often obtained about the nature of the relationship between the parents, as well as about the child's symptoms.

It is helpful to discuss the symptoms in terms of the changes the parents seek. If the parents complain of the child's behaviour at mealtimes, ask how they would like the child to behave. If they want a certain behaviour to stop — for example hitting a sibling — ask how the parents would like the child to respond in circumstances in which hitting occurs.

The development of symptoms, their duration and frequency, whether they are getting better or worse or are staying the same, and how the parents have tried to deal with them — and with what success — should then be explored.

The next step is to enquire about areas not yet covered. The principle ones are:

1. *Digestive system:* eating habits, pica, nausea, vomiting, abdominal pains, constipation, diarrhoea, faecal soiling.
2. *Urinary system:* bedwetting, wetting by day, over-frequent micturition.
3. *Sleep:* problems of going to bed and of sleeping, nightmares, night terrors.
4. *Circulatory and respiratory systems:* breathlessness, cough, palpitations.
5. *Motor system:* restlessness, overactivity, underactivity, clumsiness, tics, abnormal gait, motor weakness, whether right- or left-handed.

6. *Habitual manipulation of the body:* nail biting, thumbsucking, nose-picking, head banging, rocking and similar habits.
7. *Speech:* over-talkativeness, mutism, faulty speech of any type, including late development of speech and stuttering, comprehension of what is said.
8. *Thought processes:* poor concentration, distractibility, disordered thought, day dreaming.
9. *Vision and hearing:* any defects, evidence suggesting hallucinations.
10. *Temperamental traits:* rhythmicity, approach/withdrawal, adaptability, intensity of reaction, quality of mood, persistence/ attention span, distractibility, reaction threshold, activity level (Chapters 1 and 2).
11. *Behaviour:* follower or leader, relationship with siblings, parents, teachers, friends. Fearfulness, sensitiveness, tearfulness, sulking, irritability, temper tantrums. Obedience/disobedience, co-operativeness/negativism, constructiveness/destructiveness, truthfulness/untruthfulness, stealing, wandering from home, staying out late, group or gang membership, smoking, drinking, drugtaking. History of court appearance, probation or placement away from home.
12. *Mood:* whether mood is appropriate or child is depressed, elated, angry, fearful or showing evidence of other mood disturbance. Does the mood vary a lot? If so is this related to environmental circumstances or not?
13. *Sleep:* any problems in sleeping, nightmares, night terrors, sleep walking, excess sleepiness.
14. *Fantasy life and play:* the sort of games the child plays. Content of play. Does he/she have a lot of imagination? Dreams? Fantasy friends, transitional objects. Content of fantasy expressed through the foregoing, or in drawing, painting, conversation.
15. *Sex:* sex instruction given, sexual attitudes, masturbation, heterosexual or homosexual experiences, onset of menstruation, dysmenorrhoea.
16. *Attack disorders:* epilepsy, fainting, other alterations of consciousness, breath-holding attacks.
17. *School:* attitude to school, behaviour at school, progress in school work, social adjustment at school.

Do not look only for problems, but also note areas of strength and healthy function. Ask for examples of both strengths and symptoms, and note duration, frequency and severity. Observe also how parents describe symptoms: do they try to make light of the child's problem behaviour, or describe it in over-dramatic or rejecting terms, and so on? Interviews conducted in this way have been shown to be generally reliable, the main exception being in the area of relationship problems.

A series of studies of interviewing techniques has recently been published. These studies assessed the effectiveness of different approaches in eliciting facts and feelings from the parents of children referred for psychiatric assessment at the Maudsley Hospital (Rutter and Cox, 1981; Cox, Rutter et al., 1981; Hopkinson et al., 1981; Rutter, Cox et al., 1981; Cox, Holbrook et al., 1981). Left to themselves mothers raised most key issues, but suitable specific questioning was necessary to obtain 'good quality factual data'. An active, structured approach, used sensitively and while the interviewer is alert for clues to the presence of unusual symptoms, is best for eliciting facts. It is often important to establish the absence of certain symptoms as well as discovering which ones are present.

In eliciting feelings, the use of 'open' questions, a low level of talk by the interviewer, direct requests for the expression of feelings combined with interpretations and expressions of sympathy, seemed to be most helpful.

Some non-verbal behaviour was studied, but the results were not clear-cut; it is probable that this is important however (see Barker, 1981a, page 30).

The child's developmental history from the time of conception up to the date of the interview should be obtained. Information should be sought about the pregnancy; the child's birth and neonatal condition; subsequent progress; and any illnesses and injuries. It is useful to have a description of the child's behaviour as a baby, as a toddler, over the period of starting school and so on, up to the present date. Particular points are the acquisition of motor skills and of speech; toilet training methods and the child's response to them; past family and peer group relationships; and adjustment to school experiences.

Examining the Child

There is no set routine for the psychiatric examination of children. Much depends on the child's age, capacity and willingness to talk, and personality. In children below the age of about five, contact usually has to be largely through the medium of play, though even pre-school age children can sometimes reveal a lot about themselves in conversation. Older children, and especially adolescents, can often be examined rather as adult patients are. In the intermediate age range a mixture of play and conversation is used.

It is seldom the child who is complaining of symptoms, but an adult, usually a parent or teacher, who is either complaining on the child's behalf or more probably is objecting to some feature of the child's behaviour. So it is usually unwise to start the interview by discussing the presenting complaints. Indeed this can be a serious error; it can cause the child to identify the' person carrying out the assessment with other disapproving adults, and so develop a guarded or frankly suspicious attitude. A trusting relationship will be more difficult to establish.

The first step is to gain the child's confidence rather than to ascertain facts. The child must come to feel respected and valued, with a point of view and opinions that are important to the interviewer. The atmosphere in the consulting room should be relaxed and friendly, but not condescending. Toys, play materials and painting and drawing materials, appropriate to the child's age, should be available and in view. Younger children are best seen in a playroom. It is preferable not to have a desk between child and interviewer. To do so puts the child at a distance and makes *rapport* more difficult to establish.

It should be made plain to younger children that the materials and toys are there for them to play with and use as they choose. Some children do not at first wish to engage in conversation. This must be accepted and they should be allowed to play for a while. A conversation can then often be started while the child plays.

It is best to start talking with children on topics well away from symptom areas, such as how they got to the clinic, their interests and hobbies, games they like to play, any recent birthday, school, friends, siblings and ambitions for the future. If Christmas, Easter, Thanksgiving, a holiday or other such events have occurred recently, they can be discussed. Direct questioning about the symptoms is usually best avoided. The subject may well come up as the interview proceeds; if not, it often does not matter. This is especially so with children who have been engaging in 'antisocial' acts, such as stealing. There is little point in asking, 'Did you steal such-and-such?' If the question is answered at all, the child must say yes or no. If yes, the interviewer is none the wiser; if no, the child has been forced into the position of withholding information, which may damage the developing relationship with the interviewer and erect a barrier to communication. Still less should one say 'Why did you steal?' Such a question is futile. It tends to put the interviewer in the same category as other authority figures who may have been questioning, lecturing and perhaps punishing the child for whatever the problem may have been. While one wishes to understand why the child has been stealing it is naive to suppose that this can be done simply by asking. Often the child does at some point speak about the particular acts which have led to the referral, but this is a different matter.

The early part of the interview, sometimes the whole of the first session, is thus spent gaining the child's confidence. Once this has been achieved, at least in some measure, it is justifiable to ask, in a general way, what has brought the child to the clinic. An accurate reply is often given, but if not the subject should not be pressed.

Once *rapport* has been established with the child, particular areas may be explored. This should be done gently, using words and in a manner appropriate to the child's age and personality. It is not a matter of asking a series of direct questions; such an approach seldom gives the desired result. It is more a matter of saying, 'Lots of people have dreams when they are asleep at night . . . I wonder if you do?' The child who admits to having dreams can then be invited to recount one, and then perhaps asked whether they are mostly nice dreams, or mostly nasty ones. The child who denies having or remembering dreams may be told, 'Often when people who don't have dreams come to see us, they like to make up a dream . . . to pretend they've had one . . . perhaps you'd like to do that?' This is one way of exploring children's fantasy lives. Another method is to ask them to imagine that they have three magic wishes: what would they then most like to happen? One can then go on and say something like, 'Now I'd like you to pretend you were all alone on a desert island (or in a boat) and you could choose one person to be with you . . . anyone you like but just one person . . . I wonder who you would have?' It is then possible to get the child to choose a second, then a third person.

The interviewer should enquire for fears, worries, and somatic and other symptoms, in a similar way. Conversation about family, friends (whom the child can be asked to name and describe) and school is also encouraged. Throughout this process the interviewer must respond appropriately to what the child is saying, trying to share the child's sorrow at the loss of a pet or pleasure at being a member of a winning football team. Above all it is important to convey interest in the child's point of view. This does not necessarily imply approving of what the child does or thinks.

All children who have not reached adolescence should be invited to draw, paint and/or play with some of the toys. This enables their concentration, attention-span, distractibility and motor dexterity to be assessed. The content of their play frequently gives helpful information. Adolescents may or may not wish to paint, draw or play but it can usually be judged whether or not it is appropriate to suggest such activities.

By means of an interview such as has been described it should be possible to make an assessment of the following points about the child.

General Appearance
Are there any abnormalities of facial appearance, head, body build or limbs? State of nutrition? Is there any sign of bruises, cuts or grazes? Mode of dress and appropriateness for the climate and time of year? Does the child look happy or unhappy, tearful or worried? Attitude to the examiner and the consultation? Size in relation to age?

Motor Function
Is the child overactive, normal or underactive? Motor activities carried out? Are they done normally or clumsily, quickly or slowly? Are there any abnormal movements such as tics? Right-handed or left-handed? Can the child distinguish right from left? Is the gait normal, and if not, in what way is it abnormal? Can the child write, draw or paint? (If possible any productions should be preserved for future reference.)

Speech
Articulation, vocabulary and use of language should be noted. Does the child speak freely, little or not at all (as in mutism)? Is there any stuttering? Receptive and expressive language should be assessed, as well as the child's capacity to read and write.

Content of Talk and Thought
What does the child talk about? How easy is it to steer the conversa-

tion towards particular topics? Are any subjects avoided? Does the child's stream of thought flow logically from one thing to another? Is there any abnormal use of words or expressions? Any delusions or hallucinations?

Intellectual Function
A rough estimate of intelligence should be made, based on the child's general knowledge, conversation and level of play. (This may later be supplemented by administration of intelligence tests.) Knowledge of time, day, date, year, place and people's identity, compared with what is normally expected of a child of the age concerned.

Mood and Emotional State
Happy, elated, unhappy, frankly depressed, anxious, hostile, resentful, suspicious, upset by separation from parents and so on? Level of *rapport* which can be established with the child. Has the child ever wanted to run away, or to hide, wished to be dead or contemplated suicide? Does he or she ever cry? If so what about? Specific fears and if present how are they dealt with? Appropriateness of emotional state relative to subject being discussed.

Attitudes to Family
Indications during conversation about family members or during play.

Attitudes to School
Does the child like school? Attitudes towards school work, play, staff, other pupils? Child's estimate of own abilities and progress in school.

Enquiry into Fantasy Life
What would the child's three magic wishes be? Who would be his most desired companions on a desert island? What sort of dreams are recounted or made up? What is the worst thing — and the best thing — that could happen to the child; Ambitions in life? . . . and so on?

Sleep
Does the child have any difficulty in getting to sleep, with waking during the night or with disturbed sleep of any sort? This can often be enquired about when dreams or nightmares are being discussed.

Behaviour Problems
Does the child reveal anything about behavioural problems, delinquent activities, illicit drug or alcohol use, running away, sexual
activity or problems, or appearance in Court?

Placement Away From Home
Has the child been placed away from home? If so where, when, for
how long and why? Child's reaction to such placement.

Attitude to Referral
How does the child see the referral, and the reasons for it? Is he or
she aware of a problem and if so what?

Indications of Social Adjustment
Number of friends, hobbies, interests, games played, youth organisations belonged to and so on. Does the child feel a follower or a
leader, or bullied, teased or picked upon? If so, by whom?

Other Symptoms
Do any other points come up in conversation, for example, worries,
pains, headaches, other somatic symptoms, school problems, relationship difficulties and so on?

Play
A general description of the child's mode of play. What is played
with and how? To what extent is play symbolic? Content of play.
Concentration and constructiveness?

Children's behaviour should always be described as objectively as
possible. A useful concise description of how to go about this is
provided by Savicki and Brown (1981, Chapter 15).

It is often not possible to obtain all this information at the first
interview and more is usually obtained in subsequent sessions.
Clearly many of the points do not apply in non-speaking children.

Unless the child's physical state has already been assessed or is
being investigated by a colleague other than the interviewer, a physical examination should next be carried out. A convenient time to do
this is at the end of the first diagnostic interview. With younger
children it is helpful to ask the mother to come into the room during
the examination and if necessary help undress and dress the child.
This has the additional advantage of providing an opportunity to
observe interaction between child and parent.

Useful books on interviewing and examining children have been written by Simmons (1981) and by Goodman and Sours (1967). Rutter and Graham (1968) have investigated the reliability and validity of a procedure for interviewing children.

The Family

While the history is being taken, the background of each parent should be explored and at least a brief account obtained of the parents' origins and childhood experiences. The latter greatly influence the way parents bring up their own children. An assessment should be made of each parent's personality. It can be useful to ask each of them to make a self-assessment and also to describe their spouse's personality. Enquiry should be made about any psychiatric or physical illness in the family.

If the parents are interviewed together the way they interact should be noted. Is one of them dominant? If so, to what extent? Are they united about their children or are the children the subject of disagreement between them? What is the nature of the marital relationship?

Parental attitudes are very important. An estimate must be made of how far they are accepting or rejecting, anxious or relaxed, consistent or variable, protective or uninterested, tolerant or intolerant and, above all, loving towards their children.

Family Interviews

Increasing use is being made of interviews in which all family members are seen together, usually by one therapist but sometimes by two 'co-therapists'. This approach is the one normally used by family therapists although it need not necessarily be followed by family therapy. The assessment of families is discussed more fully in the companion volume *Basic Family Therapy* (Barker, 1981a).

Most family therapists view the family unit as a system (see Chapter 2) and are concerned mainly with current family functioning. The key to solving the problem, they believe, is to discover how the present situation is being *maintained,* and to understand what it is about the functioning of the family system that makes it necessary for one or more family members to have symptoms. Thus the focus is away from the historical development of the disturbed individual and away also from the intrapsychic processes; instead it is on the individual's current social situation. This makes sense in that most of the symptoms with which children present are *interpersonal,* that is they are concerned with how they relate to others.

In order to assess how a family system functions it is necessary to join it and participate in its transactions (Minuchin, 1974). A family cannot describe its system. The system can best be experienced by the interviewer who at the same time must not lose a sense of object-ivity, nor become emotionally involved with the family. This might cause the therapist to become an ally of or sympathiser with one or more members, or a critic or antagonist of others. It is helpful to approach the process in stages (see Haley, 1977).

1. *The greeting stage.* This consists of a period during which the family are greeted, and made to feel at home in a courteous, friendly and relaxed fashion. Haley recommends, however, that the therapist should note carefully the behaviour of the family, its seating arrangements, and mood, who tells whom to do what, who speaks and so on, while at the same time keeping con-clusions tentative.
2. *Setting the interview in context.* The interviewer shares with the family his or her understanding of the purpose of the interview, mentioning any contact there has been with the referral source, as well as explaining about anyone (supervisor or student) who may be watching through a one-way screen. If the interview is being recorded on audiotape or videotape, this also should be mentioned and permission obtained.
3. *The problem stage.* The first two stages will have taken a few minutes at most. This next stage is longer and involves asking the family what the problem is. It is often better to ask, 'What are the changes you want to achieve?' It is usually best to ask the parents first, then the children. By the end of this stage the therapist should have sought everyone's opinion on each issue that has been raised and enquired how they have tried to bring about the changes they seek. The therapist should also observe how people talk, who takes the lead and non-verbal as well as verbal behaviour.
4. *The interaction stage.* The therapist now drops out of the conver-

sation and allows the family to interact among themselves. It is sometimes necessary to encourage the family actively to do this by giving them a subject to discuss or a task to perform. It is better if they can act out their problems as well as talk among themselves. The family's 'structure' and way of functioning will usually become clearer during this period.

5. *Defining the changes that are wanted.* The therapist now reviews with the family the changes desired, and sets up a contract to work towards achieving these changes. It is helpful if all family members assent to the plan including the identified patient.

6. *Bringing the inverview to an end.* The interview ends with the setting of the time for the next appointment, if there are to be more, or discussion of any further investigations or measures that are suggested. The family should leave knowing what is to happen next, including who is to attend any therapy sessions and at what intervals of time. In addition many therapists give the family a task to do; this keeps them involved with the therapist and enables therapy to continue between sessions.

It is often possible to complete all the above stages in a single interview of an hour or so, but a second session will sometimes be necessary.

Many other schemes exist for the assessment of families. Minuchin (1974) lists six aspects which should be considered when families are assessed.

1. The family 'structure'. This consists of the arrangements which govern the transactions between members. It is discussed further in Chapter 16.

2. The flexibility of the family's patterns of functioning, and its capacity for change.

3. The family's 'resonance'. This is its sensitivity to the actions of individual members. At one extreme is 'enmeshment', that is, very high sensitivity, where the whole family at once reacts to counter any behaviour that deviates from the family pattern; at the other extreme is 'disengagement', where the sensitivity of the family system is low and there is little or no family reaction to behaviour in one member which deviates from the family pattern.

4. The family's life context. This consists of the sources of support and stress in its environment — the extended family, neighbours,

housing, work and school environments of family members and so on.

5. The family's developmental stage (see Chapter 1).
6. The ways in which the identified patient's symptoms are used to maintain the family's preferred way of functioning (its 'transactional patterns').

The McMaster (Epstein *et al.*, 1978) model of family functioning covers six aspects of family functioning and is another useful scheme for assessing families.

1   *Problem solving*

This concerns the way the family deals with problems serious enough to threaten its 'integrity and functional capacity'.

Problems are divided into two types: instrumental and affective. Instrumental problems concern such things as the provision of food, shelter and clothing for the family and also the family's financial stability. Affective problems are concerned with feelings; examples are serious hostility or distrust between family members. Some problems have instrumental and affective features, so that there is overlap of the categories. If instrumental problems are present there are nearly always affective problems also, but the reverse is not necessarily so.

The authors of the McMaster model list a series of stages in problem solving as follows:

(a) The problem must be identified.
(b) Its existence must be communicated to whoever needs to know about it, whether inside or outside the family.
(c) Various alternative plans of action need to be considered.
(d) Next, one of the alternatives must be selected and the decision taken to use it.
(e) Appropriate action should follow.
(f) The action taken should be monitored to ensure that what has been decided upon is properly carried out.
(g) Finally, there should be an evaluation of how successful the solution has been. The therapist will want to know whether the family learns from the success or failure of its problem solving efforts.

2. *Communication*

The McMaster model considers only verbal exchange. While the authors acknowledge the great importance of non-verbal communication they have not incorporated it into the model because of the practical difficulties of measuring and collecting data on non-verbal content.

Communication is subdivided according to whether it deals with instrumental or affective issues. Problems with affective communication are usually associated with problems concerning instrumental communication, but again the reverse is not necessarily the case.

Communication is also assessed in two other ways:

(a) Is it clear or masked? Or how clearly is the message stated?
(b) Is it direct or indirect? In other words is the message spoken directly to the person for whom it is intended, or does the speaker seek to convey the message through others? Here again there is a continuum between the two possible extremes.

3. *Roles*

These are the habitual patterns of behaviour that the members of a family display, and through which a family's various functions are carried out. Once again there are instrumental and affective aspects of family roles. In addition the family functions are broken down into:

(a) Necessary family functions: these include the provision of resources (an instrumental function); nurturance and support of family members and the sexual gratification of the marital partners (affective functions); and life-skill development and the maintenance and management of the family system (which have instrumental and affective aspects).
(b) Other family functions: these are functions unique to a family, such as the 'scapegoating' or idealising of a family member.

Other aspects of family roles are role allocation, the assignment of responsibility for certain family functions to particular members, and role accountability, which is the process of holding members accountable for the functions that have been allocated to them.

4. *Affective Responsiveness*

This is the capacity of family members to respond to stimuli of an emotional nature with feelings which are appropriate in both quality and intensity.

Two classes of response are recognised: 'welfare feelings' and 'emergency feelings'. Welfare feelings include love, tenderness, happiness and joy; emergency feelings include fear, anger, sadness, disappointment, depression and other related emotions.

5. *Affective Involvement*

This is a matter of the extent to which family members are involved in and value each other's interests and activities. A range of possible degrees of involvement exists. Epstein and Bishop list the following:

(a) Lack of involvement.
(b) Involvement devoid of feelings.
(c) Narcissistic involvement. This is involvement designed primarily to bolster the subject's own feelings of self-worth.
(d) Empathic involvement, based on a realistic understanding of the needs of those with whom the subject is involved.
(e) Over-involvement.
(f) Symbiotic involvement, seen only in seriously disturbed relationships.

6. *Behaviour Control*

This is the family's pattern for handling behaviour in three types of situation:

(a) Physically dangerous situations.
(b) When psychobiological needs and drives require to be met; this covers the control of behaviours such as eating, sleeping, elimination, sex and aggression.
(c) When there is a need to control the social behaviour among family members, and between family members and those outside the family.

Behaviour control obviously covers the control of children, but controls are necessary for all family members and satisfactory methods may or may not be in use.

Four styles of behaviour control are recognised by the architects of the McMaster model:

(i) rigid, with roles having very constricted and narrow standards;

(ii) flexible, where there is a reasonable standard and flexibility around it;

(iii) *laissez-faire,* where there is total latitude and 'anything goes';

(iv) chaotic, in which the style of control switches, usually unpredictably, from rigid to flexible to *laissez-faire*, so that no-one ever knows what to expect.

The Choice of Assessment Procedure

A fully comprehensive assessment will include both individual and family interviews. In some cases, however, one or other approach may be all that is necessary. Children being assessed away from their families, as in residential institutions or schools, may be best approached through individual assessments. When a child living at home is referred, especially if the presenting problems are being manifested in the home, a family approach may be more appropriate. In such cases individual interviews with child or parents may be needed later. This will certainly be true if there is evidence of severe psychopathology in one or more of the family members. Conversely, when individual interviews are done first, it may often become evident that an assessment of the whole family will be needed later. A well-trained clinician should be able to consider problems from both points of view and to carry out both individual and family interviews.

The Formulation

When the assessment of a child and family is complete, a formulation should be made. This is even more important than putting the child's disorder into a particular diagnostic category. In clinics and treatment centres where staff function as a team, the formulation is usually worked out at a conference attended by all members of the team; the same process should also be carried out by a practitioner working alone.

The formulation is a concise summary of the case in the light of all the information available. It should start with a brief statement of the current problem. This is followed by a description of how the clinician understands the case. It is helpful to look at:

(a) *Predisposing factors:* what factors in child or family predisposed to the development of the disorder? Constitutional (including genetic) factors and environmental factors should each be
considered.

(b) *Precipitating factors:* did anything precipitate the onset of the
problem, if so what? Here again constitutional, physical, temperamental and environmental factors should be considered.

(c) *Perpetuating factors:* what is maintaining the condition? Again
the four categories need to be covered.

(d) *Protective factors:* what are the child's and the family's strengths?
What factors are limiting the severity of the disorder and assisting
in healthy functioning?

The formulation is not just a listing of factors, but a description of
their interplay and relative importance. It should be a clearly written,
logical, dynamic explanation of the case, leading to a plan of treatment, management or further assessment. It should also give an
indication of the expected outcome. It is important that strengths
are mentioned as well as weaknesses. Where a 'problem-oriented' or
'goal-oriented' system of clinical recording is used, the formulation
should be the basis of the problem and strength lists. It is a good idea
to update the formulation from time to time during treatment. A
therapist's view of a case usually changes as treatment proceeds. The
following is an example of a formulation.

> Angela is a reserved, anxious twelve-year-old girl with a three-year history
> of failure to attend school despite three changes of school arranged by her
> mother at Angela's insistence. She is a physically fit, pubertal girl who
> apparently has from birth been a quiet child, slow to adapt to change and
> overdependent on her mother. The latter has long been unable to resist
> Angela's demands, and behaves similarly towards Angela's nine-year-old
> sister who seems, however, to have a more self-assertive personality than
> Angela, and is developing more independence than her sister. Before the
> onset of school refusal Angela did well at school and she appears to be of
> above average intelligence. Non-attendance was precipitated by a change to
> a stricter, male teacher and a period of illness in mother. Now attempts to
> get Angela to school result in panic and an acute exacerbation of anxiety
> symptoms. She has, however, a keen interest in horses and attends riding
> school on her own.
>   Mother and the two daughters have a close enmeshed relationship with
> each other; there is a clear boundary between their family subsystem and

father, who makes little contribution to the bringing up of the children and said little during a family interview. He spent part of his childhood in a group home. The whole family needs support over sending Angela to school. At the same time the relationship between the parents requires to be strengthened, and boundaries must be delineated between the parents on the one hand and the two daughters on the other.

Although the problem is a longstanding one, the parents are strongly motivated to receive help and are concerned about Angela's prolonged lack of education. Father seems to want to become more involved in the parenting process but at present lacks the necessary skills. In addition Angela is a physically healthy girl of above average intelligence whose progress when in school is good. She also has some interests outside the home, notably horse-riding. With treatment, which will have to deal with the family as a whole as well as with Angela's school attendance problem, substantial improvement seems possible. Angela may require some individual therapy and it is possible that a period of inpatient treatment will be of help.

Using the multi-axial classification described in Chapter 2 the diagnosis would have been as follows:

1st Axis: Neurotic disorder: anxiety state
2nd Axis: No specific delay in development
3rd Axis: Normal intelligence
4th Axis: No associated medical condition
5th Axis: Familial over-involvement (referring to the over-involvement of mother and Angela)
Inadequate or distorted intrafamilial communications (referring to lack of communication between parents).

Using DSM—III Angela's disorder would probably be classified as follows:

Axis I   309.21 Separation anxiety disorder
Axis II   V 71.09 No diagnosis on Axis II
Axis III   None
Axis IV   Psychosocial stressors: change of teacher; illness in mother.
Severity: 3
Axis V   Highest level of adaptive functioning in past year: 5 – Poor.

It will be seen that the formulation gives considerably more information than even a five-axis diagnostic scheme. On the other hand,
being a free-flowing literary vignette, it is not suitable for statistical
analysis nor for grouping disorders together for research or clinical
purposes.

Some of the inadequacies of the DSM—III are evident from the
above example. First, the term 'separation anxiety disorder' has
aetiological implications: although Angela's disorder meets the
diagnostic criteria for this disorder, it is an unfortunate oversimplification to regard Angela's symptoms as due entirely, or even mainly,
to separation anxiety. Another problem is that the DSM—III diagnosis gives no indication of the child's intellectual level, except by
omission.

CHAPTER FOUR

Conduct Disorders

Definition

Conduct disorders are characterised by antisocial behaviour. The *International Classification of Diseases* (World Health Organisation, 1977a) defines 'disturbances of conduct not elsewhere classified' as being disorders 'involving aggressive and destructive behaviour and involving delinquency'. The behaviour should not be part of some other psychiatric disorder such as a neurotic disorder (see Chapter 5) or a psychosis (Chapter 6), but 'minor emotional disturbance' may be present.

A useful definition of conduct disorder is that of Wardle (1974). He uses the term for disorders in which:

(a) The behaviour is socially disapproved.
(b) The behaviour includes 'acting-out' against people or property.
(c) The behaviour is persistent and fails to respond to normal sanctions.

The DSM–III (American Psychiatric Association, 1980) states that the 'essential feature' of a conduct disorder 'is a repetitive and persistent pattern of conduct in which either the basic rights of others or major age-appropriate societal norms or rules are violated. The conduct is more serious than the ordinary mischief and pranks of children and adolescents'. These disorders are divided into four subtypes by DSM–III:

(i) The undersocialised types. Here there is a 'failure to establish a normal degree of affection, empathy or bond with others'.

These are described as children who lack concern for the feelings, wishes and well-being of others. Their behaviour tends to be callous and they generally do not show guilt or remorse. They are egocentric children, lacking deeply felt emotional relationships with others.

(ii) The socialised types. These children show evidence of attachment to others but may be 'callous or manipulative' towards those to whom they are not attached. They lack guilt when 'outsiders' are made to suffer.

(iii) The aggressive types. These children show 'a repetitive and persistent pattern of aggression', violating the rights of others. The aggression may take the form of physical violence — assault, mugging, rape, homicide — or theft outside the home involving 'confrontation with a victim'. Thefts may involve extortion, purse-snatching or hold-ups.

(iv) The non-aggressive types. Here there is no physical violence against others, nor robbery outside the home with confrontation with a victim, but there is 'a persistent pattern of conduct in conflict with norms' for the subject's age. This may include repeated violations of important rules at home or school, persistent truancy, substance abuse, running away, persistent serious lying, vandalism, fire-setting, and stealing when it does not involve confrontation with a victim.

The DSM—III then gives diagnostic criteria for five categories:

(a) Conduct disorder, undersocialised, aggressive.
(b) Conduct disorder, undersocialised, non-aggressive.
(c) Conduct disorder, socialised, aggressive.
(d) Conduct disorder, socialised, non-aggressive.
(e) Atypical conduct disorder — defined by exclusion of categories (a)–(d).

The usefulness of the DSM—III's subdivision of conduct disorders is at present unclear. The distinction between 'socialised' and 'unsocialised' children probably is useful, though there is a continuum between the two extremes and the distinction is not always clear-cut. A study of disturbed boys, however, showed that those who were 'unsocialised aggressive' had fathers with antisocial personalities significantly more often than those who were not (Stewart et al., 1980), a finding which confirmed those of earlier studies.

Prevalence

Conduct disorders are the largest single group of psychiatric disorders in older children and adolescents. Satisfactory epidemiological data are lacking for younger children. In the Isle of Wight Survey (Rutter *et al.*, 1970) nearly two-thirds of the 10- and 11-year-olds with psychiatric disorders had conduct disorders. When the children with mixed neurotic and conduct disorders were included, the prevalence of conduct problems was 4 per cent. In the London borough studied later it was 12 per cent (Rutter, 1973). Leslie's (1974) survey of adolescents in Blackburn showed prevalence rates of 13 per cent for boys and 6 per cent for girls, on the basis of the sample seen by the psychiatrist.

As the prevalence figures indicate, conduct disorders are commoner in boys than in girls, and this is reflected in referrals to psychiatric clinics, appearances in juvenile courts and numbers in residential treatment and correctional settings.

Causes

Conduct disorder may represent a failure of the child to reach a normal adjustment within the family, or the family may be one that has itself failed to make a satisfactory adjustment in the wider community of which it is part. Children who lack a permanent family group, or its equivalent, are also particularly at risk. For example, those who have been moved repeatedly from one home to another, or who have lived in large impersonal orphanages, are likely to have special difficulty in acquiring socially desired standards of behaviour. This is partly because they lack consistent, permanent and stable parent figures with whom to identify. It has been shown that children who have been 'in care' earlier in childhood show significantly more deviant behaviour later in childhood, and that this most often takes the form of antisocial behaviour (Wolkind and Rutter, 1973).

It has been suggested that failure of early 'bonding' between mother and child may be a factor in causing the later development of antisocial behaviour. Since the development of socially acceptable behaviour is thought to be dependent on the development of secure, loving relationships between children and their parents (or parent-substitutes), the possible role of early bonding failure has been much discussed. Bowlby's theories concerning attachment (see Chapter 1), and the work of Winnicott, Dockar-Drysdale and Balbernie (Chapter 8) are relevant here. Rutter (1972) has also discussed helpfully the formation of bonds and the ways in which failure to form them may cause disorders in children.

Factors in the child are important too. Some children are easier to bring up than others. An extreme example of a child difficult to bring up to behave in an entirely socially acceptable way would be one who was seriously brain-damaged and mentally retarded. Such a child would not have the neurological capacities needed to become a normally socially adapted individual. The vast majority of children with conduct disorders do not, however, show evidence of either brain damage or mental retardation. But, as mentioned in Chapters 1 and 2, there are constitutional and temperamental differences between children, which affect how easy they are to raise (Thomas and Chess, 1977). The compatibility of a child's temperament and the temperaments of the parents is probably also important.

Antisocial behaviour *is* commoner in children with brain damage and with epilepsy, though in epileptic children the reaction of others to the fits, and the effects of medication (especially phenobarbitone – Chapter 16), seem sometimes to be the main factors. Thus when one child develops a conduct disorder and another does not, the reason may not lie entirely, mainly or even at all in different upbringing or parental attitudes. Too great an effort to explain the differences in terms of the children's respective environments may lead to an incorrect assessment and formulation.

Enviornment is none the less very important. The more stable, secure, accepting and consistent the family, the greater the chance of the child identifying with the parents and behaving as they wish – and as they do. Within the family, desired behaviour is normally encouraged verbally or in other ways, while undesired behaviour is discouraged or punished. Very often it is a matter of a smile or word of approval, or a frown or expression of disapproval. Sometimes more forceful methods, including corporal punishment, are used. The important points are that there should be consistent responses from people with whom the child has a warm relationship; a prompt response is helpful too. The younger the child, the more important promptness seems to be.

The type of reward also matters. Normally the parents' attention or approval are effective ways of reinforcing behaviour, while the withholding of attention and approval have the reverse effect. This seems to be because the parents' attention and smiles have become associated early on with more basic — or primary — reinforcers such as food. With children who have had unusual backgrounds, for example those who have lacked a constant mother-figure, social training may be more difficult. Nevertheless their behaviour is governed largely by the responses their actions stimulate. It may be that they only get consistent, approving attention from members of a delinquent gang when they indulge in antisocial behaviour. This influence may be stronger than that of an unstable, disorganised family.

Rejecting attitudes are often found in the parents of children with conduct disorders. These children have also been found to come from broken families significantly more often than neurotic children. Indeed broken homes have been found more often in the grand-parents' generation too (Wardle, 1961), and parents tend to bring their children up in the same way they themselves were brought up as children. Their own childhood experiences provide their internal model of parenthood. Rejection, lack of love and instability all militate against effective social training and against conscience forma-tion in the child. The process can be self-perpetuating, the child's antisocial behaviour causing the adverse parental attitudes to be intensified.

Other factors can contribute to the development of aggressive and antisocial behaviour. Fatherless households, in which are to be found one-tenth of the children in the USA, tend to be associated with aggressive and antisocial behaviour in boys (Biller, 1970). This may be due to the mechanism of reaction formation in boys who are concerned about their masculinity. Even in institutionalised boys, it seems that lack of contact with the father makes antisocial behavi-our more likely, whereas in girls a more important factor seems to be prolonged early experience of residential care (Wolkind, 1974). Large family size is also associated with an increased probability of anti-social behaviour in the children (Rutter et al., 1970). There is an association with social class, and even at age seven, lower class children have been shown to be more aggressive and destructive than middle class children (Newson and Newson, 1976). This may be due in part to different child rearing patterns. Neighbourhood and school also play their part. The existence of 'delinquent neighbourhoods' where antisocial behaviour is the cultural norm is well established. It is also clear that, even allowing for differences in intake, some schools have a much higher prevalence of antisocial behaviour in their pupils than others (Power *et al.*, 1972; Rutter, 1980a). This seems to be a function of their qualities as social institutions.

The development and maintenance of conduct disorders can also be undersood on the basis of systems theory as outlined in Chapter 2. This seeks to explain the behaviour of individual family members in terms of the functioning of the family system, that is its boundaries, rules, subsystem patterns and other features. An example of a severely dysfunctional family is the following.

> Robin aged eleven, had had long periods of treatment in two child psychiatric units because of his aggressive, disobedient, restless and generally difficult behaviour. When he, his two brothers, his sister and his parents were seen as a group, chaos was evident. Everyone spoke, or more usually shouted, at once and nobody seemed to be listening to what anybody else was saying. Instructions by the parents were ignored by the children: the mother was more active in issuing orders than father, who seemed to be in semi-retirement from the fray, but neither parent appeared to expect to be obeyed. All family members competed on apparently equal terms. There was no differentiated parental system, and no clear boundary between parents and children. Robin had become the identified patient perhaps because, as a big, strong, active and outgoing boy for his age, his antisocial behaviour was more threatening than that of the others. But the behaviour of the other children was little different. Only if the family changed could Robin or the others, change – unless they were removed to live long-term elsewhere, that is, in a different system.

When the family is investigated as a system, antisocial behaviour in one member may emerge as an important factor in keeping the family, or the parents, together. It may be found that the identified patient's misdeeds are the main topic of conversation and the principal focus of mutual concern. The symptoms are thus needed to maintain the family's precarious stability. There may however be severe problems in such areas as communication, role behaviour, organisational control or affective involvement; if these can be cleared up the identified patient's symptoms often disappear.

A 'systems' diagnosis and the types of causes listed earlier are not mutually exclusive. For example, a boy with certain temperamental characteristics may be better suited to the role of 'scapegoat' than the other children, or a dysfunctional family system may be more likely if father is absent. Similarly where the family, or part of it, is also part of a dysfunctional school or neighbourhood system, disorder in one of the children may be more likely.

The value of a systems approach is that it offers a rational and practical method of treatment. A therapist can often, by joining the system, and then helping change its way of functioning, bring about improvement. On the other hand, the elucidation of some other causes, while no less valid, may be less useful as a basis for therapy.

Description

The symptoms of a conduct disorder most often start within the family group. Early symptoms may be stealing, lying, disobedience and verbally or physically aggressive behaviour towards other family members. As the condition worsens these symptoms may spread and be manifest outside the family, notably at school but also in the neighbourhood. The child may be truant from school, stay out late, engage in frank delinquency (housebreaking, stealing from shops and cars and so on), run away from home and commit acts of vandalism and physical aggression. Failure in school work often accompanies conduct disorders, the child's hostile attitude to the adult world manifesting itself in refusal to take part in the activities of the school.

Conduct disorder symptoms do not always appear first within the family group. In adolescence especially they may appear when the child becomes involved in the activities of an adolescent gang. But even when symptoms are mainly, or entirely, manifest in such a setting there are often relationship difficulties within the family.

Both ICD–9 and DSM–III distinguish 'unsocialised' and 'under-socialised' from 'socialised' conduct disorders. The latter were first described by Jenkins (1969) who used the term 'group delinquent reaction'. Both the ICD–9 and DSM–III have adopted this concept, the DSM–III also dividing these disorders into aggressive and non-aggressive types, according to the type of activity in which the subjects engage.

ICD–9 includes, as symptoms of 'unsocialised' conduct disorders, disobedience, quarrelsomeness, aggression, destructive behaviour, tantrums, solitary stealing, lying, teasing, bullying, disturbed relationships with others and sexual misconduct. DSM–III further divides this group into aggressive and non-aggressive types. Running away is common in unsocialised delinquents and is discussed in Chapter 13.

There is an association between delinquent behaviour and drug abuse (Kraus, 1981). It seems that when the two behaviours co-exist the former usually precedes the latter. Kraus' findings did not support the view of delinquency as commonly arising out of economic necessity in those wanting money to buy drugs.

Truancy often accompanies other antisocial behaviour. It is different from school refusal, in which neurotic anxiety prevents the child getting to school. The truant is not prevented by anxiety, but by a stronger desire to do something else — for example, play in the park or just sit at home playing or watching television. In one common form the child leaves home, and returns there, at the appropriate times, but without having attended school. The parents think he is at school, and the school staff often conclude he is sick. It is surprising how long this can sometimes continue. If both parents work during the day the child may sit at home unknown to them, ignoring anyone from the school who comes to the house, and even destroying letters from the school. Some parents show little interest in ensuring that the child attends school, and do not regard school and its benefits as important. Sometimes parents actively encourage the truancy, perhaps to have help with housework or shopping, or with feeding the baby. Most truants are poor pupils at school (unlike school refusers who usually have good academic records), and their consequent failure to get satisfaction from school work is an additional factor in discouraging attendance. They tend to come from materially and culturally impoverished homes, a further contrast to school refusers, though some are rebellious teenagers from materially well-off homes.

Stealing is another common symptom. Like other features of conduct disorders, it only becomes abnormal when severe and persistent, and particularly when it is resistant to parental attempts to stop it. Certainly the vast majority of children take other people's property at one time or another. Persistent failure to respect the possessions of others is, however, a sign that psychological development is not proceeding smoothly. It is often associated with rejecting, inconsistent or indifferent parental attitudes.

Aggressive behaviour is a common cause of referral to child psychiatric clinics. It often occurs along with other conduct disorder symptoms. It can complicate the hyperkinetic syndrome, of which poor impulse control may be a feature (Chapter 7). Aggression often presents as temper tantrums.

Disapproved sexual behaviour may be one symptom, or even the main one, of a conduct disorder. Masturbation is so common as to be normal, as is sexual curiosity and an interest in the anatomy of the other sex. These may both be present in exaggerated form, or they may be manifested in a socially unacceptable, and perhaps unduly public, way. Sexual intercourse at an early age is another manifestation of failure to accept the pattern of behaviour laid down by the adult world. In many countries it is a criminal offence to have sexual intercourse with a girl who is below a certain age, usually between 14 and 18. While there may be no abnormality of psychosexual development, when boys or girls below the legal age are discovered to have had intercourse it is often regarded as indicating the need for special care or treatment.

There is a marked association between retardation in reading and antisocial behaviour in children (Rutter *et al.*, 1970). This applies to reading retardation generally but also to specific reading retardation, that is retardation greater than would be expected taking into account the child's age and intelligence quotient (see Chapter 14). In the Isle of Wight study one-quarter of the children with specific reading retardation showed antisocial behaviour, a very significantly larger percentage than in the general child population. The reasons for the association are not certainly established, but it is probable that many of the factors leading to antisocial behaivour also predispose to failure to learn to read — that is large family size, deprived and disturbed families and adverse temperamental factors in the child. In addition, failure in as basic a subject as reading may adversely affect a child's school adjustment; and conversely disturbed and antisocial behaviour in school may impair the learning process.

The following is an example of a severe conduct disorder, which had led on to frank delinquency, by the time of first referral for psychiatric assessment.

Paul was referred at the age of ten. He was reported to be one of a group of boys who had been staying out late, damaging public telephones, stealing from cars and breaking into shops and a school. He had also been truanting from school. His school attendance had been poor for two years, and his academic progress was well below average. He was usually badly dressed and dirty and he was considered a hostile and unco-operative pupil.

A few weeks earlier he had been placed in the care of the local authority by the juvenile court as beyond his parents' control.

At interview Paul answered questions guardedly and made no spontaneous conversation. He spoke in a matter-of-fact way and showed little emotion. He said he did not like either of the schools he had attended, and referred quite freely to his truancy and to having stayed out for periods of up to two days and nights, during which he said he and his friends slept rough. He showed little evidence of any affection for his parents, though he looked perhaps a little unhappy when speaking of how they argued. He said that on a desert island he would have three of his friends. His 'three wishes' were to go to London, to have a bicycle and go to Blackpool. His only ambition seemed to be membership of a pop group. Testing him showed him to be of low average intelligence, with marked retardation in both reading and arithmetic.

The parents' marriage had been far from happy. The parents had been separated for several short periods following rows. Father had also served a short prison sentence a few years previously. During this period mother had lived with another man and become pregnant by him, though this boy (aged four when Paul was referred) was accepted into the parents' household. An older brother had been educated in a residential school for disturbed children since the age of eight; he had been placed there because of repeated stealing and truancy.

Throughout Paul's childhood the parents' marriage had been precarious, he had no secure and consistent background for his emotional development and the parents had failed to set for him, or to demonstrate, any clear example of socially acceptable behaviour. Little interest was taken in his schooling, and indeed the parents were so preoccupied with their own problems that they had little time at all for Paul, who grew up insecure and without any strong relationship with anyone. He came to get most satisfaction from relationships with a delinquent gang, but mainly he lived for the moment. After full investigation, a recommendation was made that he should be placed in a residential school, to return to live at home during school holidays. Simultaneously a social worker undertook to try to give some help and support to the family, though the difficulty of doing so was recognised.

Comment

Paul had throughout his childhood been deprived of a stable, dependable background. He had lacked the relationships needed for normal psychological development. Apart from his rather dull intelligence (perhaps in part a consequence of his deprived background) there was no evidence of constitutional abnormality to account for his deviant development. In a more stable family he would probably have developed more normally, and indeed response to the treatment outlined above was good. His was a case of unsocialised conduct disorder. On the DSM–III Paul's order would be classified as a 'conduct disorder, undersocialised, non-aggressive'. Paul has now left school and, at follow-up, was well settled working in a factory.

Juvenile delinquency has already been referred to as a more severe form of conduct disorder. The point of progression to delinquency is arbitrary. Delinquency is usually taken to mean the commission of acts which are against the law and which could thus lead to police action. Alternatively, it has been defined as behaviour actually leading to appearance in court; but with the tendency to revise upwards the age of 'criminal responsibility', and the increasing use of other methods of dealing with children who break the law, this definition is of diminishing usefulness. Moreover, only a small proportion of individuals committing offences are brought to the attention of courts (Hood and Sparks, 1970).

Most boys who will later be convicted of delinquent acts can be distinguished by their trouble-making behaviour when aged between 8 and 10. Those who do fall foul of the law seem to be a special group distinguished, among other things, by the persistence of their delinquent behaviour.

Vandalism, the wanton damage to or destruction of property, is a form of delinquency that seems to be on the increase. It is often a group activity of adolescents. Whether done by a group or by an individual, it is usually a means of expressing hostile, aggressive feelings towards the adult world. These feelings often stem from a similarly disturbed relationship with the parents. In the child whose emotional development is following a healthy course, aggressive instincts are channelled into constructive activities (or 'sublimated'). Failure of such sublimation tends to be due to faulty relationships and identifications. Social factors may operate also; in many areas, especially urban ones, there are too few outlets available for the energies of young people. The influence of antisocially inclined groups can be important, the pressure to conform causing some of their number to commit destructive acts in which they would not otherwise engage. Closely related to vandalism is the raising of false alarms, for example sending for the fire brigade to attend non-existent fire. All these behaviours are common in socialised disorders of conduct but may occur also in the unsocialised variety.

Fire-setting or *fire-raising* is a less common but serious symptom.

Many children go through a phase of playing with matches and lighting fires but this usually responds to parental training and precept. Children who instead progress to starting fires at home, at school or elsewhere, are often expressing severe, deep-seated feelings of aggression arising from disturbed relationships with their parents.

One study of 860 child psychiatric outpatients showed that fire-setting occurred in 2–3 per cent (Vandersall and Wiener, 1970). Most of the children were referred because of impulsive behaviour such as stealing and disruptive behaviour at school. Their peer relationships were poor, the families tended to be severely disturbed and father absence was common; indeed in no case was a stable, effective father present in the home.

Similar findings have been reported by Gruber and his colleagues (1981) who also provide a bibliography on fire-setting in children. About 9 out of 10 fire-setters are boys. Gruber et al. comment on the 'tragic' life experiences of these children whose fire-setting however usually ceases when they are placed in residential homes providing good quality care. They suggest that earlier intervention in these families by child welfare agencies would be beneficial. Strachan (1981) found fire-setting to be predominantly a group activity.

ICD–9 also includes a sub-category of conduct problems, described as 'mixed disturbance of conduct and emotions'. Children with this group of disorders show conduct disorder symptoms, combined with considerable neurotic anxiety, expressed either overtly or through any of the other symptoms described in Chapter 5. In the Isle of Wight study (Rutter et al., 1970), it was shown that these 'mixed' cases had more in common with the antisocial group (most of whom had some neurotic symptoms) than with the neurotic group (who mostly did not have antisocial symptoms). This applied to sex ratio, family size and association with reading retardation. It probably applies also to treatment needs and results. Nevertheless, these children may be especially handicapped in that they have, very often, neurotically anxious families as well as unstable, disorganised or rejecting ones.

Treatment

As far as they are reactions to unfavourable and unhappy social, especially family circumstances, conduct disorders should ideally be treated by alteration of such circumstances. The problem is thus more one of work with the family, than of treatment of the child. This is well illustrated by the case of Paul, mentioned earlier, where the limitations of an approach confined mainly or wholly to treatment of the child are obvious. Paul's was a family problem, and if he was to change the family needed to change also.

Because of the complex causation of many conduct disorders, careful assessment is necessary to identify the important social, educational, medical and psychological factors in child and family.

In deciding upon the treatment needed, the structure and functioning of the family, the parental attitudes towards the child, the prospects of altering the family, the presence of psychiatric disorder in the parents (depression is often present), the role of temperamental and educational factors in the child and the duration and severity of the problems are important points. The less disturbed and better functioning the family, the greater the need to look for factors in the child, including possible associated problems like depression, neurotic disorder, epilepsy or brain damage. Another crucial matter is the degree of active co-operation which can be obtained from the family. Finally, the child's personality development to date, and the quality of his relationships and identifications, are important.

Having made such an assessment the treatment needs are usually fairly clear. Many milder problems require only a minor intervention. Indeed some conduct disorders subside without treatment. They may be little more than a testing-out of the limits of behaviour which are allowed. Commonsense advice to the parents about consistent and firm, but accepting, treatment may be all that is needed. On the other hand, the repairing of family relationships in severe cases may be a difficult and/or even impossible task. The parents may be emotionally immature, unhappily married and of limited intelligence, making effective help difficult to give. Many families are also burdened with other problems like poor housing and an inadequate income. There is a continuum from the family with only minor problems requiring brief counselling, through to those that are most severely socially and emotionally handicapped.

Where family problems are prominent, an approach by family therapy may be the best way of helping the child. This is especially so when assessment of the family suggests that the child's antisocial behaviour can be understood as a symptom of a dysfunctional family system. This is very often the case.

Individual psychotherapy for children with conduct disorders has generally poor results, though in some individual cases, where there is evident psychopathology in the child, it appears to help.

Behaviour therapy does seem to have a useful role in treatment. The persistent positive reinforcement of acceptable behaviour, combined with no response, or in some programmes a negative response, to undesired behaviour can be effective at home and in school classrooms, day treatment programmes and residential settings. Patterson (1971, 1976) has done valuable work in developing behavioural treatment programmes for children with conduct disorders.

Group therapy may be of help, and in socialised disorders of conduct treatment programmes which use peer pressure are often beneficial. The concept of a therapeutic community, which can be used in day and residential treatment programmes, aims to bring group pressure to bear on individuals displaying deviant behaviour. Related to this are programmes using 'positive peer culture' (Vorrath and Brendthro, 1976).

When a conduct disorder is severe and persistent, the child's development is going seriously awry, and treatment of the family is impossible or ineffective, residential placement away from home may be best. This should never be decided on lightly or without careful assessment, but sometimes a period in a residential treatment centre or a residential school, group home or foster home, or special therapeutic family placement offers the best prospect for the child.

In the treatment of truancy similar considerations apply. If the wider family problem can be solved the child will return to school; but if it cannot, or if it can only be expected to improve slowly, specific efforts must be made to get the child back to school. Indeed a direct, energetic attempt to overcome the truancy is usually advisable. Increased pressure to attend should be brought to bear directly on the child, and through the parents. Close liaison between school and parents is vital so that further absence is discovered at once and prompt and vigorous action taken. The threat of court proceedings, or their actual institution, may be justified and helpful. In some cases, however, the truancy is unconsciously or consciously motivated by the child's desire to get away from an unhappy situation. Antisocial behaviour which is so motivated may continue until this is achieved. If there is an associated educational problem, as there often is, this too should be tackled. If special help over seriously retarded reading or arithmetic is being given, the child's interest in attending may be much increased.

The treatment of severely deprived children presents special problems. Some children who have suffered severe emotional deprivation in early childhood, or through a long period of their childhood, lack the capacity to form deep and satisfying emotional relationships. Neither psychotherapy nor a simple change of environment is likely to be effective. The best hope of cure sometimes lies in a long period of treatment in a specialised residential setting. Theoretically a good foster home might be better still, but few foster parents have the resources to cope with such children, from whom they may get little response over a long period. Moreover, failure and rejection from the foster home would be a further adverse experience for the child. Some schemes have, however, been specially devised to select suitable alternative families, who are given continuing professional and group support (Hazel, 1977; Rubenstein, 1977; Barker et al., 1978). These schemes seem to offer a prospect of helping some children.

Drug treatment has little part in the treatment of conduct disorders, unless there is an associated condition such as epilepsy, depression, severe anxiety or hyperkinetic behaviour. Occasionally tranquillisers may be needed to control acutely disturbed or violent behaviour in these children, on a short-term basis.

The various treatments referred to in this section are discussed more fully in Chapter 16.

Outcome

Most minor, and some major, conduct disorders clear up without psychiatric or other treatment. Much depends on the stability of the family, parental attitudes, the willingness of the family to participate in treatment, the child's personality and capacity to form relationships and identifications, and any physical, intellectual or educational handicaps affecting the child. Children with severe conduct disorders, if not successfully treated, tend as adults to have a high incidence of psychiatric illness and often show antisocial and criminal behaviour (Robins, 1966; Rutter, 1980b). Such individuals often have difficulty in making stable marriages and thus put the next generation at risk also.

CHAPTER FIVE

Neurotic Disorders

Definition

Neurotic disorders are morbidly anxious reactions to stress, though sometimes the stress is slight. They are not associated with disordered perception of, or relation to, the environment as in psychosis. The concept of neurosis derived originally from the study of disorders occurring in adult patients, and some authors, for example Hersov (1976a), prefer the term 'emotional disorder'. DSM–III prefers 'anxiety disorders'.

The ninth edition of the *International Classification of Diseases* (WHO, 1977a) has a category for 'neurotic disorders' and another for 'disturbance of emotions specific to childhood and adolescence'. The latter are defined as 'less well differentiated emotional disorders characteristic of the childhood period', and there are the following sub-categories:

(a) With anxiety and fearfulness.
(b) With misery and unhappiness.
(c) With sensitivity, shyness and social withdrawal.
(d) Relationship problems.
(e) Other or mixed.

The DSM–III (American Psychiatric Association, 1980) has a section entitled 'anxiety disorders of childhood and adolescence'. These comprise:

Separation anxiety disorder.
Avoidant disorder of childhood and adolescence.
Over-anxious disorder.

In the adult section of this classification there are also codes for 'anxiety disorders' namely:

Phobic disorders (or neuroses) — 'agoraphobia', with or without panic attacks, 'social phobia' and 'simple phobia'.
Anxiety disorders (or neuroses) — 'panic disorder', 'generalised anxiety disorder' and 'obsessive—compulsive disorder'.
Post-traumatic stress disorder — which may be 'acute' or 'chronic or delayed'.
Atypical anxiety disorder.

Yet another section of DSM—III covers 'somatoform disorders'. These are divided into:

Somatisation disorder.
Conversion disorder (or hysterical neurosis, conversion type).
Psychogenic pain disorder.
Hypochondriacal (or hypochondriacal neurosis).
Atypical somatoform disorder.

Finally, DSM—III lists 'dissociative disorders' (or 'hysterical disorders, dissociative type'). These are divided into:

Psychogenic amnesia.
Psychogenic fugue.
Multiple personality.
Depersonalisation disorder.
Atypical dissociative disorder.

Most psychiatrists would probably agree that all the above categories describe expressions of anxiety, whether direct, as in panic disorder or generalised anxiety disorder, or indirect, as in obsessive—compulsive, conversion or dissociative disorders.

All of us are anxious from time to time, and it is natural for a child to be anxious for example, when going to a new school or meeting an unfamiliar adult. The normal child in such circumstances shows anxiety no greater than the situation merits, and is not over-whelmed by the anxiety. The neurotic or emotionally disordered child, by contrast, shows excessive anxiety which is severe and persistent and interferes in some way with his or her adjustment in society. It is often indirectly expressed, being dealt with by the various mental mechanisms or defences mentioned in Chapter 1.

Prevalence

Epidemiological studies show that neurotic disorders are the second commonest group of psychiatric disorders of childhood. In the Isle of Wight study (Rutter *et al.*, 1970) a prevalence rate of 2.5 per cent was found in the 10- and 11-year-olds studied, about half the rate for conduct disorders. In the Inner London Borough later studied, a prevalence rate twice that in the Isle of Wight was found (Rutter, 1973). In Leslie's (1974) study of teenagers in Blackburn conduct disorders occurred twice as commonly as neurotic disorders among boys, though a slightly larger number of the girls were diagnosed as neurotic.

Causes

The threshold for the development of neurotic anxiety varies from individual to individual. Some people develop neurotic symptoms only under great stress. Others develop them in response to everyday living. This variation in vulnerability is due in part to constitutional factors; previous experience is also important in determining a child's level of emotional development and tolerance of emotional stress. Relevant questions are: how much has the child been allowed to mix with other children or to make decisions for himself or herself? Has too much been done and decided for the child? How secure is the relationship with the rest of the family? These, and other related factors, all affect children's capacity to cope with particular situations. Some children are brought up by anxious, worrying parents, perhaps themselves suffering from neuroses. Children of parents who themselves see the world as an anxious, insecure place will tend to see it that way too.

The concept of emotional maturity is helpful. At any particular age, the normal child has learnt to cope with a range of emotionally stressful situations, and the extent to which a child can deal with stress without becoming excessively anxious is one measure of emotional maturity. Childhood should be a process of progressively decreasing dependence on parents, as the child learns to cope with more and more challenges without outside support. When this process has been slowed up, halted or even reversed, a neurotic disorder is likely to appear. Children who are faced with more anxiety and stress than they can cope with may regress to an earlier stage of development. The symptoms often express the child's conflicts in a symbolic way. 'Fixation points', a concept discussed more fully by Anna Freud (1966), are points at which psychosexual development is held up. This may result from excessive frustration, excessive gratification or a traumatic experience. The point at which fixation occurs depends on development to date: fixation will normally occur where a developmental phase has not been successfully negotiated nor the relevant conflicts resolved.

According to psychodynamic theory, consciously felt anxiety is always due in part, and often almost entirely, to causes of which the subject is unaware at the conscious level. The repressed conflicts are considered to be concerned with difficulties over the handling of sexual, aggressive and other impulses. Such difficulties are likely to arise in children who have experienced unsatisfactory and insecure relationships with their parents, especially during their first five years. The normal processes of development outlined in Chapter 1 have been distorted. The anxiety and guilt aroused by the Oedipal conflict, for example, are more easily, quickly and satisfactorily overcome in the context of secure relationships with the parents. If these relationships are tainted by anxiety and unpredictable gross changes of parental mood, the child will not overcome anxiety arising from the Oedipal situation and the various other demands of growing up. Not being able to depend on and trust his parents, the child may come to see the world as a threatening and hostile place. Parental factors are thus important in the genesis of neurotic disorders in children, but the reaction of children to them varies greatly. Some children seem able to cope with much more anxiety and instability in their families than others — probably because of constitutional and temperamental factors.

There are other views of the causes of neurotic symptoms. The 'behaviourists', among whom Eysenck (1959) is prominent, believe that neurotic symptoms constitute learned behaviour and are themselves 'the neurosis'. There are no underlying causes. Indeed the behaviourist of extreme views believes that all behaviour, 'normal' or 'abnormal', has been brought about by the effects on individuals of environmental contingencies. This view is not as much at variance with dynamic views as it might at first seem to be. Psychodynamic theories see neurotic (and other psychiatric) symptoms as having been learned as a result of the quality and nature of the intimate relationship between child and parents during infancy. An examination of the environmental contingencies operating then might show that they explained the development of the neurotic symptoms; and an examination of the contingencies operating during psychoanalysis (see Chapter 16) might explain how this process can remove neurotic symptoms. From a practical point of view, therapy based on learning theory appears to be of value in monosymptomatic or relatively uncomplicated neurotic states, such as specific phobias, but is less helpful in neurotic disorders with extensive symptoms.

The importance of the family in the causation of neurotic disorders has been mentioned, and some psychiatrists believe that often the whole family group is the basic unit suffering from the neurosis, and therefore the unit to be treated. For example Skynner (1976), in discussing school refusal, has emphasised the advantages of a family-centred approach over more traditional methods. Thus where the individual psychotherapist will examine the child's intrapsychic processes to find a cause for the neurotic symptoms, so the behaviour therapist will look at his or her learning experiences in terms of environmental contingencies, and the family therapist will look at the functioning and structure of the family as a whole. All have something to contribute to the understanding of these complex disorders. The family group approach is discussed further in Chapter 16.

Description

The capacity to cope with stress without developing a neurotic reaction varies with age. While infants can develop anxiety (as indicated in Chapter 1) in various circumstances, the term neurosis is not usually applied at this stage of development. It is probably best not employed until the use of mental defence mechanisms is established. It has been pointed out that children aged four to five often show many irrational fears (of flies, birds, dogs, earthworms, wind, the dark and so on). In older children or adults, however, they would not be normal and might be symptoms of neurosis, so that in diagnosis the patient's age, and the normal stress tolerance for that age, must be taken into account.

Neuroses in children tend to be less fixed and chronic than in adults so that the prognosis and response to treatment are on the whole better. They usually disturb the whole family and people in the patient's environment as much as the child himself; in this respect neurotic children differ from many neurotic adults, who live their lives without causing distress to others.

Neurotic disorders may be subdivided into the following subgroups:

(a) Anxiety states.
(b) Phobic states.
(c) Obsessive—compulsive states.
(d) Hysteria.
(e) Neurotic—depressive conditions.

How the various subgroups identified in both ICD—9 and DSM—III can be fitted under one or other of these headings, will be explained below. In children clear-cut examples of the types of neurotic disorder found in adults are less common than shifting clinical pictures; in these, obsessional, phobic, hysterical and depressive symptoms may replace each other, or alternate with one another, all against a background of anxiety. The value of subdividing these disorders into too large a number of categories is therefore questionable.

Anxiety Neuroses (or Anxiety States)

In anxiety neurosis the anxiety is directly expressed. These children may be shy, timid and clinging, emotionally immature, overdependent upon their parents, and poor at mixing with other children. They may fear loss of family, or death or some other disaster. They may have difficulty in getting to sleep, and sleep may be disturbed by dreams, nightmares or frequent waking. There may be free-floating anxiety, anxiety which comes to be associated with any situation the child may be in. Such anxiety is often perceived as arising from within rather than from the environment. Distractibility and impaired concentration accompany a feeling of apprehension. Common somatic manifestations of anxiety are loss of appetite, nausea, abdominal pain, diarrhoea, vomiting, headaches, dry mouth, rapid heart beat, cold and clammy hands, dizziness, sweating, sleep disturbance, poor concentration, tension, restlessness, increased frequency of micturition and palpitations. Most subjects in this condition would probably meet DSM—III's criteria for 'generalised anxiety disorder'.

Panic attacks may occur in the course of an anxiety state They are characterised by the sudden onset of extreme fear, sometimes with a sense of impending doom, often with such physical symptoms as shortness of breath, palpitations, sweating, faintness and trembling or shaking. Weekly attacks of panic over at least a three-week period constitute 'panic disorder' in the DSM—III scheme.

'Separation anxiety' is anxiety which is manifest on separation from, usually, parents but sometimes other attachment figures. 'Separation anxiety disorder' has been made a disorder in its own right in DSM—III. Separation anxiety is a feature of many cases of school refusal and will be discussed later in this chapter. Sometimes anxiety causes children to shrink from contact with strangers. This also has been given the status of a disorder (avoidant disorder of childhood and adolescence) by DSM—III. Children who worry excessively about examinations, meeting deadlines, athletic achievement, performing chores and the like and cannot relax, while tending to seek reassurance, are considered to be suffering from 'over-anxious disorder' by DSM—III, if the symptoms have persisted six months.

Most of these disorders would be classified as 'disturbances of emotions specific to childhood and adolescence — with anxiety and fearfulness', on the ICD—9 system. The important thing is to recognise them as excessively anxious reactions which require to be understood in the light of the possible causative factors mentioned above.

Phobic States

In phobic disorders there is persistent and irrational fear of a specific object, activity or situation. This leads to avoidance of the object or situation. The fear may be due to the defence mechanism of displacement. This means that it is transferred from its true (unconscious) source to the phobic object. Thus the individual who is afraid of going out of the house (agoraphobia, the fear of open spaces) is effectively preventing himself, or herself, from coping with a great many stressful situations which might be met with away from the security of home. The phobic object or objects may change during the course of the illness. While they may dominate the clinical picture, phobias are often but one feature, even a minor and transient one, of an anxiety state. There is an almost infinite variety of phobic objects. They include buses, dogs, cats, doctors, heights, enclosed spaces open spaces, shops, crowds, insects and so on.

Monosymptomatic phobias, called 'simple phobias' in DSM—III, are occasionally encountered in children. In these conditions the child has a severe and often seriously handicapping fear of one particular object or situation. The isolated phobias may differ in their causation from other neurotic disorders. They are not usually accompanied by general emotional immaturity. Their development is more easily understood on the basis of learning theory than are other neurotic disorders. Moreover they respond better to behaviour therapy. The treatment of a case of snake phobia is described in Chapter 16. DSM—III also distinguishes agoraphobia, with and without panic attacks, and 'social phobia', in which the subject has a fear of being subject to scrutiny by others.

'School phobia' is probably not, in most cases, a true phobic condition but a variety of anxiety neurosis. It is better called 'school refusal' and is described below.

Fuller discussions of phobias in childhood are provided by Berecz (1968) and by Miller *et al.* (1974).

Obsessive—Compulsive Neuroses

Obsessive—compulsive neuroses are characterised by obsessions — intrusive thoughts and ideas of which the individual cannot be rid despite conscious awareness of their unreasonableness and resistance to them. Compulsions are actions resulting from such thoughts. They are repetitive, ritualistic activities which may seem purposeful — for example hand-washing — but are carried out needlessly, because of a 'magical' belief they will prevent some undesired event from happening or otherwise influence the course of events. Obsessions and compulsions are unwelcome, unpleasant and disturbing to the individual. Psychodynamic theory regards them as manifestations of a mental defence mechanism against unconscious anxiety, a sort of 'magical' means of coping with the underlying problem.

Just as mild degrees of anxiety are a normal feature of childhood, so also are obsessional ideas and actions arising from normal anxiety. Examples are avoiding cracks in pavements, touching lamp-posts as they are passed and many feeding, dressing and bedtime rituals. In an obsessive—compulsive neurosis the symptoms are more severe and persistent, and interfere with the child's life. Complex rituals are sometimes observed. One boy had to shut the dining-room door three times, and then touch each corner of the table before he could start his meal. Obsessional symptoms are sometimes found in children who also show some degree of overt and free-floating anxiety. It will be noted that Tracie, whose case history is outlined later in this chapter, showed compulsive washing before admission. This continued also for a few days after admission, but disappeared as her anxiety lessened. Severe, chronic neuroses involving compulsive washing, such as may occur in adult patients, are not often seen in childhood, and present difficult treatment problems when they are. It may be however, that children who appear abnormally clean and tidy have mild degrees of this condition. An emotionally healthy child is as a rule a none too clean one!

Barry was referred at age nine. He was said always to have been fussy about cleaning his hands, which he washed unduly frequently. For six months he had been avoiding 'imaginary' lumps in the carpet. He would take a long time saying his prayers at night in case something went wrong or because he thought he might have made a mistake and so had to start again; and there were other obsessive—compulsive symptoms. Barry acknowledged that these ideas and actions were irrational and tried to resist them, but without success.

After outpatient treatment had failed, and because Barry was becoming increasing depressed and withdrawn, as well as expressing fear of dying, he was admitted for inpatient care. On admission he was tearful and communicated little with other children. He was always clean and well dressed, but quiet and unassertive. It soon became clear that his whole life was ruled by certain rituals. For example he had to get his clothes out of the locker without touching the locker; he had to cut his food into very small pieces before he could eat it; when getting his books out of his 'tidy box' in school he had to bring them backwards and forwards, four times, across the side of the box; and he could only walk across the dining-room by a particular route. He also had complicated rituals for getting up and going to bed.

Eventually Barry told us that the reason for most of his habits was that he was afraid something would happen to his parents if he did not carry them out. He was an intellectually bright boy, but reluctant to say much about his feelings or to talk about family relationships.

Barry proved a difficult boy to treat by psychotherapy because of his passive, uncommunicative behaviour at interview. A behaviour modification approach to be applied both in the clinic and at home during weekends, was instead worked out. This had considerable success, over a period of months, in reducing his symptoms almost to none. His parents were co-operative, middle class people and the family seemed stable, though mother was unduly anxious about Barry and had probably tended to 'infantilise' him long after he had ceased to be an infant.

Comment

This is an example of a severe and quite chronic obsessive—compulsive neurosis in a prepubertal child. Treatment was difficult and extended, with outpatient treatment following Barry's stay in hospital, over more than two years.

While severe obsessive—compulsive neuroses are not common in children, transient obsessional symptoms occur quite frequently in the course of neuroses with other symptomatology. Adams (1973) in an important review and study, reported that obsessive children made up about 1 per cent of referrals to a child psychiatry clinic. Reporting on 49 such children (29 boys, 20 girls), he found that symptoms usually started about age 6, with referral coming on average about 4 years later; and more than half the children also had phobias. He states that the outcome is usually good for a first attack of mild obsessional symptoms. It appears though that chronic, long-established cases can be among the most difficult neuroses to treat. However he relied on dynamic psychotherapy, while there is reason to believe that the behaviour therapy technique of 'response prevention' (Stanley, 1980) may yield quicker results. Elkins and his colleagues (1980), in a more recent review, point to evidence, as yet inconclusive, that biological factors may play a big role in these disorders, which seem to have a strong familial basis.

Obsessive—compulsive symptoms should be distinguished from 'impulsions', as originally described by Bender and Schilder (1940). Impulsions include behaviour such as constantly looking at or handling an object, drawing the object, being preoccupied with an object in fantasy or in thought, hoarding things, counting repeatedly and being preoccupied with numbers. The behaviour is similar to compulsive behaviour but there is little or no conscious resistance to it. Impulsions are commoner in younger children (aged four to ten) while obsessive—compulsive phenomena are more often found in prepubertal children, adolescents and adults. Some older children and adolescents who present with severe obsessive—compulsive neuroses have shown impulsions when younger. Impulsions and compulsions are sometimes present together around puberty.

Hysteria

Hysterical states may be divided into two groups, neither of them very common in childhood:

(1) Conversion hysteria, called 'conversion disorder' and classified as a 'somatoform disorder' in DSM–III;
(2) Dissociative states or disorders, which are given a major section of their own in DSM–III.

In conversion hysteria there is a loss or alteration of physical functioning. The physical manifestations may represent the 'conversion' of anxiety into the symptom or symptoms, or they may be a means of avoiding an anxiety-provoking situation. The symptoms may be motor (paralysis, or weakness or inability to speak except in a whisper) or sensory (lack of sensation to pain or touch in some part of the body or the presence of pain, discomfort or other sensations). Mild, often transient, hysterical symptoms occur fairly often in the course of other neuroses, but severe, established hysteria is uncommon in childhood. In a survey of Maudsley Hospital case material Caplan (1970) found an incidence of only 0.3 per cent of diagnosed 'hysteria' in pubertal children. In pubertal and pubescent children the incidence was 1.8 per cent. Another interesting finding was that 46 per cent of the cases were found to have an organic illness related to the presenting symptoms, either at the time or at follow-up four to eleven years later. The symptom most likely to be wrongly diagnosed as hysterical was deterioration of eyesight.

Joan, aged 13, was anxious about leaving home to go to school. Despite superior intelligence and a place at the top of the form, her relationships with other children in the school were poor. One Monday morning she complained of pain and weakness in her legs. The doctor was called and advised aspirin and a few days rest in bed. The symptoms subsided. They recurred on the first day of school after the half-term break. This time Joan was sent to a paediatrician who could find no evidence of physical illness. After two weeks off, Joan again appeared well and she returned to school and completed the term.

On the first day of the next term Joan was again unable to go to school because she could not walk and had painful legs. A psychiatric cause was now considered by the parents, and the family doctor. Joan had to be carried into the psychiatric consultation, but despite her inability to walk she showed a bland indifference to her symptoms. Her social difficulties at school and her fear of leaving mother soon emerged in discussion, and after three sessions she understood her physical symptoms as a means of avoiding school. It appeared that she had unconsciously seen them as the only way of avoiding school acceptable to her very ambitious parents. Her problems were tackled by a series of psychotherapeutic interviews, while a social worker saw the parents and helped them recognise their part in the situation.

The hysterical symptoms did not recur but Joan remained anxious about school and it was about ten weeks before she was able to return. She then did so, without recurrence of pain or paralysis.

It will be seen that in this case the 'conversion' symptoms were partly a way of expressing anxiety, but also a means of preventing Joan from getting into a situation which was anxiety-provoking for her. She had some conscious appreciation of her desire to remain at home rather than cope with the other children at school. Initially, however, she did not recognise that her physical symptoms were unconsciously motivated in the way they turned out to be. Her 'choice' of symptoms was probably related to her father's long-standing limp and pain, the result of a war wound.

While the abdominal pain, sickness and other physical symptoms occurring in many neurotic conditions arise in a similar way, in practice the term 'conversion hysteria' is usually confined to conditions where anxiety has been largely repressed and replaced by physical symptoms. Because the symptoms serve the purpose of reducing anxiety, the patient often shows little or no concern about them, despite what may appear to be a crippling disability. This so-called *belle indifférence'* was well displayed by Joan who, when first seen, expressed little or no concern about her inability to walk unaided, and smiled when describing the severity of her pain.

A rare hysterical symptom in children is *hysterical aphonia*, in which the voice is largely lost so that the subject can speak only in a whisper.

Caution should always be exercised in diagnosing hysteria as there is a real danger of misdiagnosing organic disease as hysterical. In one study of neurological disease presenting as child psychiatric disorder it was found that falling-off of school performance, loss of vision, disturbance of balance and variability of symptoms were common features (Rivinus *et al.*, 1975). An extensive review of conversion states in childhood is that of Turgay (1980), who points out that the incidence of conversion reactions varies greatly in different cultures; in Turkey, where Turgay has studied these conditions, it is apparently more common than in western countries. This paper also points out the considerable limitations of our knowledge of these disorders.

Hysterical dissociative states, which DSM—III classifies separately as 'dissociative disorders', comprise psychogenic memory loss, psychogenic fugue, depersonalisation disorder and multiple personality. All are rare in childhood, at least in western society, but rather more common in adolescence. Multiple personality, in which the subject displays two or more distinct personalities at different times, is very rare.

The mechanism of the development of these disorders seems to be similar to that underlying conversion symptoms; but instead of physical symptoms there is either loss of memory for a particular period of time (hours, days, weeks, rarely months), or a period of travel away from home or place of work with inability to remember the past (hysterical fugue), or episodes of depersonalisation or derealisation. Depersonalisation is a feeling of altered perception or experience of the self, with lost or altered experience of one's own reality. Derealisation is a similar alteration in the perception of one's surroundings.

Neurotic—Depressive Conditions

ICD—9 includes a category, 'neurotic depression' under 'neurotic disorders' and under 'disturbance of emotions specific to childhood and adolescence', a category 'with misery and unhappiness'. There are also codes for depression associated with acute reaction to major stress, adjustment reaction and manic-depressive psychosis, together with one for 'depressive disorder, not elsewhere classified'. This variety of diagnostic categories reflects the confusion and varied opinions about the diagnosis of depression, especially in childhood and adolescence (Graham 1974, 1981; Orvaschel et al., 1980). Nevertheless it is clear that children may experience depressive symptoms of varying severity, and that a smaller number show what many psychiatrists regard as depressive disorders. In these, depression is frequently accompanied by anxiety, with the anxiety often coming first.

The predominant clinical feature in these cases may be depression, the child having attacks of weeping, lacking normal interest in things and being unable to concentrate and despondent about the future. There is often disturbance of sleep and appetite. The child may express the desire to be dead, or to run away from the family, a wish which is sometimes acted out. The depression is not of psychotic intensity in that there is no disordered contact with reality. Indeed many children with neurotic—depressive conditions are found to be facing considerable environmental stress, most often due to tensions or disturbance in the family. The details are almost infinitely varied. The loss of a loved family member through death or other circumstances is a possible cause, but much more often the stress does not involve break-up of the family. Serious depression or other psychotic illness in one or other parent may be a factor; so may neurotic illness in a parent. Or the child may be unable to meet the parents' desires and expectations, for example academically at school. Physical illness in any member of the family (including parent) is particularly likely to cause anxiety or depression in the child. Disharmony between the parents has a similar effect. These circumstances, and others like them, do not necessarily cause depression. Other forms of neurotic reaction may occur, or the child may not react by neurotic breakdown at all. However, depression is particularly likely to occur when there has been chronic, long-standing stress of the varieties mentioned above.

George, an only child born to a single mother, was referred for psychiatric assessment at the age of eleven, after he had run way from home and been picked up by the police in a town about sixty miles away. His chronically depressed mother had had three periods in a psychiatric hospital during the previous two years, each for treatment of an exacerbation of her depression. George, his mother and a large dog lived an isolated existence. Mother did not mix with the neighbours and said they looked down on her because she was an unmarried mother. She lived on social security payments but from time to time bought George surprisingly expensive presents (a tape recorder and an electric organ were examples). She and George doted on the dog, for whose affections there was some rivalry between them. George was discouraged from mixing with other children and was frequently warned by his mother against friendships with neighbourhood families. On each of the three occasions when his mother had been in hospital he was placed in a foster home. At school he was considered a bright pupil but his work was patchy and unreliable. He ran away after leaving a note 'bequeathing' all his possessions, except the few things he chose to take with him, to his mother.

When first seen George was found to be very depressed. He spoke of his long-standing anxiety about his mother, who would from time to time threaten suicide, and the restrictions placed by her on his contacts outside the family. He said he ran away with the intention of going to stay with an aunt he knew slightly who lived in another part of the country. Intelligence testing showed him to be of superior intelligence, but in tests of attainment in basic school subjects he was performing at a level about average for a child of his age but not up to the standard appropriate to his intelligence. In later interviews he spoke of his desire to meet and know more of his father, of whom mother had never spoken to him.

George was at once admitted to hospital where his depression rapidly lifted without any drug or physical treatment. It was decided he would be best discharged to a residential school, a suggestion which he accepted readily. He did well there, returning home to his mother for school holidays. Meanwhile mother was supported by visits from a social worker, and seemed to benefit greatly from this.

Comment

George had been chronically anxious for many years, but had maintained a precarious adjustment until the approach of adolescence. Following three separations from mother he became increasingly worried and then depressed. He perhaps ran away more to draw attention to his plight than for any other reason. (In children, running away from home may be motivated in a way similar to some adult suicidal attempts.) The depression was almost severe enough to be called psychotic but a diagnosis of psychosis was not made in this case as the symptoms could be understood in terms of the difficulties George was facing. They were, moreover, effective in causing an improvement in his life situation through his placement in a residential school. The diagnosis was therefore one of a neurotic–depressive state

DSM–III has no special category for depression in childhood, but 'dysthymic disorder (or depressive neurosis)' may occur in children: its diagnosis requires 'either depressed mood or loss of interest or pleasure in all, almost all, usual activities . . . of at least one year's duration'. Depression, including 'major' and 'psychotic' depressive disorders in childhood, is discussed further in Chapter 6.

School Refusal

School refusal is a reluctance to attend school associated with anxiety and, often, depressive mood (Hersov, 1976b). It is sometimes called school phobia, because the child appears frightened to go to school. Such a fear can certainly be a feature of the condition, but it is often not the primary one, though at first it may seem to be. Fear of leaving home may be more important, though the importance of separation anxiety varies greatly from case to case. School refusal is distinct from truancy (Chapter 4), which is the wilful avoidance of school. If attempts are made to force the child with school refusal to go to school, increased distress usually results — though sometimes this is the best treatment, the child learning to overcome his distress. Physical symptoms, such as poor appetite, sickness, pains and diarrhoea, may occur, especially at breakfast time. These often disappear once the time for going to school has passed. This may lead parents or school staff to believe, wrongly, that the child is malingering. In the more severe cases symptoms persist at other times, but are exacerbated when the child is faced with pressure to attend school.

These children cannot cope with life at school. They often find relationships with other children difficult and become acutely anxious away from what they feel is the safety and protection of home and family. School attendance may finally cease in response to a minor additional stress, like a change of teacher, bullying by other children or transfer from primary to secondary school. The emotional immaturity of these children is often manifest in their covert aggressiveness. Having grown up in an anxious and probably indulgent atmosphere, they have not learnt to channel their aggressive drives into socially useful and constructive paths. (That is, there has been a failure of sublimation of these drives.) Their anger may seldom have been consciously aroused as they have always been given their way. When this situation is challenged they may become not only panic-stricken but also very angry. So they are anxious away from, but also angry with, their parents. The anger may be expressed verbally, or physically through tantrums or even physical violence towards the parents, or silently by refusal to speak or co-operate (sometimes with the psychotherapist as well as with the parent). Either anxiety or anger may dominate the clinical picture. Anger and hostility are often particularly marked in adolescents, being exacerbated by the normal rebelliousness of this age period, and also by the individual's feeling

of inability to fulfil the role appropriate to his or her age. In the
following case anxiety dominated the picture, and there was an
element of depression:

Tracie, aged 10, was referred because of school refusal. Her symptoms
dated back two months, to the start of a new school term. At first Tracie
became very anxious about her school books, worrying disproportionately
about small mistakes in her work. Then after being coaxed by other children to eat a horse chestnut in the playground, she became acutely fearful
that she was being poisoned. Afterwards she would eat only if her mother
ate the same food with her. She was also washing herself unduly frequently,
despite acknowledging that it was unnecessary when mother spoke to her
about it.

During the month before she was first seen, Tracie became very over-
dependent on her mother, to whom she confided frightening fantasies and
and dreams. Her mother responded to this by reassuring and comforting
her. Tracie frequently wept for her father and any attempt to get her to go
to school caused an acute state of panic. At night she would not go to
sleep until she knew her mother was in bed. She sucked two of her fingers
almost all day.

Four years previously Tracie's father had died of a subarachnoid
haemorrhage, after a short illness. Tracie, the sixth of eight siblings, was
said always to have been her father's favourite child. After father's death
she cried bitterly for days and she continued over the ensuing four years
to cry for him whenever upset. Mother also was depressed after father's
death, but did her best to comfort Tracie. This led to a mutually over-
dependent relationship between them. Tracie seemed to have made little
progress in becoming independent of mother during the ensuing four years.

Tracie was admitted to an inpatient unit for treatment. On separation
from her mother she was very upset, crying constantly and insistently
demanding that she must go home. For a few days she required constant
attention, but it was not difficult to get her to go to the unit school where
she worked well and made steady progress. At first she was reluctant to
mix with the other children but her relations with them became gradually
more normal. After eight weeks in the unit she was able to spend weekends
at home and return without upset. Towards the end of her three-month
stay in the unit she was able to go out each day to an outside school.

During the early part of her stay in hospital Tracie declined to see her
own doctor as she was invited to do daily. Instead she hung around the
building sucking her fingers. This was accepted, but later she agreed to be
seen on her own. She then began to talk about the obsessive thoughts
which previously had distressed her so much, but she seemed to feel guilty
about them and would give few details of their content. She spoke also of

her relationships with her mother, her siblings and various friends, including another girl in the unit with whom she developed a rather ambivalent relationship. She also played out scenes in the doll's house, the figure of father being always left out.

While Tracie was in hospital her mother was seen weekly by a social worker. She responded well to discussion of Tracie's difficulties and her own part in them. She was able to become less protective towards Tracie, and to handle her firmly, despite her own strongly felt desire to 'baby' her.

Tracie was discharged after three months' inpatient care and was seen as an outpatient. At follow-up 3½ years after admission she was attending school regularly, and making good progress, without showing signs of anxiety or any other symptoms. The whole family seemed to be functioning at a much better level.

Comment

This case is unusual in that father was dead, and the anxious over-protection of Tracie by mother was due to the reaction both showed to father's death. Nevertheless, the combination of an anxious and overprotective mother with a weak, passive, ineffectual or absent father, is common (Skynner, 1976). The child becomes increasingly emotionally immature and sooner or later develops overt neurotic symptoms; in Tracie's case these consisted of school refusal coming on following a minor stress, namely the start of a new school term with a new teacher. Very little fantasy material emerged during interviews with Tracie, and this is often the case in children with school refusal. A period of skilled treatment in hospital nevertheless enabled her to overcome her problems.

School refusal is probably the commonest presentation of the DSM—III's 'separation anxiety disorder'. Berney *et al.* (1981) found separation anxiety to be 'moderate to marked' in 87 per cent of 51 children between 9 and 15 with 'school phobia'. It is clear, though, that it is only one factor. Sometimes, especially in adolescents, stress in school appears a more important factor.

Other Neurotic Syndromes

Sometimes particular symptoms such as poor appetite with weight loss may dominate the picture, and many cases of *anorexia nervosa* (see Chapter 10) are neurotic disorders. *Elective mutism* (Chapter 8), in which there is refusal to speak to people outside the family circle, is also often a neurotic condition.

Treatment

This is usually psychotherapeutic, and in most cases parents and child or the whole family should be involved in the treatment. In many of the milder cases, this can be quite short-term and the interviews infrequent. The contact with the child may or may not involve the working through of unconscious conflicts. If the parents are over-anxious about the child, or over-protective, they will need help and perhaps even a period of psychotherapy. Family therapy is often of value in such cases, and in adolescents with school refusal (where the family psychopathology is often more complex and chronic) it can be particularly valuable. Skynner (1976) believes that non-involvement of the father is important aetiologically, and reports good results from family-centred treatment. Where anxiety-producing environmental circumstances are important, at home, in school or in the course of peer-group relationships, it is sometimes desirable to try and remove or reduce the stress in the early stages of treatment and then gradually reintroduce it. This process bears a relation to behaviour therapy as used in the treatment of specific phobias.

Other types of treatment are possible. A temporary reduction of anxiety may be secured by means of sedation with small doses of benzodiazepine drugs such as diazepam or chlordiazepoxide (see Chapter 16). Children living in particularly insecure or anxiety-provoking home environments may benefit from daypatient or inpatient treatment in a children's psychiatric unit, combined with help for the family.

It has been suggested that treatment with tricyclic antidepressants is of benefit in school refusal, but the one controlled trial which found imipramine to be of value (Gittelman-Klein and Klein, 1971) has not been replicated. A more recent trial of clomipramine, a related drug, failed to demonstrate any significant short-term effect (Berney *et al.*, 1981).

While children with severe and long-standing neuroses need specialist help, many milder cases can often be treated in the community. Un-hurried interviews with child and parents, or with the whole family, are usually necessary, perhaps supplemented by drug therapy and/or by adjustments of the child's environment. The latter may be achieved as a result of discussion with the family or through change in the child's school environment.

In the treatment of neurotic school refusal it is necessary to consider carefully the stage at which efforts should be made to get the child to return to school. If the child is still attending school, even with great difficulty, efforts to make the school environment temporarily less stressful and to provide support for the child while attending, are well worth-while. In mild and early cases an early return to school is advisable, and usually leads to good results (Kennedy, 1965). This should be firmly presented to the child after the agreement and co-operation of school staff and parents, and anyone else who may be involved, have been obtained. Sometimes it can be agreed at a family interview at which a member of the school staff is also present. If the situation is handled firmly and calmly most children return to school. Any necessary treatment can then be offered to the family. The parents and/or child may ask for a change of school and, while this can be helpful, it is seldom in itself adequate; it often represents an attempt by both child and family to deal with their anxiety, and perhaps guilt too, by attributing the difficulties simply to events at school. Attempts to force severely anxious or depressed children, or children who have been having panic attacks, to school tend to aggravate the symptoms. In such cases, psychotherapy must usually be started first and it may be some months before the child can return to school. In severe cases, however, admission to a child psychiatric inpatient unit may be helpful and education can be continued in this setting (Barker, 1968).

The various treatment methods mentioned are discussed more fully in Chapter 16.

Outcome

The outcome in childhood neurotic conditions is generally favourable. Neurotic symptoms, even severe ones, frequently clear up even without psychiatric treatment and without being followed by any observable psychiatric disability. Such an outcome is more probably in children whose emotional development has been satisfactory and also where the neurotic symptoms occur in response to marked environmental stress. In other instances neurotic symptoms persist, especially in the absence of suitable treatment. Emotionally immature children, who are often overdependent on their parents, tend to do less well. Constitutional predisposition, which may be shown by a positive family history and by the appearance of symptoms with little apparent environmental cause, may also be associated with a poorer response to treatment.

If psychiatric disorder persists, the type of disorder diagnosed in adult life is likely to be a neurosis or an affective psychosis (Robins, 1966). This contrasts with conduct disorders which, if disturbed behaviour persists into adult life, are more likely to be followed by antisocial or criminal behaviour.

CHAPTER SIX

Psychotic Disorders

Psychotic disorders are characterised by altered contact with reality. The psychotic child is attempting to adapt to a subjectively distorted concept of the world. This contrasts with neurosis in which the child is adapting in a morbid fashion to his or her real life situation.

In infants and young children it can be hard to be sure whether psychosis is present, because the child's concept of the world can only be inferred from observed behaviour. An important point is the present of withdrawal from, or failure to make, normal emotional contact with people.

Another difficulty is that the onset of psychoses in early childhood, and especially in the first year or two, seriously distorts personality development and intellectual functioning. Since intelligence is manifested mainly through learned behaviour (such as speech and motor skills) children who have failed to learn such behaviour because of withdrawal and failure to make social contacts cannot give evidence of their intelligence in the normal way. Thus it can be difficult or impossible to decide what level of cognitive functioning they might have achieved had they not become psychotic. This makes the distinction between psychosis and mental handicap difficult. A further complication is that mental handicap and psychoses may co-exist.

The classification of childhood psychoses is hampered by the difficulty in assessing the state of mind of young children and by uncertainty about the causes of these conditions.

The ninth edition of the *International Classification of Diseases* (World Health Organisation, 1977a) divides psychoses with origin specific to childhood into the following categories:

(a) Infantile autism.
(b) Disintegrative psychosis.
(c) 'Other': atypical forms of infantile psychosis which may show some of the features of infantile autism.
(d) 'Unspecified': includes 'schizophrenia, childhood type' and 'schizophrenic syndrome of childhood'.

In addition altered contact with reality occurs in *acute* and *subacute confusional states* (which the ICD classifies under 'transient organic psychotic conditions'), in certain forms of *dementia* which, rarely, occur in childhood and in *affective psychoses*.

The DSM—III (American Psychiatric Association, 1980) does not use the term psychosis for severe disorders occurring early in life, in the belief that these conditions 'bear little relationship to the psychotic disorders of adult life', though it does not explain why psychoses of infancy should resemble those of adult life. Instead it has coined the term 'pervasive developmental disorder', since 'many basic areas of psychological development' are affected simultaneously and severely. The disorders are subdivided into:

(a) Infantile autism, which may present as the 'full syndrome' or as a 'residual state'.
(b) Childhood onset pervasive developmental disorder, which also may exist as the 'full syndrome' or as a 'residual state'.
(c) Atypical pervasive developmental disorder.

The 'disintegrative psychoses' of ICD—9 are classified as dementias in the DSM—III.

Infantile Autism and Other Infantile Psychoses

In 1943 and 1944 Kanner described a group of severely disturbed children and named the syndrome they presented *early infantile autism*. This term, often shortened to infantile autism, has continued in use, sometimes being applied to children with disorders conforming precisely to Kanner's description, and sometimes being used more loosely. Many other terms have also been applied to psychotic disorders of early childhood, for example *infantile psychoses, childhood autism, childhood schizophrenia, schizophrenic syndrome of child-*

hood and *symbiotic psychosis*. Since there is evidence (Kolvin *et al.*, 1971; Rutter, 1976) that psychotic disorders of infancy and early childhood are distinct from schizophrenia as it occurs in adulthood or later childhood, terms which imply that these disorders have a relation to schizophrenia are best avoided. If the term *infantile psychosis* is used, implying a severe disorder starting in the first 2 or 3 years of life with evidence of altered reality contact, infantile autism becomes a form of infantile psychosis — the one with the most clear-cut clinical description.

Prevalence

Epidemiological studies in both Middlesex, England (Lotter, 1966) and Camberwell, London (Wing, 1980) agree on a prevalence rate for autistic conditions of between 4.5 and 5.0 per 10 000 children. In both studies, rather less than half the children identified were considered as falling into the 'nuclear group' — that is those with the full syndrome; the remainder had autistic features but not the full picture. A boy:girl ratio of between 3 and 4 to one was found. Although Lotter's (1966) study suggested a bias towards the higher socio-economic classes, this was not confirmed in Wing's (1980) research. In Lotter's (1966) study the apparent social class bias may have been due to factors affecting referral and diagnosis.

Lotter (1978) also found 'autistic-like' conditions in 2–3 per cent of 300 mentally handicapped children in nine African cities, indicating that the condition is not confined to western societies.

Causes and Associated Factors

The causes of infantile psychoses are uncertain. Genetic, environmental, constitutional and organic cerebral causes have all been suggested. It is, however, established that there are associations between infantile psychosis and both mental handicap and language disorder.

There is evidence that genetic factors play some part in causing autism. Folstein and Rutter (1977), studied 21 pairs of same-sexed twins, one or both of whom had autism. Eleven were monozygotic (MZ) and 10 dizygotic (DZ). Four of the MZ pairs but none of the

DZ pairs were concordant for autism. In addition 6 non-autistic co-twins (5 MZ and 1 DZ) showed a serious cognitive disability — speech delay, IQ below 70 or scholastic difficulties. Thus there was 36 per cent concordance for autism in MZ twins against none for DZ twins; and 82 per cent concordance for cognitive disorder in MZ pairs, against 10 per cent in DZ pairs. Both differences are statistically significant. The findings could not be explained on the basis of brain damage at birth, but it did seem in some cases that the disorder resulted from an inherited cognitive defect plus brain damage.

Environmental, especially family, factors have been blamed. Kanner (1943, 1944) asserted that the parents lack emotional warmth and are detached and of obsessional personality. There is no firm evidence of this, though parental personality attributes could conceivably contribute, given certain biological factors in the child. Alternatively, reported parental attitudes could be reactions to the children's conditions.

Brain damage is certainly present in some psychotic children, and occasionally a child with the clinical picture of infantile psychoses turns out to have a neurological disorder such as a cerebral lipidosis (see below). But most brain-damaged children are not psychotic, and many psychotic children show no evidence of brain damage. Nevertheless a surprising number — 29 per cent in one study (Rutter, 1970a) — of non-epileptic psychotic children later develop epilepsy. This is much greater than the incidence of epilepsy in the general population.

Autistic behaviour is sometimes seen in children with various forms of brain damage and metabolic disturbance (Cohen, 1980). Chess (1977) reported 10 cases of 'the complete autism syndrome' among 243 children with congenital rubella; another 8 showed a 'partial syndrome'; these represent prevalence rates some 200 times those in the general child population. Cohen (1980) has also pointed out the many similarities between infantile autism and the Gilles de la Tourette syndrome (see Chapter 8). He distinguishes 'primary childhood autism' which 'eludes aetiologic classification', and 'secondary disorders' in which autism is secondary to another disorder. Many of the latter conditions would fall in the category of 'disintegrative psychoses' of ICD-9 (see below).

While brain damage may be a contributory factor in autistic children, it is quite unclear what part of the brain is involved (Rutter, 1976). There does however seem to be reason to regard the syndrome as a central disorder of language and cognition (Rutter *et al.*, 1971).

The association of infantile psychosis with mental handicap is strong. A majority of a group of 'autistic' children studied by Rutter and Lockyer (1967) obtained IQ scores in the 'mentally handicapped' range, though about a quarter fell in the 'normal' range. In most cases the low IQ did not appear to be due to the psychotic process, and it tended to remain at about the same level even following recovery from the psychosis.

The association with language disorder is important. Speech and language retardation are almost invariable in infantile psychosis. There is usually a severe receptive language problem and also a profound defect of inner language. This affects not only verbal language but language function generally, so that there is a failure to use gesture, which most children with developmental language disorders (see Chapter 9) use extensively.

There is little evidence for the view that infantile psychosis is a form of schizophrenia coming on early in life. Studies by Kolvin and colleagues (1971) of psychoses starting in infancy, and those commencing later in childhood, showed that the two groups of conditions differ in sex incidence, social background, family history of schizophrenia, intellectual level, cognitive function, presence of delusions and hallucinations, and course.

Description

Kanner (1943, 1944) in his original accounts of autistic children, described four main features: autistic aloneness, delayed or abnormal speech development, an obsessive desire for sameness and onset in the first two years of life. These are still widely regarded as the basis for the diagnosis of infantile autism, though other infantile psychoses are recognised in which the clinical picture does not conform precisely to Kanner's description. DSM—III, however, has dropped the requirement that an obsessive desire for sameness is necessary for the diagnosis of infantile autism.

Autistic aloneness refers to failure to form normal social relationships with people. Attachment behaviour is lacking and instead of relating to individuals as people, psychotic children tend to treat them as inanimate objects. Their parents find them unresponsive; they do not seem to want to be kissed or cuddled and may resist parents' attempts to give them physical affection; and they often fail to assume the posture appropriate for being picked up or nursed. They do not distinguish between parents and strangers, approaching either indiscriminately. A related behaviour is gaze avoidance, the failure to make eye-to-eye contact with people. While autistic children may at times look at people, they usually fail to do so when appropriate, for example during conversation. Also they may appear more fascinated by a person's spectacles, or facial contours, than with facial expression as a normal child would be.

Delayed, absent or *abnormal speech*, is an invariable feature of infantile psychosis. Speech may not be acquired at all, or it may develop very late. Less frequently it develops normally for up to 2 or 2½ years but is then partially or completely lost. The failure to speak is but one manifestation of a severe, and often profound, defect of language function (Bartak *et al.*, 1975). This is shown in non-verbal as well as verbal behaviour. Thus there is an absence of symbolic or imaginative play, toys not being used as the objects they represent: a psychotic child may use a toy telephone to bang on the floor or to swing to and fro but will probably not imitate adults' use of a telephone as other children do. There is a failure to imitate and use gestures. In younger autistic children play tends to be repetitive, stereotyped and at a basic sensori-motor level.

As these children grow up some language skills usually develop, and about half of them acquire some useful speech. Language usually remains seriously impaired however. Pronominal reversal is common. Asked, 'Do you want lunch?', the child will reply 'You want lunch', or may repeat the whole question. Use of 'I' and 'me' is often absent, or comes very late. Echolalia, the repeating of words and phrases spoken by others (of which the repeating of questions is an example), is common. Sometimes the echolalia is delayed, the words or phrases being repeated after a lapse of minutes, hours or days. This leads to the use of words and phrases, often highly stereotyped ones, totally out of context. Later still the child may be able to talk quite well about concrete, factual matters but have great difficulty with abstract ideas, producing no creative or imaginative ideas. Some of these children are greatly preoccupied with mechanical things like train or bus timetables, highway routes and their numbers and the like. Speech may be stilted or monotonous, without the usual intonations and inflexions. Associated with these problems there are usually some continuing difficulties in understanding speech, especially abstract ideas, or in following the plot of a story.

The *obsessive desire for sameness* tends to show itself through a 'fierce resistance to change', manifested either by severe distress if any article of furniture is moved from its accustomed place in the home, or if a different car route is followed to a familiar place. The child may restrict food intake to a few similar articles; and the similarity may even be in shape, for example sausages, fishsticks or chips only (Rees, 1974). Some psychotic children show strong attachments to particular objects which seem to have special importance to them (Marchant *et al.*, 1974). Others have rituals for dressing or undressing and may insist on wearing certain clothes.

In many cases the child's behaviour and development appear to have been abnormal from birth. In a minority of cases, however, there is a clear history of normal development for anything up to about 2 to 2½ years, followed by development of psychotic behaviour; Elaine, described below, is an example.

Other symptoms frequently present are poor concentration, distractibility, overactivity (sometimes also periods of underactivity), sudden and apparently unprovoked anger or fearfulness, and outbursts of aggressiveness. These children tend to show a lack of fear about realistic dangers (fire, heights and so on) and resist learning new behaviour or skills. They often choose to examine objects, and people, by touching, tasting or smelling them, rather than by visual inspection. In infancy, feeding and toilet training problems are common. In place of normal play these children often engage in activities such as rocking, head-banging, flapping the hands up and down or whirling round and round.

Children with infantile psychosis often look healthy and intelligent and may also show limited areas of normal or even precocious intellectual function, while functioning at a retarded level in other respects. Their memory is sometimes remarkable. It may be combined with great musical skill, so that the child can reproduce accurately long and complicated pieces of music. Some children show special facility in mathematics, and are found to perform at a standard well ahead of their age. Patchy performance in intelligence tests is common.

Not all children with infantile psychosis present clinical features which conform precisely to Kanner's description of infantile autism, and the severity of the condition varies. The feature most often missing, or not well marked, is the preoccupation with sameness, which may be why it is not included in the DSM—III criteria, except as one example of 'bizarre responses to various aspects of the environment'. These children do not show delusions, hallucinations or the forms of thought disorder encountered in schizophrenia.

Elaine was born at full term following a normal pregnancy. Her birth weight was 2.5 kg. She appeared a healthy baby but feeding was difficult. Breast feeding was abandoned after two weeks, but even on the bottle she was difficult and fractious. She was an active baby and slept only for relatively short periods. Her parents considered her a quick and active baby and her motor development during the first year was if anything ahead of normal. She said her first words at ten months, and was reciting nursery rhymes by eighteen months. She was very musical and by this age could sing several songs. At just over twelve months Elaine had frequent breath-holding attacks and one of these was followed by a major convulsion. She was put on phenobarbitone, but as it made her worse she was taken off it after a few weeks. She had no more seizures.

When aged about twenty-one months, towards the end of her mother's second pregnancy, Elaine's behaviour began to cause the parents concern. She repeatedly and often inappropriately made remarks like 'I don't like Mummy poorly' and expressed her dislike of various other people.

Her condition deteriorated following the birth of her sister. Elaine was then twenty-three months old. Her speech regressed further and she started repeating people's questions instead of giving replies. She no longer talked to people. She spent long periods rocking and took little notice of people. Episodes of severe temper and screaming developed, but she retained her musical skill. At two years and six months a neurologist diagnosed her as 'autistic'.

At age three she was taken to a child guidance clinic but twelve weeks of weekly attendance brought no benefit. She had by this time lost most of her speech. She remained hyperactive and difficult to manage at home.

Elaine was seen at age four years and six months. Her parents described her as being hyperactive, impossible to communicate with, obsessed with food and unpredictable in mood, quiet periods being succeeded by severe tempers. She would not go on her own to the toilet, as she had done, and often wet, and occasionally soiled, herself. But she was considered intelligent, had a good memory and knew where everything was. She now had no speech. Her hearing had been tested and pronounced normal. She was considered agile and good with her hands.

At this time Elaine appeared an attractive, well-dressed, overactive child. She ignored the examiner and engaged in a manneristic dance from time to time. At other times she moved restlessly and apparently aimlessly round the room. Her main interest in toys was putting them into her mouth, but she did not play with any of them in a conventional way. She made no response to speech. She vocalised a few sounds, but produced no recognisable words. She laughed once or twice but for no obvious reason. Otherwise she showed little emotional reaction. The presence in the room of three unfamiliar adults did not seem to affect her behaviour at all.

Elaine's parents were both university graduates, father a university lecturer, mother a secondary school teacher. Both were deeply concerned about Elaine and were prepared to go to great trouble to help her and obtain treatment for her. The family appeared a stable one and there was no family history of psychiatric illness.

Comment

This is a case of psychotic illness coming on in the second year, not conforming precisely to the classical picture of infantile autism in that there was no marked preoccupation with 'sameness'. It fits the DSM—III criteria for the 'infantile autism' category of 'pervasive developmental disorder'.

Differentiation from Other Conditions

The conditions with which psychosis of early childhood is most likely to be confused are deafness, mental handicap and developmental language disorders. The question of whether or not there is also brain disease, for example cerebral lipidosis, can be hard to decide; thorough neurological investigation is usually advisable.

In most cases there is good evidence, from the history and as a result of clinical examination, that the child can hear and is failing to respond to people, rather than failing to hear. It is wise in all cases however to have audiometric assessment carried out. Electroencephalographic measurement of evoked responses to auditory stimuli is sometimes of value in deciding whether the stimuli are reaching the cerebral cortex.

While mental handicap may co-exist with psychosis, retarded children usually relate freely with people, are not preoccupied with sameness and are more generally retarded, whereas the retardation of psychotic children is often patchy. The psychotic child also has a specially severe form of impaired understanding of speech, in the use of gesture and in the understanding of grammatical structure, disabilities which have been shown to be relatively more severe than in normal or mentally handicapped children of the same mental age (Hermelin and O'Connor, 1970).

Developmental language disorders are described in Chapter 9. The main point is that there is no withdrawal, and language disordered children are usually normally responsive and communicate freely by non-verbal means. Echolalia and pronoun reversal are commoner in psychotic children. Preoccupation with sameness and other bizarre behaviours are not a feature of the behaviour of language disordered children. Severe receptive and central language difficulties are of course themselves features of infantile psychosis.

DSM–III includes a category called 'infantile autism, residual state', for disorders in children who once met the criteria for infantile autism, but no longer do so. As autistic children grow older some of their symptoms lessen or disappear, leaving an odd, emotionally under-responsive, sometimes ritualistic, concretely thinking individual who may be excessively preoccupied with the rote learning of lists, mathematical processes or other concrete things. At the same time there is often poverty of abstract thought.

Treatment of Children with Infantile Psychoses

Many treatment methods have been tried. The results of psycho-therapeutic approaches have been disappointing, though psycho-therapy can be helpful to some psychotic children at particular points in the development of the disorder. Psychotherapy is discussed extensively in Szurek and Berlin (1973).

Nowadays autism and the other 'pervasive developmental disorders' are no longer seen as the withdrawal into psychosis of basically normal children (Rutter, 1976). They are rather regarded as bio-logically handicapped children, particularly in the area of central language processing. So treatment is designed to promote more normal development and to assist these children in the development of language. Emphasis is also placed on helping families deal better with these difficult children.

Behaviour therapy seems to be the most effective approach to the treatment of these children. It is clear that their behaviour can be changed by operant conditioning techniques (Currie and Brannigan 1970: Lovaas et al., 1973), which can also be used to teach speech. While conditioning techniques cannot overcome a severe biological defect in the capacity to use language, they can ensure that whatever language potential the child has is realised, and as neurological maturation proceeds the child's potential may improve. Yet sometimes conditioning techniques do no more than teach the child simple receptive language, like obeying commands or responding to simple questions, and perhaps making simple statements or requests. Whatever the level of function of the child, however, these techniques appear the most hopeful of those currently available. It also seems that changes brought about by treatment in an institution away from home may not always be accompanied by similar changes when the child goes home or to a school in the community (Lovaas *et al.*, 1973). Treatment located in the home and school seems to be of more benefit, and parents and teachers should be actively involved in it.

When these children grow up most require special schooling, usually in the form of skilled, small-group teaching. Special day units for autistic children and those with similar disorders are increasingly being provided. A few residential schools also exist, but it is probably better, in most cases, not to remove these children from their homes; sometimes however geographical considerations leave no choice but residential schooling.

Residental treatment may be required if the severity of the behavioural disturbance is greater than can be coped with at home, or if there are severe problems in the family. It should always be kept as brief as possible, with the family being involved in the treatment as much as possible These children are particularly susceptible to institutionalisation because of their tendency to withdraw and their failure to communicate normally. For this reason long-term residential care is to be avoided whenever possible.

Drug treatment may be of symptomatic benefit. Haloperidol appears to reduce stereotyped behaviour and to render autistic children more susceptible to behaviour therapy, especially those over about 4½ (Cohen *et al.*, 1980).

Help for the families is often needed, since the stresses caused by having a psychotic child in the family can be great. If possible the parents should work closely with the professionals treating the child. It is also helpful, as well as true, to make it clear to the parents that they are not the cause of the disorder. Any guilt they may feel can be further reduced by the process of making them 'co-therapists', as is the practice in many behaviour modification programmes.

The various treatment methods mentioned are discussed further in Chapter 16.

Outcome

Many of these children show a measure of improvement, starting most commonly about age four to six, though it may be later. Much probably depends on whether, at this stage, they are in an environment in which their slowly improving language skills, and increasing capacity to form relationships, are exploited to the full. Some 10 to 20 per cent of children with psychoses of early childhood recover or show marked improvement, sufficient to enable them to attend an ordinary school or to work. A further, probably similar, percentage can live at home under sheltered conditions and can attend a special school or training centre. Fifty to sixty per cent do not make any substantial improvement and ultimately require long-term institutional care.

Children who do improve often show residual signs of the psychotic process. They may be emotionally cold and aloof, and unaware of, and so insensitive to, the feelings of others. They may be preoccupied with train timetables, spotting the makes of cars and other things. There is often continuing evidence of the underlying language disorder, with poor comprehension of speech and of abstract ideas. Speech may be stilted, mechanical, repetitive or echolalic, or any combination of these, or it may be absent, despite relatively good adjustment in other spheres. Hyperactivity and aggressiveness tend to lessen and have often disappeared by puberty, but epilepsy develops in up to 29 per cent of cases. It is commoner in individuals with low intelligence quotients.

The outlook is related to whether any useful speech has developed by the age of five. If not, later development of speech is less likely and the outcome generally poorer. The results of intelligence testing carried out early in the illness also tend to correlate with speech development. The lower the intelligence quotient obtained, the worse the outlook.

Disintegrative Psychoses

ICD–9 defines disintegrative psychoses as those in which 'normal or near-normal development for the first few years is followed by loss of social skills and of speech, together with a severe disorder of emotions, behaviour and relationships'. The loss of speech and social skills usually occurs over a period of a few months. Overactivity and repetitive, stereotyped behaviour are common, and intellectual impairment is a frequent, but not invariable, part of the clinical picture.

DSM—III does not use the term 'disintegrative psychosis', suggesting instead that these disorders should be classified as dementias.

Causes

Disintegrative psychoses are often due to organic brain disease, though cases occur in which no evidence can be found of organic disorder. Sometimes evidence of underlying brain disease emerges much later, even at post-mortem examination (Creak, 1963). Cases due to brain disease can be divided into two groups according to whether or not they are associated with progressive cerebral disorders (Corbett *et al.*, 1977). Non-progressive causes include various forms of encephalitis (in which there is either cerebral infection or a reaction in the brain to a generalised infection) which results in damage which does not progress once the infection has cleared up. Infantile myoclonic epilepsy, and lead poisoning (once exposure to lead is terminated) are other possible non-progressive causes.

Progressive causes include tuberous sclerosis, hepato-lenticular degeneration, Huntington's chorea, lipidoses, diffuse cerebral sclerosis and subacute sclerosing panencephalitis. Each of these is described briefly below. Fuller accounts are given by Norouha (1974) and Wilson (1974).

Description

The clinical picture of disintegrative psychosis is quite varied. The essential features are a severe, prolonged disorder, with loss of reality contact, occurring in the absence of any other family disturbance or, if there is family or other psychosocial stress, of a severity out of proportion to the stress. Other features include relationship difficulties, usually withdrawal, ritualistic and manneristic behaviour, delusions, hallucinations and a deterioration of educational or social behaviour, or both. In progressive cases the intelligence quotient may drop, the performance score being first affected, and neurological signs indicating focal lesions in the nervous system may appear. The electroencephalogram (EEG) often becomes abnormal, and serial examinations may reveal deterioration. When psychotherapy or behaviour therapy are tried in progressive cases they are either unsuccessful or only have short-lived effects.

The history and clinical picture vary according to the cause and the following are brief summaries of conditions which may underlie disintegrative psychosis.

(a) Non-Progressive Causes

Encephalitis following measles, mumps, influenza or other infectious diseases may be followed by psychotic symptoms such as those described above. There is usually a history of an attack of the infectious disease, followed by such indications of encephalitis as loss of consciousness, seizures and specific neurological signs. Examination of the cerebrospinal fluid in the acute stage usually provides evidence of cerebral involvement. Sometimes the evidence of encephalitis is less clear-cut, and when a psychotic child presents for assessment, it may be hard to be sure whether there was any brain damage at the time of an earlier infectious disease. The worldwide epidemic encephalitis which occurred after the 1914–1918 war led to many cases of severe post-encephalitic psychotic disorders and most of the earliest inpatient psychiatric units for children in the U.S.A. were opened primarily to deal with children suffering from post-encephalitic conditions (Barker, 1974). Since then cases have been mainly sporadic.

Infantile myoclonic epilepsy (infantile spasms, salaam attacks) is a form of epilepsy with onset usually in the first year of life. It often leads to a psychotic state and dementia (Jeavons and Bower, 1964; Jeavons *et al.*, 1970). The attacks, which consist of a sudden flexion of the arms while the head simultaneously drops forward, may be frequent at the height of the condition, when there may be scores or even hundreds of attacks per day. They usually die out during the second year of life. The end result is usually a severely mentally retarded child, but some of these children present with a psychotic picture. The degree of withdrawal may resemble that seen in infantile psychoses, though the history usually distinguishes the conditions. The withdrawn behaviour sometimes leads to the suspicion that the child is deaf.

There are various known causes of infantile spasms, including brain damage at the time of birth, reaction to immunisation, and such other conditions as tuberous sclerosis, inborn errors of metabolism and cerebral agenesis; but in many cases no cause can be discovered, and the condition comes on after a period of normal development.

Treatment using adrenocorticotophic hormone (ACTH) appears to be of value and lessens the chance of the child being left with severe brain damage.

Lead encephalopathy results from the ingestion of excessive amounts of lead. It may cause brain damage and mental retardation. In children it is often associated with pica, the eating of substances not normally regarded as edible; old lead paint is the commonest danger. The use of lead, or lead paint, in toys does not normally occur nowadays, though it occasionally happens in error. Lead is also used in car batteries, in the structure of buildings and in industry, and lead poisoning has been known to occur in children playing with materials on rubbish dumps and in old buildings. Lead can be absorbed through skin and lungs as well as through the gastrointestinal tract.

In mild cases there may be a behaviour disorder with irritability, restlessness, inability to concentrate and loss of interest in things. In severe cases the behaviour disorder may be of psychotic intensity. Loss of appetite, vomiting, abdominal pains, constipation, headaches and sleeplessness may occur. There may be pallor due to the anaemia lead poisoning causes. Lead poisoning may lead to dementia, sometimes sufficient to cause severe mental handicap.

The diagnosis is supported by finding basophilic stippling in the red cells, and increased density on X-rays of the ends of long bones, but these may be absent even though there are behavioural symptoms due to lead intoxication. Raised levels of lead are found in blood and urine, and there is excretion of coproporphyrin in the urine. Lead poisoning should be treated in a specialised centre; all sources of lead must immediately be removed and the excretion of lead promoted by chelating agents. In the absence of treatment and if exposure to lead continues, the condition is of course progressive.

(b) Progressive Causes

Tuberous sclerosis (or epiloia) is a rare condition due to a dominant autosomal genetic trait. Sporadic cases also occur. Multiple tumours and malformations in the brain are associated with epilepsy and mental deterioration. There may also be behavioural symptoms, and withdrawal, of psychotic intensity. A characteristic rash develops on cheeks, nose, chin and forehead.

Hepato-lenticular degeneration (or Wilson's disease) is inherited as an autosomal recessive trait and is a disorder of copper metabolism. Various parts of the body are affected; the damage to the brain may cause a psychotic syndrome or milder psychological symptoms. Involuntary movements, emotional lability, fits and a dementing process are characteristic features. These children can sometimes be helped by restricting copper intake, and by administration of penicillamine to increase the excretion of copper.

Huntington's chorea is a degenerative disease of the nervous system which is inherited as a dominant trait. Onset is usually during adult life, but may occur in childhood. The first symptoms tend to be involuntary choreiform movements, or a dementia. In the early stages, however, disturbed behaviour may dominate the clinical picture, there being emotional lability, hyperactivity and excitement, irritability and delusions as well as intellectual deterioration. No treatment is known which cures the process but anti-Parkinsonian drugs such as benztropine or orphenadrine may control the involuntary movements.

In the *disorders of sphingolipid metabolism* (lipidoses) fatty substances (sphingolipids) accumulate in the brain and other parts of the body. These disorders are usually inherited and due to recessive genes. Various different lipids may be involved. A variety of neurological symptoms occur, for example blindness and fits. Onset may be at any time during childhood with progressive deterioration, leading eventually to death, occurring over a period which may be months or years. Sometimes the condition presents, not with neurological symptoms, but as a progressive disintegrative psychosis; or it may closely resemble infantile psychosis. Deterioration may be slow and cases are on record in which the diagnosis was unsuspected until revealed by post-mortem examination upon death some years later (Creak, 1963). Tay-Sachs disease (or amaurotic family idiocy) and metachromatic leukodystrophy are particular forms that may present with psychiatric symptoms, and eventually progress to dementia and death.

Diffuse cerebral sclerosis (Schilder's disease) describes a group of conditions in which the white matter of the brain degenerates. Some forms, the leukodystrophies, are genetic in origin. The myelin sheaths of the nerve fibres are lost (demyelination) and this is followed by the growth of fibrous tissue (gliosis). Several forms have been described, with onset from infancy onwards. In the early stages there may be bizarre, unpredictable and variously disturbed behaviour, often with apparent loss of contact with the environment. Cortical blindness or deafness, in which the brain is unable to make normal use of the nerve impulses reaching it, may also occur. A falling-off in the performance of school work may be the presenting symptom. Labile and inappropriate emotional responses are sometimes early features. The course is progressive and the early symptoms are followed by profound dementia. No treatment is known which will arrest the disease process.

Subacute sclerosing panencephalitis (von Bogaert's disease) is a rare form of virus infection affecting the brain cells. It may present with a psychotic picture, or with deteriorating performance at school. Personality change, intellectual deterioration, memory loss and withdrawal may be followed by epilepsy, leading to a state of profound dementia and ultimately death. The EEG findings are characteristic and diagnostic. The condition is thought to be due to a virus which cannot be distinguished from that which causes measles, though the disease itself is quite different in its manifestations and pathology.

Dementia infantilis (Heller's syndrome) is a term first used by Heller in 1930 to describe a dementing process, often associated with disturbed, restless, psychotic behaviour, starting at about the age of 3 or 4 (Heller, 1954). The term is little used nowadays and the cases Heller described appear to have been examples of progressive disintegrative psychosis.

Treatment of Disintegrative Psychoses
In few cases is it possible to affect the underlying disease process although, as indicated above, in lead poisoning the lead present in the body can be removed, sometimes with clinical improvement. Otherwise treatment is mainly symptomatic and palliative; measures which may help in particular disorders have already been mentioned.

Non-progressive cases often benefit from the treatment methods which are helpful in infantile psychoses. Considerable recovery may occur after encephalitis: improvement may continue to be evident for as long as a year. The normal processes of growth and maturation also continue.

Epilepsy may complicate organic disorder of the brain; anticonvulsants should be used to achieve as complete control as possible. Hyperactive behaviour should be controlled using either a phenothiazine drug or haloperidol. Drug treatment may also be needed for sleep disorder.

These families usually require much help, but in the case of progressive disorders, long-term residential care may eventually become necessary. Special education is often required. The various treatments mentioned are discussed more fully in Chapter 16.

Outcome
In non-progressive disorders the long-term outlook depends largely on the severity of any brain damage. Social and language skills may improve with maturation, combined with behavioural treatment and an appropriate educational programme. Progressive cases seem to be commoner, however, and have a poor outcome. In many cases a state of dementia, often becoming severe, develops, followed by death — though this may not occur until well into adult life. The rate of deterioration varies widely.

Schizophrenic Psychoses of Later Childhood and Adolescence

In later childhood, and particularly in adolescence, there occur psychoses which more clearly resemble schizophrenia as it is seen in adult patients (Rutter 1976; Vrono, 1974).

Prevalence
Childhood schizophrenia is rare. In child psychiatric practice, children with such psychoses are seen less often than children with psychoses of earlier onset, and in only very few adult schizophrenic patients does the disorder date back to before puberty. Onset before age 7 is very uncommon. After puberty, however, the incidence increases greatly and the fifteen- to twenty-year age range is a common period for the onset of schizophrenia.

Causes
The causes of childhood schizophrenia are not known but genetic predisposition plays a part, as in adult schizophrenia. No metabolic or biochemical abnormality has as yet been shown to be causal, nor have any psychological factors or environmental stresses been proved responsible, though it has been suggested that certain patterns of family behaviour can contribute to the development of schizophrenia (see Barker, 1981a, Chapter 11).

Description
The clinical features resemble those of adult schizophrenia. Many

of these children are reported to have been odd (shy, diffident, withdrawn, timid or sensitive) before the development of the psychotic symptoms. There is a history of delayed development, especially of speech, in nearly half (Fish, 1977), but this contrasts with infantile psychosis in which this is almost invariably present.

At the onset there is a change of personality and an alteration of the contact the child makes, on an emotional level, with the environment. There may be progressive withdrawal from contact with people, with a violent reaction if attempts are made to counter this, but the degree of withdrawal is less marked than in infantile psychosis. Emotional reactions to people and situations may be inappropriate, or flat. Thinking tends to become loose and woolly, with a falling-off in the standard of school work as an early manifestation. This thought disorder is a major symptom of schizophrenia and takes various forms. There is often loosening of the constraints normally present on thought association. Thus the subject may when talking turn from one subject immediately to another apparently unrelated one (the so-called 'knights move'). Various other disorders of the form and stream of thought such as thought blocking, when thoughts suddenly come to a stop, or thought insertion, when the subject experiences the insertion of what are felt to be alien thoughts into the mind, may be present.

There may be abnormalities of motor function with underactivity or overactivity, but especially with bizarre movements and posturings. Also evident may be disturbances of volition such as passivity and lack of drive, stubbornness, negativism, or impulsive outbursts of aggressive or in other ways inappropriate behaviour. Delusions are often present but may be difficult to distinguish from fantasies. Hallucinations, usually auditory, are common and they, and delusions also, probably account for many of the preoccupations of these children (with people's spectacles, the time, motor vehicles and so on).

There is a lack of agreement among psychiatrists about the precise criteria which should be used in making a diagnosis of schizophrenia. There are considerable variations between different centres and different countries. Schneider, a German psychiatrist, described certain 'symptoms of the first rank', each of which he believed was diagnostic if it occurred in clear consciousness. These were conveniently summarised by Kendall (1972):

1. Auditory hallucinations taking any one of the specific forms:
    (i) Voices repeating the patient's thoughts out loud or antici-
        pating them.
    (ii) Two or more hallucinatory voices discussing, or arguing
        about, the patient who is referred to in the third person.
    (iii) Voices commenting on the patient's thoughts or behaviour,
        often as a running commentary.
2. The subjective experience of alien thoughts being put into the
   patient's mind by some external agency, or of own thoughts
   being taken away (thought insertion or withdrawal).
3. The experience that the patient's thinking is no longer confined
   within his or her own mind, but is instead shared by or accessible
   to others (thought broadcasting).
4. The experience of feelings, impulses or acts being carried out
   under external control, so that the patient may feel like a robot
   or like someone who is hypnotised.
5. The experience of being a passive and reluctant recipient of bodily
   sensations (haptic, thermic or kinaesthetic) imposed by some
   external agency.
6. Delusional perception — arising fully fledged on the basis of a
   genuine perception which would be regarded as commonplace by
   others.

Although these symptoms are reliable as indications that a diagnosis
of schizophrenia is appropriate, they are absent in 20 per cent or
more of cases. Moreover they can be hard to elicit in withdrawn
children.

The behaviour of schizophrenic children is often changeable and
unpredictable. Thus impulsive and overactive behaviour may alternate
with withdrawn and underactive behaviour. Behaviour may also
become socially inappropriate, with sexual exposure or talking or
shouting at people inappropriately. Regressive behaviour such as
wetting, soiling and infantile behaviour at mealtimes may also appear.

Paranoid schizophrenia (in which the patient falsely believes he or
she is being persecuted) is seldom seen in childhood, but becomes
commoner in adolescence.

While schizophrenic psychoses may occur in mentally retarded
children, most schizophrenic children are of average intelligence,
some higher. They continue to perform in intelligence tests at or
above the average level long after the onset of their illness, but

usually become increasingly retarded educationally because in their disturbed state learning is impaired.

Treatment

Symptomatic improvement, with reduction in the severity of symptoms such as impulsivity, aggressiveness and hallucinations, can often be obtained by administration of phenothiazine tranquillisers such as chlorpromazine, fluphenazine and perphenazine. Haloperidol is also sometimes helpful. Supportive psychotherapy may help and it may be possible to find an educational regime (perhaps in a special school or hospital unit) from which the patient can gain benefit. Family therapy has been advocated for schizophrenia. Its role is unclear but is discussed further in *Basic Family Therapy* (Barker, 1981a).

Outcome

It is doubtful whether any of the above measures alter the long-term course of the disease, which is usually progressive. Symptomatic improvement on phenothiazine drugs may be considerable however, and with maintenance treatment some patients can live a useful life in the community. Occasionally remission occurs but more often there is deterioration which may lead to the need for long-term care in hospital. There have, however, been few long-term follow-up studies of schizophrenic children and data are scanty.

Affective Disorders

Affective disorders are conditions characterised primarily by a deviation from normal of the mood (or *affect*). This may be in the direction of depression or of elation (as in *mania*). In adults, disorders sometimes occur in which there are periodic changes in mood between psychotic depression, normality and psychotic elation. In certain cases the gross periodic mood changes occur regularly and with little apparent relationship to environmental events. This condition, *manic-depressive psychosis*, or *bipolar affective disorder* as DSM—III calls it, is very rare before puberty, though a few cases have been reported (Puig-Antich, 1980). Indeed mania, and its lesser form hypomania, are rarely seen in children. Depression is more common, though not as a feature of manic-depressive psychosis. Clear-cut depressive and manic psychoses are commoner in adolescence, though even in this age range manic conditions are rare.

Depression of mood frequently occurs in children faced with environmental stresses. When the depression can be understood in terms of the stress the child is facing, a diagnosis of psychosis is not appropriate. When the depression is disproportionately severe, however, and is not appropriate in terms of the reality the child is facing, the condition may be termed 'psychotic depression'. Thus the differentiation is a matter of clinical judgement involving assessment of both the child's mental state and his life situation. George, the boy whose case is described in Chapter 5, was close to the borderline between neurotic depression and psychosis. Had he attempted suicide instead of running away from home he might have been called psychotic.

In clinical practice the question of whether a particular depressive state should be called a 'psychosis' is relatively unimportant. A detailed assessment of the subject's mental state, especially the severity of the depression, and of any suicidal risk, is what is most necessary. Mania and depression are discussed here for convenience. Neurotic depression is also discussed in Chapter 5. DSM—III does not distinguish these types of depression; instead it codes the various forms of mania and depression as 'affective disorders'.

Causes

Manic-depressive disease appears to have a biological cause, and sometimes periods of depression and mania alternate regularly for many years, regardless of the subject's environmental circumstances. The underlying causes are not fully understood, but biochemical changes in the brain are involved. It may be that similar processes can cause attacks of depression, without mania, but how often this happens in children is not known. What is clear, however, is that most depressed children are facing considerable stress. There is often an unhappy family situation, a lack of security, and an atmosphere of instability and pessimism among family members. Sometimes there is gross parental strife or a broken home. Parental rejection or scapegoating of the child is common. Difficulties at school or in relationships with other children may contribute. Genetic factors may also play a part.

Description

Until recently there has been uncertainty about whether depression equivalent to the 'major depression', as defined in DSM—III, occurs in children as well as adults. Some thought that childhood depression most often presented through 'depressive equivalents', such as boredom, restlessness, poor concentration, behaviour problems, running away, delinquency, promiscuity or truancy. While depressed children no doubt may show such symptoms, the tendency nowadays, especially in North America, is to use adult diagnostic criteria. Thus the DSM—III criteria for major depression comprise depressed mood, together with at least four of the following present for at least two weeks: poor appetite or 'significant weight loss'; sleep disturbances; psychomotor agitation or restlessness; loss of interest in usual activities; fatigue; feelings of worthlessness, self-reproach or inappropriate guilt; poor concentration or slowed thinking; and recurrent thoughts of death or suicide. Poznanski (1982) uses similar criteria in a helpful discussion of the clinical picture of childhood depression.

Puig-Antich (1980), in his valuable review of the field, also points to the use of adult criteria for the diagnosis of 'major depression' in both children and adolescents. He suggests that the child interview is assuming greater importance in making the diagnosis, that there seems to be a high prevalence of affective disorder and alcoholism in the biological relatives of depressed children, and that between 10 and 27 per cent of 'unselected child and adolescent patients' may suffer an affective disorder.

Children's moods tend to be more labile than those of adults, but in the depressed child there is a more long-standing and continuous mood of sadness, though some fluctuation from day to day, or at different times of day, may occur. Self-blame and expressions of guilt are common. One depressed 12-year-old said that her 'nervous state' was responsible for her father's difficulties at the office, mother's anaemia and general ill-health and the bad behaviour of the brother and sister. She also had difficulty getting to school and entertained suicidal thoughts.

Depression can also occur as an accompaniment of other disorders. Graham (1974) advocated caution in making the diagnosis and pointed out that in the Isle of Wight epidemiological study sadness and misery occurred in roughly equal proportion in both the children with conduct disorders and those with neurotic conditions. 'Pure' depression was found in only three children in the population studied, a rate of less than 0.2 per cent.

The term *anaclitic depression* was coined by Spitz (1946) to describe a condition of misery, crying, withdrawal and failure to thrive in babies and young children suffering from severe deprivation of parental care. This was apparently an environmentally determined reaction to a lack of care, and probably nothing to do with the depressive psychoses of later life.

Depression in adolescence is discussed further in Chapter 13.

Differentiation from Other Conditions

Depression must be distinguished from the sadness or unhappiness which affects all children from time to time, especially following a loss or disappointment. Here the DSM—III criteria, mentioned above, are helpful; it is also useful to consider whether or not the degree of unhappiness is proportional to the severity of the loss. Depression must also be differentiated from the chronically low self-esteem found in many children who have been brought up in rejecting, hostile and unstable family settings. In a sense these children are deeply depressed, but low self-esteem has often become a part of their personality structure. Having been brought up to look upon themselves as worthless, they often act accordingly, doing poorly at school or dropping out of it altogether, adopting an antisocial lifestyle or resorting to drugs or alcohol to alleviate the bad feelings they have about themselves. While seriously in need of help these children — and many adolescents in the same position — often do not fit the DSM—III criteria for major depression, presenting rather with conduct disorders. Theirs is a chronic disorder of personality development (see Chapter 8) rather than a more specific depressive condition.

Treatment

The treatment of depression in childhood requires full assessment of the child's condition and environment. Where the condition is a reaction to an obvious stress, this should be removed, if possible, or modified. In many cases the cause of the depression lies in the family, for example when a child is scapegoated, and an approach by family therapy is required. In other circumstances the child benefits from psychotherapy.

There is reason to believe that antidepressant drugs may be helpful in depressed children. Although in a controlled trial of imipramine Puig-Antich (1980) found a response rate of 60 per cent in both imipramine- and placebo-treated children, the blood level findings were interesting. When the children receiving imipramine were subdivided according to whether the blood levels were above the median level (152 ng/ml), it was found that there was a 100 per cent response in the high plasma level group but only a 33 per cent response in the low plasma level group. This area requires further research, but it is clear that blood levels of imipramine vary a lot in children even when weight-related doses are the same, and this may be an important factor in explaining their varying response to antidepressant drugs.

The various treatments mentioned are discussed further in Chapter 16.

Suicide in Children

Suicide is rare in pre-pubertal children. Shaffer (1974) obtained information about all the recorded suicides in children aged 10 to 14 in England and Wales over a seven-year period and found none below age 12. On the other hand, some authors believe that there is under-reporting of childhood suicide (Garfinkel amd Golombek, 1977). They assert that death by suicide in childhood is often reported as accidental to avoid the stigma attached to suicide. While this may be true in North America, Shaffer cites good evidence that this is not the case in England and Wales.

In Shaffer's study there were 21 boys' and 9 girls' deaths. This is an annual suicide rate of 1 child out of every 800 000 in the 10- to 14-year age range. The commonest method of suicide was coal-gas poisoning, followed by hanging and drug overdose. Shaffer noted two personality stereotypes in the series. One consisted of children who had led a solitary existence, were of superior intelligence and appeared to have been culturally distant from their less well educated parents. Their mothers were mentally ill. Before their death they had seemed depressed or withdrawn, and some of them had stolen or stayed away from school.

The second group, which included several of the girls, consisted of children judged impetuous or prone to aggressive or violent outbursts, as well as being suspicious, and both sensitive to and resentful of criticism.

In most of the cases there had been prior antisocial behaviour and in 46 per cent previous suicidal behaviour was reported. The commonest precipitant was a disciplinary crisis.

Shaffer and Fisher (1981), reviewing the epidemiology of suicide in children and adolescents, conclude that, in the United States as in England and Wales, suicide is very rare before age 13, though apparently somewhat commoner than in England and Wales. It is much commoner in the 15- to 19-year age range (with a US rate of 7.6 per 100 000 adolescents), and seems to be increasing.

Suicidal attempts and threats are much more common than completed suicides. Attempted suicide should be regarded as serious and always justifies careful psychiatric evaluation of the child and the family situation. Often there is an element of depression though this may clear, usually only temporarily, after the attempt, if the child is in hospital and is being treated solicitously by the family. Attempted suicide has been found to be associated with severe disturbances in children's emotional and family relationships; parental rejection is common. Long and difficult treatment involving the whole family may be needed and repeated suicidal attempts often occur (Connell, 1971). Suicidal behaviour becomes much commoner in adolescence. Adolescent suicide is discussed in Chapter 13.

Outcome
Most depressed children recover either with treatment or spontaneously, though the depression may last several weeks or months, especially if suitable treatment is not instituted. The outlook is closely related to how far it is possible to remove or lessen whatever environmental stress the child is facing. If there is chronic, severe stress or family relationships are grossly disturbed and cannot be repaired, the outcome may depend on whether the child can be found a happier place in which to live. If the stress continues the depression may become chronic, with serious risk to future personality development.

Acute and Subacute Confusional States

In these conditions there is diffuse impairment of brain function with a state of delirium or confusion. Episodes are generally short-lived. The condition is usually reversible following the removal of the cause, though irreversible changes may occur.

The commonest causes are systemic infections, intracranial infections, metabolic disturbances, acute brain injury and chemical intoxications caused by drugs or other toxic ingested substances. Similar states are sometimes seen in epilepsy. Children, especially in their first few years of life, are particularly prone to develop delirious states during an illness causing a high fever. Common examples are pneumonia, measles (and other acute infectious fevers) and meningitis, but in all these antibiotics have greatly reduced the incidence of psychiatric complications. All sedative drugs, if taken in sufficiently high doses, may cause delirium, as may atropine and related substances. Of importance because of their illicit use by young people are amphetamine drugs, cannabis, lysergic acid diethylamide and other hallucinogenic drugs, heroin, other opiates and cocaine.

The main symptoms of delirium are clouding of consciousness, confusion, disorientation (for time, place and person) and vivid, often frightening fantasies or hallucinations. Memory is impaired. Restlessness, fearfulness or anxiety, increased suggestibility and rapid variation in the state of consciousness are also common features. Orientation may be difficult to assess in children, and this criterion cannot apply in infants who have not yet achieved normal orientation for time, place and person. The vivid fantasies reflect the normal tendency for young children to indulge readily in fantasy. It is often difficult to be sure whether or not the patient is actually hallucinated. When they occur, hallucinations tend to be mainly visual.

Confusional states vary in severity and in acuteness. Sometimes the child is confused and disorientated, but the complete syndrome is not present. Convulsions are a common feature of these states in the first five years of life, but do not usually presage continuing epilepsy.

The treatment of these conditions is that of the underlying cause.

CHAPTER SEVEN

Enuresis, Encopresis and the Hyperkinetic Syndrome

Although enuresis and encopresis have sometimes been regarded as 'developmental' disorders, they are not so classified in either ICD–9 (W.H.O., 1977) or DSM–III (APA, 1980). ICD–9 classifies them under 'special symptoms or syndromes not elsewhere classified', and DSM–III as 'other disorders with physical manifestations'. In ICD–9 the 'hyperkinetic syndrome of childhood' comprises a category of its own; so the same applies in DSM–III but here it is renamed 'attention deficit disorder — with hyperactivity'!

Enuresis

Bedwetting, or *nocturnal enuresis,* often occurs on its own. It may be accompanied by daytime wetting, or *diurnal enuresis;* less commonly diurnal enuresis occurs on its own. Most children achieve day and night continence by three to four years of age, usually being dry by day before they are dry at night. Persistent enuresis beyond age 5 is abnormal.

Prevalence studies show bedwetting to be very common. About ten per cent of children still wet their bed at age five; the percentage falls to about five at age ten and one to two per cent continue during their teens. Different studies however have produced different results, partly because of variable criteria for enuresis (Kolvin *et al.,* 1973). There are also big differences between countries. In Australia and North America the rate is three times that in Sweden, where the prevalence is about 8 per cent at age 5. The British rate is thus nearer the Swedish one, rather than that of the 'bed-sodden states of America' *(British Medical Journal,* 1977). The prevalence generally drops with increasing age, but some studies have shown an increase between the ages of five and seven, especially in boys. This is presumably due to the appearance, between these ages, of cases of secondary enuresis, that is enuresis appearing after the child has become dry. The prevalence of daytime wetting is considerably lower than that of nocturnal wetting; about 2 per cent of 5-year-olds are wet by day once a week or more, though about 8 per cent are wet at least once a month. In the 7- to 10-year-old age range diurnal wetting seems to occur in about 1 per cent of children, with some excess of girls.

The *causes* of enuresis are imperfectly understood, and probably vary from case to case. Genetic factors seem to play a part. Enuresis tends to run in families and a study of twins by Bakwin (1971) showed monozygotic twins to be concordant for enuresis about twice as often as dizygotic twins. Physical causes are rare and most enuretics have no demonstrable physical abnormality except for small bladder capacity. It has been shown, however, that enuretics have on average smaller maximum bladder capacities than non-enuretics; that they pass urine more frequently than non-enuretics; and that their bladders are only functionally and not structurally small. Enuresis may also be associated with urinary infections, especially in girls, and occasionally there is a structural abnormality of the urinary tract. Other rare causes are nocturnal epileptic fits and conditions causing the production of excessive quantities of urine (for example, diabetes). Most physical causes lead to diurnal as well as nocturnal enuresis.

There is an association between enuresis and emotional disorder, though most enuretic children are not disturbed. Enuresis can, like soiling, be a part of a pattern of regression. Enuresis can also be a symptom of a more general disturbance such as neurosis, psychosis or adjustment reaction. It has been suggested that early disturbing events (family break-up, temporary separation from mother, birth of a sibling, accidents, operations, hospital admission, moving house) can cause enuresis. MacKeith (1968) believes that there is a 'sensitive' period for learning bladder control (one-and-a-half to four-and-a-half years) and that if something happens to interfere with learning or training at that time, subsequent learning will be more difficult.

Unusually deep sleep has been said to contribute to nocturnal enuresis, but satisfactory evidence that enuretic children do sleep especially deeply is lacking, though this theory, like most of the others, has not been disproved. Another theory is that delayed maturation of the nervous system (or certain parts of it), which may be partly genetically determined, is important. This would account for the findings of twin studies and the fact that there is a positive family history in up to 70 per cent of cases of primary enuresis. It might be expected that delayed biological maturation would be more likely to lead to continuing enuresis if combined with family disorganisation, inconsistent training or other stresses producing anxiety. Delay in achieving bladder control is also a feature of mental handicap, and is usually marked in the presence of severe retardation. Berg (1979), in a review of daytime wetting, points out that there is some reason to believe that wetting by day is more likely to be associated with psychiatric disorder than is bedwetting.

Enuresis, and its causes are discussed in the book *Bladder Control and Enuresis* (Kolvin *et al.*, 1973) and also by Shaffer (1976).

Most cases of nocturnal enuresis are 'primary', the child never having become dry at night. The only symptom, initially at least, is the passing of urine while asleep. Later this may be complicated by feelings of anxiety or guilt, particularly if the child is blamed or punished for the wetting. Depending on the family's attitudes towards the symptom, secondary emotional disorder may develop. Indeed enuresis causes great unhappiness and distress to some children – perhaps its main psychiatric importance. Many children are blamed for it and some severely punished. It can prevent holidays, visits to relations and friends, and participation in camping activities.

About one bedwetter in five has increased frequency of micturation by day but without day wetting. In other cases there is both increased frequency and daytime wetting. The presence of these features, however, is more often associated with the existence of other evidence of anxiety or emotional disorder. Infection of the urinary tract is also more likely if wetting occurs both by day and by night.

Investigation and treatment should go hand in hand. In primary enuresis carefully taken histories from child and parents will establish that the enuresis is the outstanding problem, and that any other emotional symptoms are a consequence of the wetting. It is important to adopt an optimistic outlook while taking the history and to let the family feel that the problem is a common one, and not too serious, despite the inconvenience it may cause. Many parents, and children, are unaware of the frequency of the complaint. The self-blame both often show must be dispelled as far as possible. The history must be considered to see whether there is evidence of any physical abnormality of bladder or urethra. The abdomen and external genitalia should be examined, and the urine tested, especially for evidence of infection. X-ray examination of the urinary tract is done routinely in some clinics, but is probably only necessary if there is evidence to suggest a physical abnormality. The latter is unlikely if the wetting is purely nocturnal.

When there is no evidence of physical or emotional disorder, as in most cases, the choice of treatment lies between drug therapy and treatment with the pad and buzzer. Either method should be combined with support and reassurance for the family. The symptom is usually best talked about as a 'delay in learning to control the bladder while asleep' (or 'when excited', etc.) rather than as a serious disease. It should be made clear that the wetting is involuntary. (Deliberate, that is consciously intended, wetting is rare and is almost always a symptom of a general disturbance such as a conduct disorder.)

The only drugs which have been shown to be effective are tricyclic drugs such as imipramine and amitriptyline. Imipramine has been shown, in controlled trials, to be effective in a significant number of cases, though the response rate falls well short of 100 per cent, and the relapse rate is high. It should be given initially in a dose of 25 mg at night, increasing if necessary to 50 mg. The mode of action of the tricyclic drugs is uncertain. They are also antidepressants, but it may be that they are effective in enuresis as a result of their side-effects on the autonomic nervous system, rather than because of their antidepressant action. It does seem, however, that some children thought not to be disturbed show behavioural changes for the better while on imipramine for enuresis, and a few show adverse psychological effects including irritabiltity and depression (Werry et al., 1975). If there is a response to medication it should be continued at least until the child has been dry for a continuous period of a month. A very cautious reduction in dosage can then be tried. Any sign of relapse should lead to an increase to the former dosage. The total duration of treatment needed is usually several months.

Conditioning with the pad and buzzer appartus is often used as the treatment of first choice (Shaffer, 1976; Dische, 1971). The apparatus consists essentially of two metal sheets, one at least being perforated, which are placed in the bed and attached to a buzzer or

Figure 1

bell. The wire gauze or foil-covered sheets are arranged so that there is a sheet (flannelette or cotton) between them, and another one on top of the upper one. If only one of the foil-covered sheets is perforated, this should be the upper one. The wires are then attached, with the metal sheets in such a position that they will become wet as soon as the child starts to pass urine. The arrangement is shown in Figure 1. The wires lead to a buzzer or bell which is best placed at a sufficient distance from the bed, preferably at the bottom, to prevent the child switching it off without getting out of bed. It is switched on when the child goes to bed, and as soon as the sheet separating the two metal pads gets wet the circuit is completed and the buzzer sounds. It is better for the child not to wear pyjama trousers; this ensures quick wetting of the sheets. The child is woken by the buzzer and should then get out of bed, turn off the buzzer, pass urine and, ideally, re-set the apparatus using dry sheets. Sometimes in the initial stages the buzzer may sound two or even three times in the course of a night. In such cases there is often a particularly quick response to the treatment. Use of the apparatus should be continued at least until the child has been dry continuously for three weeks. Even after this period relapse may occur, but relapses usually respond quickly to a second course of treatment. In occasional cases more than one further course of treatment is needed.

Certain points are important in this treatment. It is essential to get the child's co-operation. Without it treatment is seldom successful. It is best for the child to set up the apparatus, switch it on and keep a record of wet and dry nights, rather than have the parents do these things. Some children, if not adequately prepared, are frightened of the machine; others are suspicious or hostile. It is easy for a child to sabotage its use, so any feelings such as these must be explored and dealt with before treatment is started. If after a few discussions a child of seven or older does not accept the treatment there may well be an emotional disorder needing treatment in its own right.

The apparatus can seldom be used effectively in children below age six. Sometimes it is necessary to wait until a year, or even two, later before adequate co-operation can be gained. Children of six to seven may be better moved into, or near, their parents' bedroom, so that a parent can help them re-set the buzzer and rearrange the bed after they have woken.

If any relapses are treated promptly along the lines suggested, a good response to conditioning treatment is usually obtained. Success rates of 80 per cent or better may be expected. In refractory cases imipramine 25–50 mg at bedtime, or amitriptyline in the same dose, may be combined with use of the buzzer. Other measures such as restricting the amount the child drinks, or lifting during the night, should be avoided. They tend to delay the conditioning process.

Buzzer ulcers are an occasional complication of the use of the buzzer. They may occur if current passes between the electrodes through the skin. This can occur if the apparatus and drawsheet become disarranged so that the electrodes touch the skin. It can also occur when conduction through the skin is facilitated because the skin is wet with urine or, possibly, sweat. It may happen in the presence of urine if (a) there is insufficient urine to trigger the alarm so that a small current passes for a considerable time; (b) the buzzer fails to operate because the battery is partially exhausted; or (c) the child fails to wake up when the alarm sounds, so that buzzing continues until exhaustion of the battery causes the relay to cease operating, whereupon the electrodes again become live. Modern buzzer design has largely eliminated these problems, but it is important that a flat battery is never used.

Outcome: As the figures for prevalence show, there is a tendency for children to grow out of their enuresis, though the spontaneous recovery rate is not sufficient to justify therapeutic inaction. Active treatment, particularly of primary enuretics in the age range six to nine, usually gives good results. If treatment is left till later the results tend to be less satisfactory. Sometimes secondary emotional disorder interferes with treatment, though it can usually be overcome. Children with impoverished and disorganised homes, especially when they share a bed with one or more siblings, are difficult to treat. Even if the child can be got into a bed on his own, systematic and correct use of the buzzer may be hard to achieve. Drug therapy may be easier. Occasionally it is justifiable to admit children from such backgrounds to a hospital or other institution for conditioning therapy.

Encopresis

Encopresis, or faecal soiling, is the passing of faeces in the clothes. It may occur by day and at night. Children are normally 'clean', that is continent of faeces, by the age of three. Some otherwise normal children do not achieve continence until a little later, but soiling beyond the age of four is abnormal, except in mentally retarded children.

Prevalence: Bellman (1966) in a study in Sweden, found a prevalence rate at age 7 of 2.3 per cent in boys and 0.7 per cent in girls, a boy:girl ratio of 3.4 to 1. In the Isle of Wight survey of 10- and 11-year-olds, the prevalence was 1.3 per cent in boys and 0.3 per cent in girls (Rutter *et al.*, 1970). Clinical sudies also show a much higher rate in boys than girls. The prevalence falls practically to zero by age 16.

Causes: Figure 2 illustrates the various ways in which soiling can arise.

First, encopresis may be divided into retentive and non-retentive categories, according to whether faeces have accumulated in the colon and rectum in excessive amounts. This is determined by palpation of the abdomen: in severe cases the faecal masses can readily be felt in the dilated intestine. Digital examination of the rectum should also be carried out: in retentive soiling a large ballooned rectum full of faeces will be felt. There are also often faeces to be seen leaking out the anus.

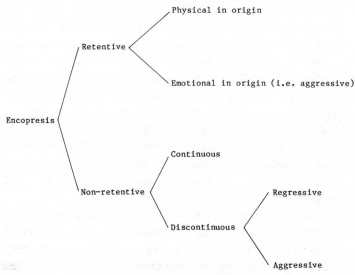

Figure 2   Types of encopresis

Retentive soiling may be due to physical or to psychological causes. The commonest cause is an anal fissure, which causes severe pain on defaecation. Because of the pain, the child may consciously hold back from passing faeces which accumulate over time. Eventually, whatever the cause, the muscle in the intestinal wall, and the sphincters controlling defaecation, lose their tone and the constipation persists, even though the original cause — such as an anal fissure — may no longer be present. Hirschprung's disease is a rare condition in which the nerve ganglia are congenitally absent from a section of the colon. This section is therefore unable to contract normally and thus move the faeces on. The colon behind it becomes loaded with faeces and dilates. In these cases, however, the rectum is normal on digital examination. X-ray examination of the abdomen may be employed to confirm the diagnosis of faecal retention and a barium enema will show whether there is an aganglionic length of bowel, as in Hirschprung's disease.

Psychologically caused retention of faeces usually occurs in the context of a disturbed relationship between child and parents, most often mother (Anthony, 1957; Pinkerton, 1958). It starts as a negativistic refusal to defaecate, often as a reaction to obsessive, coercive toilet training by parents who have a high regard for order and cleanliness and over-value early bowel and bladder control. Toilet training may have started early, even within the first few weeks of life. Success surprisingly early, perhaps in the first year of life, may be reported. It is then particularly distressing for the parent when the child later starts to soil. This however is what is intended — unconsciously — by the child, who may be, in other ways, clean, tidy and well behaved. But these children express their unconsciously felt anger through their parents' Achilles' heel, namely bowel control. It has also been reported that these children are immature and show excessive dependence on their mothers, their fathers often playing little part in the families (Hoag *et al.*, 1971). The mothers often have a great fear of constipation and may use laxatives to excess. Their preoccupation with bowel function may date back to their own childhood experiences.

As these children continue to resist defaecating, faeces pile up in the colon and rectum, which gradually become distended with masses of faeces which may ultimately become hard and impacted. Liquid faeces may pass round these masses and constantly leak out of the anus, the child no longer having any control over the process.

The end result may be indistinguishable from that occurring in physically caused faecal retention.

Non-retentive soiling may be 'continuous' or 'discontinuous'. Continuous soiling has been present from birth, the child having never been toilet trained. It is often due to lack of proper toilet training and usually occurs in children who appear in other ways poorly cared for. They are often dirty and badly dressed. There may be other evidence of poor social training. Truancy from school may be reported and progress at school is often unsatisfactory. The families usually face, or through their social inadequacy have acquired, many other problems. These may include bad housing, a burden of debt, unemployment or a criminal record. The child's soiling may be just one feature, though perhaps the most prominent and trouble-some, of a general pattern of immature behaviour. Continuous soiling may also be associated with mental retardation; these cases are readily distinguished by the accompanying general retardation of development.

Discontinuous non-retentive soiling may be either 'regressive' or 'aggressive'. Regressive soiling may occur in children from any social class. The symptom is usually readily recognised as due to some acute or continuing emotional stress. There may be regression in spheres other than bowel function. There may also be other evidence of anxiety. The anxiety is, however, understandable in the light of the stress the child is facing. (If it were disproportionate, a diagnosis of a neurotic disorder might be more appropriate. Some short-lived episodes of regressive soiling reactive to acute stress are appropriately classified as adjustment reactions.) The symptom is closely akin to the diarrhoea some adults experience before examinations, interviews and the like.

Aggressive non-retentive soiling has a similar psychopathology to that of psychogenic retentive soiling, except that, instead of refusing to defaecate at all, the child refuses to do so at the desired place and time. Like the children with psychogenic retention, these tend to be clean, often too clean, well-dressed, inhibited children who do well at school. They often appear ashamed of their soiling, and may attempt to conceal it, for example by hiding or destroying under-clothes. They may be reluctant to discuss their bowel function but may allude to it in play or drawings. In about half of this group of chidren food refusal is also reported by the parents, though these children are usually adequately nourished. There is frequently an absence of the rough play and self-assertiveness usual at the child's age. Typically, these are bright, successful pupils at school, in contrast to the typical 'continuous' soiler who usually is not.

The *clinical picture* is not always as clear-cut as the above account might suggest. Some 'aggressive' soilers, whether retentive or non-retentive, have never been successfully trained as infants. Sometimes there are both aggressive and regressive features, as in the following case in which there were factors evoking both anxiety and hostility towards the parents.

David was referred for psychiatric assessment at age eight, the main symptom being soiling. His birth had been normal, he was described by his mother as an easy baby to bring up, and she said toilet training was completed by his first birthday. He gave mother no trouble as a toddler and at five he went to school without difficulty. When David was six his sister died after a short illness. This upset both David and his mother, who had always been an anxious woman. She became depressed and was admitted briefly to hospital for psychiatric treatment.

On examination David was a quiet, inhibited, very clean and well-dressed boy. There was little spontaneous conversation or play, but he was polite and 'correct' in his behaviour.

Mother, by contrast, was a big, talkative, anxious and dominating woman. She tried to decide and control every activity of David, over-protecting him yet at times getting very angry with him, usually for minor, or even imagined, misdeeds. She did not bring father to the clinic but reported that he worked well in a steady job and was a good provider.

David was admitted to hospital for treatment. He was found to be chronically constipated and was given Senokot regularly. He settled quickly and after about two weeks became more self-assertive in his play and showed some aggressiveness towards the other children. His soiling had completely stopped within three weeks of admission. He did well in the clinic school.

Mother's behaviour was very disturbed. She visited daily for long periods, preventing David taking part in some of the activities arranged for the children. She was often highly critical both of David and of the hospital staff, yet she spoilt him by bringing him food and expensive presents. She seemed grossly over-anxious about him. Father visited less often, and was a quiet man who behaved appropriately when with David.

Despite mother's doubts about the treatment, her lack of trust in the hospital staff, and her apparent need for a mutually dependent relationship with David she allowed him to remain in the hospital for seven weeks.

David was then allowed home for a weekend, but his mother could not bring herself to let him return after this.

The mother proved a most difficult person to help. She was chronically anxious, had episodes of severe depression, was suspicious of the family and neighbours, and of the hospital staff's efforts to help her and David, and expressed much guilt about her daughter's death. She had apparently brought David up in a rigid, obsessive way. David had conformed until the death of his sister. He, and mother, then became very anxious and various types of regressive behaviour, particularly soiling, appeared. Mother reacted angrily and David could only assert himself by continued refusal to conform in the matter of bowel control.

It was perhaps a little surprising that after discharge David did not start to soil again, according to his mother's account, but it was clear that family relationships remained disturbed and the mother required further psychiatric treatment.

Investigation: A detailed history from the parents and mental and physical examination of the child are often all that is needed to establish the type of soiling. Its severity must also be ascertained. This may be anything from slight staining of underclothes to the passage of all faeces in the clothes. It is important also to discover whether or not there is any retention of faeces, as outlined above.

Diagnosis tends to be most difficult in long-standing cases, particularly when there is faecal retention and overflow incontenence. The origin of the symptom may then be impossible to discover. If it was physical, emotional disorder may have appeared secondarily, due to parental disapproval and the child's anxiety and guilt. If it was emotional, the child's negativistic refusal to defaecate may have been complicated by long-standing constipation and dilation of the colon.

X-ray examination of the abdomen may help. The most useful procedure is visualisation of the large intestine by means of a barium enema. This may show a narrow length of undilated colon with a great increase in size of the colon proximal to it, indicating Hirschsprung's disease. In psychogenic cases the whole length of the colon is dilated.

Treatment: This depends on the cause, the presence or absence of constipation or faecal retention, the age of the child and the duration of the condition. Many cases are treated by paediatricians or family practitioners, especially where constipation or overflow incontinence is present, and when the main treatment need is to provide toilet training for a child who has not been effectively trained.

Constipation, if present, must be dealt with. It often responds well to regular administration of a laxative such as Senokot. One to four tablets daily are usually required. If there is also much retention of faeces enemas and/or suppositories may be needed. In the more severe cases of retentive soiling, the child is usually best admitted to hospital for treatment (Pinkerton, 1974). This is certainly so if physical treatment other than the oral administration of laxatives is needed. Even then, enemas and suppositories should only be given after a good relationship with the child has been established by the nurse, and after due explanation of the treatment to the child. Otherwise the treatment may be regarded, unconsciously at least, as a further aggressive attack. Thus while the constipation may get better the basic emotional problem may worsen. Indeed, physical measures must only be carried out as part of a wider plan of treatment dealing also with the emotional problems. Occasionally manual removal of the faeces under general anaesthetic is necessary.

Most children who soil become clean within two or three weeks of admission to hospital, provided that if there is faecal retention, this is relieved. If the soiling continues it may be because the hospital staff are dealing with it in a punitive or hostile way, or because the disturbed interaction with the parent is continuing. For example, one boy for several weeks handed his mother soiled underpants to take home and wash, unknown to the staff.

If there is no evidence of constipation or retention of faeces, no physical treatment of the bowel condition itself is required. If there has been a failure to provide normal toilet training, the child usually responds to a period of consistent, firm and kind training. This can be done in hospital, or some other residential setting; but it is better, if more difficult, to get the parents to do it at home. The family may need intensive help, not only with toilet training their children, but also in overcoming other social difficulties. Behaviour modification programmes can be helpful in these cases (Sluckin, 1975).

Regressive soiling in the acutely anxious or insecure child does not usually require treatment in itself. It is best made light of, while attention is directed to removing the cause of the child's anxiety. If this is impossible, psychotherapy may help the child cope with the stress he or she faces. This is discussed further in Chapter 16, as is drug therapy which may occasionally be helpful.

When soiling is due to a disturbed relationship with an obsessive parent, as outlined above, psychotherapy is needed. With younger children, treatment aimed primarily at altering the parents' attitude to the problems, and thus the handling of the child, may be the main need. Sometimes an approach by family therapy is helpful.

Where there is 'aggressive' soiling, with or without retention, a lot of work may need to be done with the parents. Usually the mother has the greater need. Once a trusting relationship with her has been established, the whole question of constipation and its dangers may be discussed. It can be difficult to get this viewed in proper perspective by these bowel-conscious people. When this has been done, at least partially, the discussion can go on to the child's symptoms. Ultimately the parents have to be led to an understanding of the soiling as a means of self-expression, or protest, or as a manifestation of anger, in a child who feels unable to express these feelings in other ways. Difficult as open aggression may be for these parents to accept, they need to see that its expression can be a sign of improvement. Simple explanation of these points is seldom sufficient. Discussion over a period of time, in the context of a trusting relationship with physician or social worker, is required. Group therapy can be helpful in this process (Hoag *et al.*, 1971).

Psychotherapy with the child is more often needed in older children (over 8 or 9) with chronic and well-established soiling. Such children are often less sensitive to changes in parental attitudes.

The *outcome* of encopresis depends on its type. Regressive soiling generally disappears quite quickly, especially if the child is admitted for inpatient treatment. Aggressive soiling, especially when accompanied by retention, is harder to treat and may take longer to stop. In most cases the soiling has ceased by the mid-teens (Bellman, 1966), but it appears that some of these children later show their unresolved aggressive feelings in other ways.

The Hyperkinetic Syndrome of Childhood

The hyperkinetic syndrome is described in ICD–9 (WHO, 1977) as being characterised essentially by short attention-span and distractibility. In DSM–III (APA, 1980) this condition is called 'attention deficit disorder' and is subdivided into cases 'with hyperactivity' and those 'without hyperactivity'. There is also a sub-category for use when an individual has in the past been diagnosed as having 'attention deficit with hyperactivity' but is no longer hyperactive, though other features of the syndrome persist.

While hyperactive children undoubtedly exist, as do children in whom there is lack of normal capacity for sustained attention, there is dispute about whether the condition merits the status of a disorder. Shaffer and Greenhill (1979), for example, argue that the diagnosis 'hyperkinetic syndrome' tells little about aetiology, response to treatment or longer-term outcome. Also it does not permit generalisations to be made about clinical state. It is probably because of the problems brought out in this review that prevalence studies have yielded widely differing results.

The diagnostic criteria used greatly affect the prevalence figures found, as do the ages of the children studied, the population they are drawn from and the methods of investigation used. North American prevalence rates for the hyperkinetic syndrome — which may be regarded as describing very roughly the same group of children as the DSM—III's attention deficit disorder with hyperactivity (ADD—H) — are generally higher than British ones; this is probably due to the use in most British studies of the criterion that hyperactivity must be present in the interview situation. By contrast, questionnaire and rating scale data, which have tended to be used in North American studies, give higher prevalence rates. Safer and Allen (1976), reviewing the literature, conclude that parents report 35—50 per cent of boys and 20—25 per cent of girls as hyperactive, and elementary school teachers report 40 per cent of their students as restless and one-third as inattentive. But when only 'a prominent degree of hyperactivity and inattentiveness' is considered, the prevalence falls to 5—10 per cent. If learning disability is an added criterion the prevalence is about 5 per cent. The disorder is commoner in boys than girls, ratios of 3:1 or 4:1 being quoted by Safer and Allen, though DSM—III alleges a 10:1 ratio, with a 3 per cent prevalence rate. Safer and Allen suggest that the prevalence in elementary school is: boys, 8—9 per cent; girls, 2—3 per cent. These are mainly North American figures; by contrast in the Isle of Wight epidemiological study (Rutter et al., 1970) of 10- and 11-year-olds only two cases of hyperkinetic syndrome were found in 2199 children (0.1 per cent). By this age hyperactivity has often lessened, however.

Various causes have been suggested for this syndrome. There is evidence that genetic factors play a significant role and that polygenic inheritance is the most likely mechanism (Morrison and Stewart, 1976). Some children with the hyperkinetic syndrome have an organic brain disorder (Werry, 1972), but most do not and many brain-damaged children are not hyperactive. Hyperkinetic children tend to have been very active babies (Safer and Allen, 1976) and it is possible that some are children at one end of a normally distributed range of activity levels; such children might be especially at risk if growing up with parents who react adversely to a child with that temperamental trait. Environmental factors at home and at school may also play a part in the labelling of children as hyperactive (Hartsough and Lambert, 1982).

Sometimes the terms 'minimal brain damage' or 'minimal brain dysfunction' are applied to hyperactive children and at times the terms are used almost as if they were interchangeable. Thus Wender (1971) one of the main proponents of the concept of minimal brain dysfunction (MBD), even quotes descriptions of hyperactive children when describing 'MBD'. On the other hand, he states that children with MBD may be underactive; also that many of them show no neurological abnormalities of any sort. In addition over 100 clinical manifestations are attributed to MBD, making the concept virtually useless as a diagnostic entity. It is small wonder it has been described as a 'myth' (Schmitt, 1975). Confusion is avoided if the term is not used.

Description: The hyperkinetic syndrome, or ADD–H, is character-ised by motor hyperactivity, restlessness, impaired attention and impulsivity. These children are highly distractible but attend only briefly to distracting stimuli. Onset is usually before age 3, but the disorder may not come to professional attention until the child starts school. Young children often show sustained, gross motor activity; older children and adolescents may show great restlessness and fidgetiness. As well as difficult behaviour in school, these children often fail to learn. This seems to be in part due to the failure of attention, causing inaccurate work with impulsive errors, as well as failure to attend to what is being taught; there may also be other learning difficulties. Antisocial behaviour and emotional outbursts may accompany the other symptoms. The emotionalism is often shown through temper tantrums, but other manifestations of anger, unhappiness, joy or annoyance may appear and disappear with bewildering frequency.

These children can be hard to manage at home as well as at school. Often the symptoms first become obvious when the child begins to walk. The parents then find these children are constantly on the move, concentrate poorly and are prone to interfere with furniture, ornaments, the contents of drawers and so forth, to an unusual extent. Normal methods of control are ineffective. Sleep disturbance is sometimes reported in younger hyperkinetic children, but many of them sleep well: apparently their activity has exhausted them by bedtime, though they are liable to waken early in the morning.

Assessment and Treatment: Treatment must be preceded by assessment of the type of excessive motor activity present; the situations in which it is more, or less, prominent; and any associated problems such as learning difficulties and poor school progress. It is important to discover whether there are associated perceptual or motor difficulties, or mental handicap.

This syndrome is one of the few child psychiatric disorders in which drugs can be of real value. The choice lies between methylphenidate, various amphetamine derivatives, phenothiazine drugs and haloperidol.

Methylphenidate has been shown, in well-planned clinical trials, to have a significant effect in controlling children's hyperactive behaviour. It seems however that the effects of methylphenidate and its related drugs, the amphetamines, are non-specific. Rapoport *et al.* (1978) showed that normal prepubertal boys given dextroamphetamine responded in the same way as hyperactive children.

In the short term methylphenidate in appropriate doses usually improves concentration and classroom behaviour, decreases impulsivity and makes purposeless activity more goal directed (Weiss, 1981). It also improves the quality of mother–child interaction (Humphries *et al.*, 1978), suggesting that the controlling behaviour often seen in the mothers of hyperactive children is more a response to the hyperactivity than its cause. Weiss (1981), in an excellent review article, discusses many aspects of the treatment of hyperactive children. She points out that the long-term effects of the stimulant drugs are less satisfactory than the short-term ones. Children receiving medication tend still to fail in school, develop antisocial behaviour and experience social ostracism. It is therefore important to have a comprehensive treatment plan in addition to the use of medication.

Behaviour modification programmes may help deal with associated behaviour problems and it is sometimes possible to condition attention or concentration. Remedial education may help a child overcome a learning problem. Where there is a high anxiety level in child or parents, psychotherapy, either for individuals or the whole family, may help. Indeed help for the family is as important as treatment of the child. Support and advice on management may greatly assist the parents; obsessive and anxious parents often find these children particularly difficult.

The various treatment methods are discussed further in Chapter 16.

Outcome: Hyperactivity tends to lessen with increasing age, often ceasing by puberty, but learning disorders and antisocial behaviour may continue. A follow-up study of 17- to 24-year-olds showed that poor socialisation skills and a poor sense of well-being were still present significantly more often than in control subjects. So too were scholastic difficulties and restlessness; but there was no difference between the groups in work adjustment, antisocial behaviour, non-medical use of drugs or serious psychiatric disturbances (Hechtman *et al.*, 1976).

'Attention deficit disorder without hyperactivity', as defined in DSM–III, is a less well documented condition. The features are the same as for ADD–H, except that hyperactivity is absent and 'the associated features and impairment' are generally milder.

CHAPTER EIGHT

Other Clinical Syndromes

Adjustment Reactions

Adjustment reactions are defined by ICD—9 (WHO, 1977), as 'mild or transient disorders . . . without any apparent pre-existing mental disorder'. The term is applied to circumscribed or situation-specific disorders which are generally reversible. They are usually related to major stresses, and may last a few days or up to a few months.

DSM—III (APA, 1980), defines 'adjustment disorder' as a 'maladaptive reaction to an identifiable psychosocial stressor' and arbitrarily sets a limit of three months from 'the onset of the stressor' to the reaction.

ICD—9 distinguishes three main types of adjustment reaction: those with depression (either brief or prolonged depressive reactions), those with disturbance mainly of other emotions and those with disturbance of conduct. Provision is also made for a mixed type. DSM—III has eight subtypes: adjustment disorder with, respectively, 'depressed mood'; 'anxious mood'; 'mixed emotional features'; 'disturbance of conduct'; 'mixed disturbance of emotions and conduct'; 'work (or academic) inhibition'; 'withdrawal'; and 'atypical features'. Use of these sub-categories does no more than draw attention to the predominant symptoms shown in each case.

Since adjustment disorders are defined more by their mild and transient nature and by the fact of their being reactions to environmental stress, there is no typical clinical picture.

Susan was referred at age 15, by the juvenile court. She had been born in Jamaica. Her parents had emigrated to England when she was three, but she had remained in Jamaica with her grandmother, joining her parents at age 12.

It seemed that Susan never had any problems in Jamaica where she was happy, had a warm relationship with her grandmother and progressed well at school. From the time she came to England, however, she had been unhappy. She said this was partly because she found the work and atmosphere at school different from that which she was used to, but mainly because of her home situation. Her parents had been strangers to her when she arrived but had expected love and obedience from her, which she found it difficult to provide on demand. She said of her mother, 'She treats me different, she don't like me, she treats me like a dog'. She believed she was brought over simply to look after the four younger children born in England, who seemed to have secure, warm relationships with the parents.

After some months of increasing unhappiness at home Susan ran away and was missing, and also absent from school, for two months. It transpired she had been living with a 17-year-old distant cousin during this time. Her parents reported unfavourably on her behaviour at home and she refused to return there.

On being placed in a group home Susan settled down well, behaved normally, showed no signs of emotional disorder and said she was happy.

Comment

There was no evidence that Susan suffered from any serious psychiatric disorder. Her condition was rather a transient, reversible reaction to migration from one culture to another, combined with her arrival to live with a family who did not give her the support, security and understanding she needed. Her symptoms rapidly subsided with a change in environment. Her condition is an example of an adjustment reaction with a depressive element. On the DSM—III she would be classified as showing an 'adjustment disorder with depressed mood'.

Timothy was referred by the family doctor at age 4 years 9 months. He had been showing aggressive behaviour since the birth of the only other child in the family, a sister two years younger. His mother described him as rude, fidgety and 'not a happy child – very highly strung'. The family had recently moved into a new housing development, with many houses still under construction. Father (30) was an executive in an industrial company which was going through a financially difficult time. He worked long hours, arrived home late, tired and bad-tempered, and gave mother little support. He had had an emotionally deprived family background. While mother said she came from a warm, close family all the other members of it lived in another part of the country.

At interview Timothy was a good-looking, well-dressed, friendly boy. He spoke freely, had a good vocabulary for his age and was pleasant and likeable in his attitude. In conversation he gave some indication of rivalry with his sister, but said he was happy at school, where he was nearing the end of his first term. He appeared in other respects a normal, healthy child.

The problem was formulated as that of a boy living in a socially isolated family. His mother was looking after two essentially healthy children with little help from her husband or anyone else. Consequently she had been unable to give Timothy enough support and attention, a situation which was exacerbated when the sister was born. Treatment consisted of five interviews with the parents and two with Timothy. The main work was done with the parents. It aimed to help them understand Timothy's needs and, perhaps more important, each other's. They were well-motivated people of high intelligence and seemed to be helped by these few interviews spread over six months. After this time Timothy's symptoms had disappeared, Karen, the sister, had started at a pre-school playgroup and the parents felt the problems were resolved.

Comment

This was a mild adjustment reaction, fitting best in the subgroup 'with mixed disturbance of emotions and conduct', although the problem was really the family's. Brief intervention yielded good results.

Quentin was referred at age five after his mother had been told by the school principal that he would not respond to discipline and therefore could not attend school. The school staff complained, among other things, that Quentin went into the girls' toilets in spite of being told not to and had repeatedly tried to climb over a wall, a thing which was forbidden because there was a busy road on the other side. The teachers consequently feared for Quentin's safety and were not willing to be responsible for him in the circumstances.

Quentin's mother was unmarried. Quentin was her only child and had lived what seemed to have been an isolated life with her and his maternal grandparents before starting school. He had a mild speech defect and was a little hyperactive, but the main problem seemed to be that he had been much indulged and overprotected by his mother and especially by his grandparents who had mainly looked after him. These circumstances seemed to be the main reason for his difficult behaviour on starting school.

Quentin was admitted for a short period of inpatient assessment and treatment. He showed only mildly difficult behaviour, and this quickly ceased; he made good progress in the unit school and was discharged to attend a different school.

Comment

Although this boy had been indulged and overprotected, his personality development was fundamentally sound and he was of above average intelligence. The environment in the particular school Quentin started in at age five presented problems of adjustment for such a boy. His case was one of adjustment disorder 'with disturbance of conduct'.

These cases illustrate some of the stresses that may lead to adjustment reactions. Other common stresses are the departure or return of a parent, bereavement, serious illness in a family member and social or academic difficulties at school.

Personality Disorders

Some children show seriously maladaptive personality characteristics from an early age. While many psychiatrists are reluctant to use the term 'personality disorder' in children and adolescents, who have the capacity for further development, in some instances the deviation is so pronounced and long-standing that the diagnosis is justified.

A diagnosis of personality disorder implies that the individual has developed inappropriate ways of dealing with daily tasks, with interpersonal relationships or with the handling of stressful situations. In many cases there are difficulties in all these areas.

The *causes* of personality disorder are unclear. In many cases the modelling of inappropriate parental behaviour patterns seems to be a factor, and there is often also unsuitable, inconsistent or even largely absent parenting. The relationship of these disorders to such factors is, however, by no means direct, and in many instances genetic and other biological factors are probably important. Extreme variations of temperament may play a part, as may a bad 'fit' between the temperamental style of the child and the parents' temperaments.

Dockar-Drysdale (1968, 1973) and Balbernie (1974) have written extensively about 'unintegrated' children. Their work is based on that of Winnicott (1960). They believe that many children with personality disorders have lacked 'primary experience'. Describing what he means by this, Balbernie (1974) states, 'the mother in nurturing and care, provides regular, ordered, complete experiences of well-being through which a child learns that it does survive separation'. Lacking this experience children act out their anxiety, do not feel guilt, lack regard for others' feelings and fail to value themselves. To quote Balbernie again 'the basis of well-being is the experience of a basic sense of natural order that is internalised'. This has not been provided for unintegrated children.

Several categories of unintegrated children are described including 'frozen children', whose primary experience has been interrupted when they and their mothers would be starting to separate out. They survive 'without boundaries to personality, merged with their environment and unable to make any real relationships or to feel the need for them'.

Also described are 'archipelago children' who have achieved the first step towards integration, but whose 'ego-islets' have 'never fused into a continent', that is a whole person.

Two other categories are 'false-selves' and 'caretaker-selves'. Describing the 'false-self' Winnicott (1960) writes:

> The false-self sets up as real and it is this that observers tend to think is the real person. In living relationships, work relationships, and friendships, however, the false-self begins to fail. In situations in which what is expected is a whole person the false-self has some essential lacking. At this extreme the true self is hidden.

Winnicott describes types of false-selves approaching more closely a state of health. This leads to the 'caretaker-self' which is built upon identifications. Inside the caretaker is the child's 'little self', carefully concealed. There may then, for example, be a delinquent 'caretaker' stealing, without conflict, on behalf of the 'little self'.

One particular disorder of personality in childhood has been labelled 'schizoid personality' by Wolff and Barlow (1979). Something similar was originally described as 'autistic psychopathy of childhood' by Asperger (1944). Wolff and Barlow provide a good description of the syndrome, as well as reporting a research study comparing 'schizoid' children with autistic and with normal children.

The children are mostly boys – only about 1 in 10 is a girl – and are solitary, finding group activities, especially rough games, stressful. Social adjustment problems at school are the main cause of referral. Other features are obstinacy and aggressive outbursts when under pressure to conform, especially at school; preoccupation with their own systems of ideas and beliefs – electronics, dinosaurs or space matters, for instance; emotional detachment; a lack of empathy; rigidity, at times of obsessional proportions; sensitivity, sometimes with paranoid ideas; learning problems in some cases – often despite high I.Q., and bizarre antisocial behaviour in a few cases. Crises at school often lead to referral and presenting symptoms include school refusal, running away, temper outbursts, suicidal threats, stealing and elective mutism (see below).

This syndrome seems to consist of a reasonably distinct group of children. Wolff and Barlow (1979) were able to distinguish various ways in which these schizoid children were different from the other groups they studied. Generally they were intermediate between the autistics and the normals. Like autistic children, they showed stereotypies and tended to impose patterns, and they had linguistic handicaps and lacked perceptiveness for meaning. Yet they lacked the repetitiveness and the motivation for tasks of cognition and memory of autistic children.

Schizoid personality disorder is one of the best described and studied of childhood personality disorders. These disorders have also been called 'borderline states' (Ekstein and Wallerstein, 1956; Geleerd, 1958), a term used in DSM–III but not in ICD–9. 'Borderline states' in adolescence are discussed by Masterson (1972), but these also are probably better described as personality disorders The term 'borderline' is no doubt used because these are conditions which have some characteristics reminiscent of psychotic children, but without a true psychotic picture. Thus there are no delusional beliefs, nor the three classical symptoms of autism (see Chapter 6).

Many other personality disorders are described, mainly based on work with adults. Caution is advisable in applying these labels in childhood: the younger the child the greater the caution that is warranted. Only serious, long-standing disorders, especially those which appear independently of environmental circumstances, merit such labels. Table 2 summarises the various categories of personality disorder described in the main two diagnostic schemes currently in use. In DSM–III, however, several of them, are defined as applying

TABLE 2:   CATEGORIES OF PERSONALITY DISORDER

ICD-9	DSM-III	Main features
Anankastic	Compulsive	Rigid, inflexible, obsessive, ritualistic, perfectionistic.
Hysterical	Histrionic	Over-dramatic, flamboyant, labile mood, suggestible, drawing attention to self, egocentric, dependent.
Asthenic	Dependent	Helpless, clinging, passively compliant, lacking vigour.
Sociopathic/ asocial	Antisocial	Lacking feeling for others, disregarding social norms and obligations, failing to plan ahead or learn from failure, poor work and parenting record.
Schizoid	Schizoid	Distant, cold, aloof, detached, introspective, unresponsive, few or no close friends.
—	Schizotypal	Social isolation, ideas of reference, 'magical' thinking, recurrent illusions, odd speech, suspiciousness, hypersensitivity.
Paranoid	Paranoid	Suspicious, jealous, sensitive to slight or imagined insults, affective responses restricted.
Explosive	—	Readily express anger, violence, hate, affection, either verbally or physically. May relate in shallow fashion. Demand immediate gratification.
Affective	—	Show lifelong mood deviation or alternation.
—	Narcissistic	Grandiosely self-important, with fantasies of success, power, brilliance or ideal love. Require attention and admiration, resent criticism, lack empathy and take advantage of others.
—	Borderline	Impulsive, unpredictable, with unstable but intense interpersonal relationships. Identity uncertain, mood unstable, fearful of being alone, self-damaging.
—	Avoidant	Hypersensitive to rejection, avoiding relationships, socially withdrawn, desiring affection and acceptance. Low self-esteem.
—	Passive–Aggressive	Resisting social and work demands, procrastinating, dawdling, stubborn, intentionally inefficient.
'Other' and 'Unspecified'	'Atypical, Mixed or Other'	—

only over age 18. Below 18 there is a 'corresponding diagnostic category' as follows:

Disorders of childhood or adolescence   Personality disorders

Schizoid disorder of childhood or adolescence	Schizoid personality disorder
Avoidant disorder of childhood or adolescence	Avoidant personality disorder
Conduct disorder	Antisocial personality disorder
Oppositional disorder	Passive—aggressive personality disorder
Identity disorder	Borderline personality disorder

So the schizoid child may only develop a personality disorder on his or her 18th birthday! It is also only some of the children in the above categories who will meet the criteria for personality disorder after 18. This rather confusing arrangement no doubt arose out of a commendable desire to avoid labelling children as suffering from personality disorders, in view of their potential for change.

It is evident that ICD–9 has fewer categories than DSM–III but the relative value of the two schemes, and the validity of the various categories, is at present uncertain.

It will be clear that personality disorders are a very varied group of conditions. The following case summaries can give only a limited idea of the wide range of possible ways they may be manifest.

Thomas had always been a difficult child, his mother said. His first weeks of life were interrupted by an operation for pyloric stenosis, and he was a difficult, negativistic baby and toddler. More serious, however, was his lonely, asocial behaviour. As he grew up would not talk to other children or to strangers. He violently resisted school at age five, kicking and screaming, and resisting doing anything he was asked. Transfer to a school for slow-learning children, and then a year in a children's convalescent hospital under the care of a psychiatrist did little to help him.

At age nine Thomas appeared a good-looking boy, well-dressed, but timid and anxious. He failed to respond to most questions, and the few answers he did give were either very short verbal ones or consisted of nodding or shaking the head.

During a subsequent 2-year period of first inpatient and then daypatient treatment, Thomas made little progress. He remained quiet, isolated and passively resistant, though he could become acutely physically and verbally aggressive, for example when a physician approached him to take a sample of venous blood for a test. He persistently resisted participating in psychological tests.

The family situation was difficult in that there was much marital strife, Thomas being the focus of many parental disagreements. The parents were divorced when Thomas was 11, and soon afterwards his mother remarried. Thomas, however, remained a passive, non-communicative, friendless boy without contacts outside his home.

Comment

Thomas's personality had been odd, and his relationships with his family unusual, from infancy. When he was seen for assessment a gross, long-standing disorder was present, having many of the features of the schizoid personality described above. While Thomas also showed many of the features of elective mutism (see below), his disorder involved his whole personality functioning and his social and educational development. His early experiences and family relationships seemed to have combined with biological factors to produce the problem.

Laura was first seen at age 13, at which time her mother said she could no longer cope with her. She was stealing money both in the house and outside it, lying, staying out late and associating with friends her mother had forbidden her to see. When she was asked to mind her two younger half-siblings she acted irresponsibly. She had twice run away for periods of a few days.

Laura had had many changes of home. For her first few months she lived with her mother and father. When they separated she was placed with an aunt who was later convicted of child abuse: the charges related to the aunt's own children, but Laura said she too had been beaten repeatedly. At age 5 Laura returned to live with her mother, who was now divorced. For the next eight years she lived an unstable existence. At times she was in the care of child welfare agencies, at others she was with her mother, who had a large number of brief relationships with different men. These men would live in the home from a period of a few days up to a few months, before the relationship broke up.

Laura was admitted to a residential treatment centre for assessment and treatment. She proved a difficult child to get to know. She was emotionally cold and aloof, so that staff never knew what she was thinking or feeling.

At various times she ran away, sometimes to her father. She played truant from school, stole money and other children's property and told lies. She was also suspected of having clandestine meetings with boys with whom she had been told not to associate. Staff found that the biggest problem in helping Laura was getting emotionally close to her. She seemed always to give the response that seemed most expedient. This often involved lying. It was impossible to get to the real Laura, they felt. Her life seemed to be a sort of store-front, with little or nothing behind it — or at least nothing that could be discovered. She did, however, from time to time reveal fantasies about her family, especially her father. She said that he loved her, and that only circumstances beyond his control stopped him having her to live with him. In fact he had only had about half-a-dozen contacts with her in the previous 10 years, but on two or three occasions when she had run away to him at his place of work he had given her a friendly reception and even bought her lunch.

While it proved possible to modify Laura's behaviour using behaviour therapy techniques, the changes did not persist when the therapy was stopped. Behaviour change based on her relationships with people, and on identifications, was not apparent.

Comment

The central feature of Laura's disorder seemed to be an inability to form warm, close relationships with people. Her personality problem seemed to fit best into the group with predominantly sociopathic or asocial manifestations of ICD—9, or the antisocial personality of DSM—III. It is probable that a major causative factor was her lack of a loving, stable relationship with a mother-figure during her first few years of life. She had many features of Winnicott's 'false-self' children, described above.

Terence was first referred for psychiatric assessment at the age of twelve. He had been abandoned by his mother as a baby and admitted to the care of the local authority. He spent his first five years in a residential nursery, and then moved to a group home, where there were several changes of houseparents.

The presenting problems were Terence's tendency, since age six, to spy upon female staff members when they were undressing or having a bath, and an incident in the early hours of one morning. On this occasion he went into the older girls' bedroom, got into the bed of one of them and started exploring with his hand the breasts and genitals of this girl, greatly to the alarm of the girl and the staff.

At interview Terence was a big boy for his age, in early puberty, but passive and reluctant to discuss freely the presenting problems. When confronted with his voyeuristic acts he always maintained they would not be repeated. He had learned his lesson and would discuss the subject no further. Invariably, however, the acts were repeated. Various treatment attempts, including psychotherapy and drug therapy, failed. Terence seemed lacking in any motivation for treatment.

Terence was subsequently moved to another, smaller home where at first he seemed to settle. But after a few months, similar problems again arose. He was referred back to the author at age 16, after appearing in court charged with sexually assaulting girls. He admitted that he had approached girls 'mauling them and feeling their breasts', as he put it. He was unable to make any normal contact with girls. The staff of the home where he was then living reported that they had the utmost difficulty in getting him to go to the local shops because most of the assistants were teenage girls with whom he was too shy to talk.

Terence did obtain a job in a local factory, where there were a number of girls. He dealt with this situation by having nothing whatever to do with the girls — not even talking to them. In other respects there was no evidence of psychiatric disorder.

Although Terence was successful in keeping out of trouble with the police over a period of six months, he was later convicted of further sexual offences.

Comment

This boy's psychosexual development took an abnormal course at least from the age of six. It is probably significant that he had spent all his infancy and childhood in institutions, and had been looked after mainly by female staff. How important was the lack of a normal family life and of suitable identification figures, and how major a part was played by constitutional factors, it is impossible to say. Not all boys brought up in similar circumstances show this sort of deviant psychosexual development, so constitutional vulnerability was probably important. In any event, by the age of 16 Terence showed signs of an established pattern of voyeurism, as described in DSM–III. (In both ICD–9 and DSM–III there are separate sections for psychosexual disorders, which are not listed in the sections on personality disorders.)

The *treatment* of children with personality disorders is difficult and it is likely that by the time such a disorder is established only radical, intensive long-term measures have any hope of success. Only a few therapists and treatment centres have concentrated on trying to help such children; among such centres in Britain are the Mulberry

Bush School and the Cotswold Community. For further information on this work the reader should consult especially the work of Barbara Dockar-Drysdale (1968, 1973) and Richard Balbernie (1974).

The British Department of Health and Social Security also proposed, in 1971, to set up *youth treatment centres*. These were designed for what were described as 'severely damaged boys and girls' who 'show grossly impaired capacity for making relationships and a paucity of satisfying life experiences'. The publication proposing the centres listed the following characteristics of the children they were intended to treat. They are a useful summary of the characteristics of probably the most difficult group of personality disorder, though of course some disorders take other forms, for example, withdrawal (as in the case of Thomas mentioned above) or deviant psychosexual development (as in Terence's case).

(a) They exhibit a markedly diminished sense of responsibility to an extent that staff find frustrating and alarming, since the normal capacity to respond co-operatively to help seems to be so seriously impaired.
(b) They lack restraint, inhibitions and development of the more mature reactions that are found in some measure in the majority of approved (i.e. 'training') school boys and girls.
(c) They lack concern, guilt or anxiety about the consequences of their behaviour.
(d) They are capable of explosive violence which may appear undirected and unmotivated, and they may show an altered state of consciousness with violence.
(e) They may exhibit marked symptoms of instability which are often distressing and bizarre and undermine staff confidence in handling and management.
(f) Their conduct at times may be potentially dangerous to themselves, other children, the staff and the outside community.
(g) They may present, during adolescence, acute behaviour difficulties displayed less acutely throughout childhood.
(h) They show a grossly impaired capacity for making relationships and a paucity of satisfying life experiences.

The *outcome* in children with personality disorders tends to be poor, at least unless intensive long-term treatment is available. Prevention may offer more hope and is discussed in Chapter 17.

Tics and Gilles de la Tourette's Syndrome

Tics, sometimes known as *habit spasms*, are repeated, sudden movements of muscles or groups of muscles, not under the voluntary control of the subject and serving no obvious purpose. They most often affect the face, and eye-blinking tics are one of the commonest types. A variety of facial contortions may occur and muscle groups in other parts of the body may be affected too. Thus the whole head and neck may be suddenly and briefly moved in one direction or contorted. Trunk and limbs may display similar movements. A feature of tics, as opposed to the involuntary movements seen in the various forms of chorea, is that the same movements occur repeatedly, in severe cases scores or hundreds of times a day. When they involve large movements, especially of the trunk and limbs, tics can constitute a serious handicap. Vocal tics are similarly sudden and involuntary vocalisations. They may consist simply of noises, or actual words may be vocalised.

Prevalence. About five per cent of seven-year-old children have a history of tics. They are often considered to be of 'nervous' or 'emotional' origin but in reality their cause is unknown. Causes that have been suggested include emotional tension, brain damage or developmental abnormality; explanations derived from learning theory have also been put forward. Studies by Cohen and his colleagues (1979) have suggested that there is reduced turnover of the neurotransmitters, serotonin and dopamine, in the brain and have suggested explanations based on the results of their studies (Cohen, 1980). There may well be multiple factors involved. Tics are commoner in children than in adults and in younger children than in older ones.

Description. A survey of 100 ticquers seen at the Maudsley Hospital, London, provided much information about the condition (Corbett *et al.*, 1969). Seven per cent of children seen in the child psychiatric department had tics. Boys predominated in a ratio of more than three to one. The tics most commonly started about age seven. The face was the most frequently affected part of the body. Isolated tics of other parts were less common. The ticquers showed certain emotional symptoms significantly more often than the general clinic population of disturbed children. These were 'gratification habits, speech disorders, disorders of defecation (including encopresis) and obsessional and hypochondriacal symptoms'. By contrast, tempers and aggression, truanting, fighting and depression occurred less often in ticquers. These findings could meant that the tics (and the symptoms that go with them) are means of expressing anxiety and aggression in individuals who have difficulty in expressing these emotions more directly. Moreover, many of the ticquers were found at later follow-up to be anxious even though the tics had improved.

DSM—III describes 'transient tic disorder', 'chronic tic disorder' and 'Tourette's disorder'. The first two are distinguished by their duration, the chronic disorder being present over one year and by the unvarying intensity of the chronic form.

The *Gilles de la Tourette syndrome* consists of the combination of motor tics, usually severe, with involuntary vocal and verbal utterances, often obscene (sometimes known as coprolalia). The vocal tics may take the form of impulsive enunciation of words spoken by others (echolalia). The condition starts in childhood and may persist into adult life, though it sometimes resolves. It is not certainly established that sufferers from this condition have anything other than particularly severe forms of tic syndrome, though some authors believe they do.

In the *treatment* of mild tics the general management should consist of a supportive attitude, combined with the removal or alleviation of any circumstances causing anxiety in the child. The tics should be made light of, and parents encouraged to ignore them. They should be explained as a somatic manifestation of anxiety. In the more severe and persistent cases, including Tourette's syndrome, treatment with the drug haloperidol is helpful. Doses up to 6 mg per day may be needed (Greenberg and Stephans, 1977). Psychotherapy has also been recommended, but its efficacy is uncertain; if there is serious associated emotional disorder however it may be helpful. Claims have also been made for various forms of behaviour therapy, but again their effectiveness is unclear.

The *outcome* is quite good. The Maudsley study suggests that most children's tics improve, and 40 per cent had recovered at follow-up five years after psychiatric consultation. There seemed to be a tendency to anxiety and neurosis in the patients followed up. Tourette's syndrome presents a more difficult treatment problem, but the symptoms often remain in abeyance if the subject is maintained on haloperidol.

Stuttering

Stuttering (or stammering) is the repeated interruption of the flow of speech by repetition, prolongation or blocking of sounds. In children aged two to four there are often hesitations, repetitions of the first sounds of words or phrases, and irregularities of the rhythm of speech. This is known as 'clutter' and sometimes precedes true stuttering, though in many cases the child grows out of it and comes to speak normally.

Stuttering may also appear after speech has been acquired. It is present in about one per cent of school children. It usually starts before the age of ten. It is three to four times commoner in boys than in girls. Its causes are not fully understood but hereditary predisposition, other constitutional factors (notably brain injury and mental retardation), emotional stress and anxiety may play a part. The consensus of current opinion seems to be that there is an underlying disorder of neurological maturation, and that faulty learning processes contribute also. Disturbed parent—child relationships may affect the learning of fluent speech. As a group, stutterers are late in starting to talk and below average in intelligence. There is often a family history of the condition. Nevertheless there are many exceptions to these generalisations. The syndrome was well described by Andrews and Harris (1964).

The severity of stuttering varies from occasional repetition of speech sounds to severe blocking of speech which seriously interferes with communication. The severity may vary greatly from time to time. Some children can speak freely at home but stutter at school. Some can sing freely but talk with a stutter. Some are obviously worse when anxious, but others are not. Anticipatory anxiety may be present and avoidance behaviour often develops. At first the avoidance may simply be of certain letters or sounds but it may spread to involve particular places or social situations, so that the subject's whole life pattern is affected. Sometimes stuttering children become isolated at school, and their communication difficulty may affect their ability to take part normally in lessons and other activities.

Usually stuttering is not a part of a more widespread psychiatric disorder, and in most cases the contribution of emotional disorder appears small, at least as regards the basic cause, though anxiety may exacerbate the condition. Neurotic symptoms or antisocial behaviour sometimes seem to develop as a reaction to stuttering.

The *treatment* of stuttering is usually undertaken by speech therapists. The psychiatric contribution to it is limited. Techniques intended to relieve anxiety, promote relaxation in the child and encourage self-confidence may help. Various specific techniques are recommended for the symptom, for example 'syllabic speech', in which stutterers are taught, usually in a group, to speak slowly and deliberately, syllable by syllable. Psychotherapy should probably be reserved for cases in which there is associated emotional disorder in child or family. Drugs, particularly haloperidol, may help, especially in the more severe cases (Rantala and Petri-Larmi, 1976). Approaches to treatment, and other aspects of the syndrome, are discussed by Wingate (1976).

Many children who stutter outgrow the symptom, but in some cases it persists into adult life.

Elective Mutism

In elective mutism the child refuses to talk in certain circumstances, often at school, yet talks freely elsewhere, especially at home. It is generally considered a rare condition, occurring in one per cent or less of referrals to child psychiatry clinics. No population study was on record until Brown and Lloyd (1975) published a survey of all 6072 children who enrolled in infant school in Birmingham, England one September. These were children aged about 5. Forty-two were still not speaking in class after 8 weeks in school, a prevalence rate of 7.2 per 1000 children. The number of mute children fell steadily during the subsequent four terms. At 64 weeks after starting school only one child remained silent at school. The condition is thus fairly common as an initial reaction to school, but is rare as a persistent problem. Similar findings were reported by Bradley and Sloman (1975). They found 26 electively mute children in a total sample of 6865 Canadian kindergarten children, with a highly significant excess of children from immigrant families.

Kolvin and Fundudis (1981), in a valuable review, suggest a prevalence of 0.8 per 1000 seven-year-olds, or a little lower, on the basis of an epidemiological study in Newcastle-on-Tyne (Fundudis *et al.*, 1979) and the number remaining mute 10–12 months after starting school in Brown and Lloyd's study. The causes of elective mutism are discussed by Kolvin and Fundudis (1981), from whose paper much of the following material is derived. Genetic factors are suggested by the relatively high prevalence of shyness that has been found in the parents, in whom there seems also to be an unduly high incidence of psychiatric disturbance. Electively mute children tend to be late starting to talk, and a history of enuresis and encopresis has also been found in them significantly more often than in control groups. It seems also that when these children do speak, they tend to show immature speech or other speech abnormalities.

Most of these children seem to have been shy from early in life; 'subsidiary' personality patterns reported by Kolvin and Fundudis were 'submissive'; 'sensitive and weepy'; and 'moody – aggressive, sulky and stubborn', the last named being the commonest. Elective mutes come from a wide cross-section of socio-economic backgrounds.

Elective mutism is probably a complex disorder, to which genetic, personality, emotional and family factors all play a part, perhaps with family interaction patterns contributing too. Unlike many child psychiatric disorders it is as common in girls as in boys, perhaps even somewhat more so.

The main *clinical feature* is the child's failure to talk, at school, in the consulting room and usually in most places other than home. Yet at home the child talks freely. Other behavioural abnormalities may be present. Brown and Lloyd found that children who were mute at school showed other behaviour patterns which distinguished them from speaking children: they were more likely to stop an activity when the teacher approached and to avoid playing with other children, and less likely to draw, go to the toilet or approach the teacher's table.

In the doctor's office or therapist's playroom these children usually behave as negatively non-verbally as they do verbally. They may passively decline to sit down when invited to do so, or to engage in any play activity. Some will shake or nod (usually shake) their heads in reply to questions, others deny the examiner even this response. At the same time they can usually be seen looking around the room, apparently taking everything in. They can be extraordinarily stubborn, remaining silent for session after session for months, even years. Yet given the right conditions (for them) they can speak freely. One girl who was making good, if non-vocal, progress at school was observed on closed circuit television to be talking freely and in a relaxed way when alone with her family; but as soon as a staff member entered the room she became silent and remained so as long as he was in the room.

It has been suggested that there are different types of electively mute children. Reed (1963) described four cases. Two were 'hyper-relaxed'; and made little response to any kind of stimulus, being generally negativistic and immobile. The other two showed much tension and anxiety. He thought that the first group, which could be called 'manipulative', might have learned mutism as an attention-gaining and evasive form of behaviour, while the second, which might be called 'phobic' used mutism as a fear-reducing mechanism. This is probably an oversimplification. Kolvin and Fundudis are probably nearer the mark when they suggest that elective mutism is a hetero-geneous condition including 'electively mute groups with and without personality problems in the parents', and children mute in school who may or may not show marked personality deviations. Immigrant children seem particularly prone to this reaction.

Kolvin and Fundudis found that their 24 elective mutes had a mean IQ 85 which was lower than that of 82 speech-retarded controls (mean IQ 95), which in turn was lower than the mean for a group of normal controls (101).

Treatment of the established, long-standing case can be very diffi-cult. Brown and his colleagues (1975a), in a review of treatment, list the following approaches which have been tried: suggestion, per-suasion, coercion, psychodynamically oriented play therapy, speech therapy, family therapy and behaviour therapy. All have met with only equivocal success. This does not of course apply to the mute child recently arrived at school, who is likely to start to speak within a few terms at most, but to the case which has persisted longer than this. It seems that the most effective treatment may be behaviour therapy, but only for Reed's second group, the 'phobic' cases. The 'manipu-lative' group often show a stubborn resistence to any treatment.

Outcome: Elective mutism is usually a self-limiting condition, becoming manifest when a child first attends school. Severe, chronic cases are rarer and outcome data are scanty, but total mutism apparently does not usually persist into adult life. Of Kolvin and Fundudis' 24 cases, 11 improved 'markedly' or 'moderately' while still at school, 10 of them before age 10. The 'phobic' group seem more responsive to treatment than the 'manipulative' group, but in both cases the outcome in terms of adjustment in adult life is unknown.

Epilepsy

Although epilepsy is a neurological rather than a psychiatric condition, it merits brief mention here. Disturbed behaviour may be caused directly by epileptic seizures, and in addition the psychological and social consequences of the condition can cause emotional disorder. Descriptions of epilepsy and its management are readily available in textbooks of neurology and paediatrics.

Both major epileptic seizures (*grand mal*) and minor ones (*petit mal*) may have important repercussions in a child's life (Bagley, 1971). Apart from the inconvenience of repeated loss of consciousness the child's schoolmates or siblings, or adults, may witness major fits, and become frightened, anxious or hostile. Some activities such as swimming or cycling may have to be curtailed. The condition may provoke anxiety or rejection in parents, relatives or teachers. The child may come to feel 'bad', or imperfect, or at least 'different'. Some children come to feel that the fits are in some mysterious way their own fault. These difficulties are, however, mainly due to the attitudes of others and are thus not inevitable.

In addition to the psychological repercussions of the condition, disturbed behaviour can itself be caused by epilepsy, especially of the temporal lobe variety, a form of *focal epilepsy* arising in the temporal lobe of the brain. This may cause abnormal behaviour which can sometimes be difficult to recognise as epileptic. The behaviour appears purposive and can be quite complicated, like running around, screaming and shouting. It can take the form of aggressiveness and severe temper. If consciousness is obviously altered at some point, or if the child is drowsy or has a headache at the end of the attack, diagnosis may be easier. It is in children who do not obviously show these features that the distinction between epilepsy and a conduct disorder can be hard to make. To compound the problem, the two can co-exist, as in the case of Rowland, described below.

In *akinetic attacks* (or *drop attacks*) there is a sudden, brief loss of muscle power or tone, causing the subject to fall down on to the knees. There is often no obvious loss of consciousness, and it may be thought that the person affected has just stumbled. The EEG pattern is different from that typical of minor fits. This type of seizure, like the brief lapses of consciousness in minor epilepsy – which may number hundreds per day — may be confused with psychologically caused disorders. Some epileptics have other neurological or intellectual handicaps which may add to their difficulties (though many are otherwise normal and of average or higher intelligence). Thus an epileptic child may be faced with a variety of difficulties, giving a greater risk of psychiatric disorder than in non-epileptic peers. Medication given to control fits, especially phenobarbitone, can also have unwanted side-effects, and adversely affect behaviour and cognitive function.

The following two case histories illustrate ways in which epileptic children may present with behavioural symptoms which may require joint psychiatric and neurological care.

Helen was referred at the age of six. She was said to have developed normally until three. She then had a major epileptic fit, after which she lost, over a few months, the few words she had acquired. She became noisy and hyperactive, and rocked back and forth in her chair. She ceased playing with other children.

On admission to hospital she was hyperactive, played and rocked repetitively, appeared to understand speech but did not herself speak. Four weeks later she had a series of epileptic seizures during the night. When these were controlled she was left with a spastic paralysis of the left face, arm and leg. This progressed during the next few weeks to involve the right side.

An air encephalogram (in which air is injected into the ventricles of the brain to show them up on X-ray) showed widespread degeneration of the brain tissues.

Comment

Helen had a degenerative brain disorder. This was not at first obvious, but the quite rapid progression and the investigations which were done as a result made the diagnosis plain. Her disturbed behaviour was due mainly to her cerebral condition. Her family was a stable one, and environmental factors played a minimal role in her condition.

Rowland was referred at age eleven. He complained of 'horrible feelings'. These consisted of acute, irrational fear, particularly of dying, lasting a minute or so. He would get up to ten attacks a day; they also sometimes occurred when he was in bed at night. He sometimes described the attacks as 'a fear of God'. He also had episodes, in which his face felt 'funny' and he complained of getting thoughts of dying, of being about to swear and of possible future actions which he was then unable to control. For example, he said he had thought he might fall down on the way to school which he later found he could not help doing.

Rowland's parents complained of difficult, uncontrollable, vicious and very naughty behaviour. This had been increasing in severity since the age of six. Rowland would get very angry with people, wander off and play truant from school. He once tried to strangle his younger brother. He also had nocturnal 'turns', occurring in the early morning, in which he twitched and made choking and snorting noises.

Rowland was the oldest of three siblings. The others were well. So also were the parents, physically, though they were anxious and distressed about Rowland's behaviour. Both pairs of grandparents lived near and so also did a number of aunts and uncles. Many of this extended family gave the parents advice, and also interfered in their dealings with Rowland. Thus if he were refused something by his parents he would usually get it from another relative. This appeared to have contributed to Rowland's behaviour getting out of control.

At about 5 a.m. during Rowland's first night in hospital he was observed by the nursing staff to have a typical major epileptic fit; he also had several during subsequent nights. He continued to have attacks of irrational fear by day, as well as episodes of altered consciousness lasting fifteen to twenty seconds, in which he felt unable to move. During these nothing abnormal was noticed by the staff. He was at times aggressive to other children and had violent temper outbursts. On the Wechsler children's scale his intelligence quotient was in the average range. He was about three years retarded in reading. No abnormal physical signs were found on examination and an X-ray of his skull was normal. An EEG showed abnormal electrical discharges in the right temporal lobe of the brain, more marked during sleep supporting the clinical diagnosis of temporal lobe epilepsy.

The nocturnal fits ceased, and Rowland's 'feelings' improved, when treatment with anticonvulsant drugs was started. His behaviour remained very disturbed and aggressive, however. He continued to try to manipulate the hospital staff as he had his family at home, asking one member for something which had been refused by another; or giving one member a false account of what another had said or done. When he was thwarted in this he would become angry, though over the course of a few months he began to accept firmer control, and after six months his behaviour was greatly improved.

Comment

Rowland clearly had a brain abnormality with focal discharges arising in the right temporal lobes. The problem was probably made more difficult by the five-year delay in diagnosis, during which Rowland was subject to conflicting discipline and control at home, and became progressively more disturbed in his behaviour and retarded in his school work. One reason for the delay in diagnosis was that father's sister had epilepsy; this had caused in father a great fear of the condition, and a firm denial that Rowland had it, despite the nocturnal attacks. Even after the diagnosis was made in hospital it took father a while to accept it. Earlier diagnosis and treatment, and help for the family in handling Rowland, might have avoided some of the more disturbed antisocial behaviour, for instance the truancy and aggressiveness to siblings. Thus the clinical syndrome Rowland presented was the outcome of a combination of intrinsic, organic factors and social, environmental ones.

It is of interest that an EEG done a year before admission was normal, which illustrates the important point that such a negative finding by no means excludes the diagnosis of epilepsy.

In the *treatment* of epilepsy anticonvulsant drugs are important, but as important as administering the right drugs are the support and help given to the child and the family. The nature of the disorder should be explained in appropriate terms and any queries or doubts in the minds of child or family should be discussed. This may need to be done repeatedly. There is a considerable folklore about epilepsy, some of it most alarming to those afflicted with the condition. The aim should be to enable the child to live as normal a life as possible, though some restrictions, for example on swimming and cycling, may be necessary. As optimistic a view as is justified should be taken in each case. The point that the condition is a common one should be stressed. Progress should be regularly reviewed, including the child's educational performance and adjustment in school. Medication is usually continued until the child has been free of fits for at least two years. The importance of taking the medication regularly must be stressed. Sometimes assessment or treatment in hospital is necessary, and a few epileptic children require long-term residential education (Pond, 1974).

CHAPTER NINE

Specific Delays in Development

The DSM—III (APA, 1980) has a separate axis (2) for 'specific developmental disorders'; so also does the multiaxial modification of ICD—9 (WHO, 1977) proposed by Rutter *et al.*, (undated) and outlined in Chapter 2, though it uses the term 'specific delays in development'.

These disorders consist of delayed development of particular functions relative to the child's general level of development, when not due to another disorder.

The sub-categories listed in ICD—9 are:

1. Specific reading retardation.
2. Specific arithmetical retardation.
3. Other specific learning difficulties.
4. Developmental speech/language disorder.
5. Specific motor retardation.
6. Mixed developmental disorder.

DSM—III lists the following:

1. Developmental reading disorder.
2. Developmental arithmetic disorder.
3. Developmental language disorder, expressive and receptive types.
4. Developmental articulation disorder.
5. Mixed specific developmental disorder.
6. Atypical specific developmental disorder.

In the past, other conditions have been considered 'developmental' including enuresis, encopresis and the hyperkinetic syndrome (Chapter 7). They share with the conditions dealt with in this chapter a higher incidence in boys than in girls and frequent occurrence in the absence of other psychiatric disorder.

Specific Reading Retardation

Reading difficulties are common and in societies with a high literacy level they are serious and handicapping disorders.

The *prevalence* of reading retardation depends on the age group and population studied and the criteria used to define the retardation. Reading attainment is in general related to intelligence level; brighter children tend to learn to read faster than duller ones. While the reading quotient cannot always be expected to equal the intelligence quotient (see Chapter 14), techniques exist which enable predictions of expected reading age to be calculated from a child's age and IQ (Yule, 1967). By this means *specific* reading retardation can be calculated (Rutter and Yule, 1975): it is distinct from general reading backwardness, which simply means that the child is not reading up to the level expected for his age.

In the Isle of Wight epidemiological study of 9- and 10-year-old children a prevalence of specific reading retardation, defined as a reading level 28 months or more below that expected for age and IQ, was found to be about 4 per cent. The prevalence of reading backwardness (28 months or more behind the level expected on the basis of age alone) was about 6.5 per cent. The Isle of Wight consists of rural areas and small towns, and the prevalence of reading problems appears to be higher in large cities, especially poor inner city areas. A study in inner London, using the same criteria as were used in the Isle of Wight, showed specific reading retardation to be present in about 10 per cent of ten-year-olds, while the rate of general reading backwardness was 19 per cent (Berger *et al.*, 1975). A higher prevalence of reading problems in inner city children has also been found in American studies (Eisenberg, 1966).

Specific reading retardation is considerably commoner in boys than in girls, the boy:girl ratio in the Isle of Wight study being 3.3 to 1, as opposed to 1.3 to 1 in the general reading backwardness group.

The *causes* of specific reading retardation are complex. The predominance of boys suggests biological susceptibility, perhaps genetically determined. Other factors which may contribute include difficulty in distinguishing right from left, other minor neurological disorders, delayed language development and current speech difficulties (Rutter and Yule, 1975). Social factors indirectly play a part since the condition is commoner in inner city children and there is also much variation from school to school (Berger *et al.*, 1975). An association has also been reported with large family size (Rutter, 1967a), and reading problems are commoner in the families of these children than in the general population. Thompson (1973) has reviewed the aetiology of reading disabilities, paying particular attention to the concept of maturational delay. It is not surprising that children who have had difficulty learning spoken language also find it hard to learn the associated written symbols.

How well a child learns to read or write, or to do arithmetic, depends also upon how well he is taught, how regularly he attends school and what his motivation to learn is. The latter is largely a function of his relationship with whoever is teaching him, and may also be affected by emotional factors. Frequent changes of school or teacher, especially if teaching methods change too, can contribute. Cultural factors are also involved. The child from a home in which books and written material are much valued and used is better placed than one in whose home there is a dearth of books and no interest in reading; an extreme case is the family in which the parents are illiterate. All these factors may contribute to reading delay in any child, but especially in the biologically vulnerable.

The association between reading retardation and antisocial behaviour was mentioned in Chapter 4. Sturge (1982) has confirmed that the association is a close one, but failed to demonstrate a clear causal relationship one way or the other. She concluded that the association is 'a complex one'.

The *clinical picture* of specific reading retardation is that of a child with a history of a serious delay in learning to read, perhaps following delay in the acquisition of speech and language skills, while development in other areas has been relatively normal. Writing, and particularly spelling, are also impaired, and the spelling difficulty may be more severe than the reading problem, persisting after the child has learnt to read.

Ingram (1974) has distinguished two types of reading and spelling difficulty. In the first, the child has difficulty in identifying and differentiating the written symbols, in orientating them in space and in perceiving the position of each one among the other symbols (letters or words). These are referred to as 'visuo-spatial' difficulties.

The second group consists of children with so-called 'audiophonic' difficulties. Such children have difficulty in recognising the sound symbols represented by the written material, and also in building the symbols up into meaningful words. They find spelling similarly difficult because they cannot easily identify the syllables of which a word is composed, and thus they may get the syllables in the wrong order.

A third and more handicapped group consists of children who have both visuo-spatial and audiophonic difficulties.

The term *developmental dyslexia* is sometimes applied to these disorders, but using such a term has the disadvantage that it may give the impression that the condition is a sort of 'disease', which it is not. There is no objection to saying a child is dyslexic, providing it is realised that this is just a way of saying in Latin that he has a reading problem. More important is the making of a functional diagnosis which takes account of all relevant factors, biological, social, emotional and educational.

Assessment and treatment of children with these problems are the special province of the educational psychologist and remedial teacher. Various of the tests described in Chapter 14 may be used in elucidating the nature of the child's difficulties. This is a necessary preliminary to working out a programme of remedial help. In severe cases individual remedial teaching is usually needed. Secondary emotional disorder may be present, and the child who finds he cannot read may eventually 'give up', leading to school difficulties, including truancy.

The *outcome* depends on the severity of the disorder and the help available to the child in school and at home. Many children overcome their reading problems, with or without help. Some seem eventually to reach a state of 'learning readiness', but much later than normal. Children who have had reading disability are often left, as adults, with spelling difficulties and poor writing. If reading difficulties are not correctly diagnosed and treated in good time, emotional and behavioural difficulties may appear, combined with progressive failure at school.

Specific Arithmetical Disorders

From time to time children are seen who show specific retardation in areas other than reading. Spelling difficulties have been mentioned as a common accompaniment of reading retardation, and have been reviewed by Frith (1978).

Arithmetical difficulties are probably the next most common problem. The term 'developmental dyscalculia' had been used to describe specific difficulties in the development of arithmetical skills. Slade and Russell (1971) described four adolescents who had all had severe difficulty with arithmetic from an early age such as could not be accounted for by a generally low level of intellectual functioning. Of the four basic arithmetical processes, the greatest disability seemed to be in multiplication, though all processes were affected.

Retardation in mathematics has been much less extensively studied than reading retardation; Lansdown (1978) has reviewed it and suggests multifactorial causes and gives a 'tentative description of specific mathematical retardation'.

Arithmetical difficulties are generally less handicapping than reading problems, but may also lead to secondary emotional disturbance. They also require skilled psychological assessment and remedial teaching.

Language Disorders

A baby's first sounds are undifferentiated crying. By two months this has become differentiated so that it varies according to the circumstances in which it occurs (for example, when hungry, cold, or in pain). Within a month or two the baby also starts to babble, and during the following months the variety of sounds, consonants and vowels, increases. Babbling is made up of a succession of sounds produced spontaneously by the infant. Many of these sounds will be incorporated into words when speech is acquired.

By about nine months the child's use of consonant–vowel combinations takes on a communicative function: these combinations are used for calling, for responding and for expressing intentions.

The development of language is a very complex process. The child must acquire the ability to observe objects and events in the environment before coming to understand them and express them in language. The development of language is thus closely tied up with cognitive, that is thinking, capacities. The learning of the meaning of words is closely related to concept development. Subsequently the child has to understand and learn sentence forms (syntax) and also acquire the skills necessary to request, protest, label and express other intentions (pragmatic abilities).

The first spoken words usually appear around the age of one, but children usually attempt to communicate by very simple vocalisations and gestures before that. The first words are often ones like 'dada' and 'mama', which may simply be bits of babble reinforced by the attention and approval given them by the parents. The subsequent acquisition of vocabulary is closely tied in with the child's perception, for example, of shape, and the words heard and used in relation to them. Thus at first all round objects may be labelled 'ball'. At the same time the child is trying actively to work out how language is put together, so that every attempt at communication is, in a way, a testing of an hypothesis. This applies to the acquisition of words, phrases and sentences. It is clear that even young children 'make up' new words using rules they have inferred, as when they produce words like 'sheeps' or 'gived' which they will not have heard used by others. Such errors are often corrected by parents and others with whom the child talks. Much the same applies to phrase and sentence construction, and indeed the learning of syntax starts almost from the acquisition of the first words. When a child says something and finds that it is not properly understood it is necessary to try again, perhaps after receiving some help or instruction from the person with whom he is talking. It is largely by such give-and-take that the child learns to master the complexity of verbal language. For all this there must be, of course, a background of neurological readiness.

During the second year an increasing, but relatively small, number of words is acquired, many of them the names of objects. Short phrases appear about the middle of the second year, sentences and simple questions about age two. At first small groups of words, mainly nouns and verbs, are produced, for example 'mummy come', 'doggie naughty'. 'No' and 'yes' are often incorporated into phrases like 'apple no' or 'Johnnie apple no', which express their meaning quite well in a sort of verbal shorthand. Phrases of this type are often acquired during the second year and gradually sentences with a more normal structure replace them. Adjectives are used increasingly to qualify nouns, and pronouns are used with greater correctness. Subsequently the finer points of syntax are gradually mastered, though this is a process which continues well into and through the child's primary school days. The use of adverbs, prepositions and conjunctions appears relatively late, though normally before the child starts school at five.

The child's vocabulary increases rapidly in the third and fourth years. At the same time articulation, the accuracy with which words are pronounced, improves. At first the child's attempts at many words may be poor. Parents usually understand them before outsiders do.

Vocabulary and sentence structure are culturally determined. In most countries there are regional variations in speech patterns. There are usually also social class differences, only partly determined by intelligence. Thus 'normal' speech development in a labourer's child would be likely to differ from the 'normal' for a university lecturer's child, as regards both vocabulary and syntax. In some English-speaking families the double negative ('I don't want no more tea') is accepted usage, and naturally this is what the child growing up in such a family will learn.

Between the ages of two and seven there are equally important changes in children's capacity to comprehend spoken language. This also is learnt in an organised way. Thus it appears that children at first interpret sentences by assuming that the first noun is the subject/actor of the sentence (Bever, 1970). This leads to the child learning to interpret the subject–verb–object sequence as representing actor–action–recipient. This strategy works well as in 'the boy chases the girl', but later the child must learn to refine and change the strategies used to deal, for example, with 'the boy is chased by the girl'. Gradually children learn to cope with sentences of increasing complexity, as they hear them used.

Further information on language development is to be found in the book *Language Development: Structure and Function* (Dale, 1976).

Abnormalities of Speech and Language Development
Language disorders may involve non-verbal comprehension, verbal comprehension and verbal expression. The division of these disorders into receptive and expressive types, as in DSM–III, is overly simplistic. Martin (1980), in a useful and concise article, points out that many varieties of language disorder are possible, depending on the presence and extent of difficulties in the three main functions mentioned above. Much more important than the attaching of a diagnostic label to a language disorder is the delineation of precisely what language functions are lacking and to what degree.

Generally speaking verbal expression cannot be better than verbal comprehension, nor verbal comprehension than non-verbal. Occasional exceptions to this rule are met with, as when totally deaf children are taught some verbal expressions through lip reading and highly specialised teaching methods.

While the prevalence of severe language disorders has been estimated by Rees (1974) to be one per thousand live births, the rates for milder forms are clearly much higher. Prevalence figures of course depend upon ascertainment criteria. In the Isle of Wight survey of 9-, 10- and 11-year-olds, 6.2 per cent of 147 'controls' — children without intellectual retardation or specific reading retardation — showed 'poor complexity of language'. The rates for the children with specific reading retardation were much higher (15.1 per cent) and for those with intellectual retardation higher still (63.2 per cent).

Causes: Children may fail to develop language because of deafness, severe mental handicap or gross sensory deprivation, but the term 'specific developmental language disorder' is not usually applied to such conditions. While total deprivation is rare, relative language deprivation is commoner. This may occur in large, badly run institutions such as orphanages, and also in some poorly endowed, under-privileged families, where retarded language development may be a cultural phenomenon.

In most children with specific language delay the main cause appears to be abnormality of the central nervous system. The necessary neurological apparatus has not developed normally, or at least is not functioning correctly. In the presence of such an abnormality a degree of deprivation of language experience (resulting from any of the causes mentioned above) may have a particularly damaging effect. Often the cause of the delayed neurological development cannot be discovered, but sometimes there is a history of cerebral trauma at birth or soon afterwards. In many cases there appear to be genetic factors, and a family history of late speech development, other speech difficulties, and reading and spelling problems is common.

The main *clinical feature* is that the child is late starting to talk. The first words (except perhaps 'dada' and similar items of babble) are acquired late, sentence construction is delayed and when words are produced they are abnormal. The extent to which the child can understand speech varies a lot. In severe instances there is little or no understanding of speech. This condition has also been called 'congenital auditory imperception'. It can be demonstrated by electroencephalographs that there is a normal response in the cerebral cortex to sounds, but they are not meaningful to the child. In such cases there will of course also be an expressive disorder.

Diagnosis depends on the late acquisition of speech in the presence of normal, or relatively normal, development in other spheres. Deafness and psychosis must also be considered. Audiometric examination and specialist opinion may be necessary for this. Various special tests are also available. Figure 3 shows the processes of language comprehension and expression. Any of the stages may be affected, language-disordered children having difficulty in the decoding–encoding area.

Figure 3 The comprehension and expression of language

Treatment is usually carried out by speech therapists working in conjunction with neurologists and otologists. If there is a severe receptive language problem, speech may never be acquired, though it may be possible to teach a few stereotyped phrases. Where the difficulty is mainly expressive a concentrated training programme, perhaps using operant conditioning techniques (see Chapter 16), may be of value. Fortunately many cases are relatively mild and the result of delayed neurological maturation. Such children tend to develop speech in due course and, when ready, can be helped by speech therapy (Lahey and Bloom, 1977). Their language capacity may, nevertheless, remain somewhat impaired so that they have difficulty learning to read and write.

Articulation Disorders

Developmental disorders of articulation are given a special category of their own in DSM–III, according to which they occur in 6 per cent of boys and 3 per cent of girls, of school age. Abnormal articulation may be due to a neurological condition affecting the control of the muscles responsible for speech, as in cerebral palsy; it may be due to a structural abnormality of the larynx, palate or tongue; it may be a developmental condition (and indeed is always present along with severe language disorder); or it may have emotional causes.

The latter two groups are the main ones of psychiatric importance, though severe dysarthria from any cause may have psychiatric consequences.

Developmental articulatory disorders are often simply the persistence of infantile modes of articulation beyond the period of life at which they usually disappear. They may be due to delayed neurological maturation; the frequent combination with language delay tends to support this.

The *clinical picture* is of a child who speaks freely and appears to understand speech normally (unless there is also a language disorder), but is hard to understand because of the use of ill-formed words. Longer words are more difficult than shorter ones, parts of words (often the ends) may be missed out, and consonants tend to be more affected than vowels. The later acquired speech sound (t, sh, th, f, z, l and ch) are most often affected. Usually the parents can understand the child better than can outsiders. Indeed the parents, being used to the child's mode of pronunciation, may not realise the severity of the disorder.

Treatment is primarily the sphere of the speech therapist, though paediatrician, otologist and psychiatrist may all have something to contribute in the management of the more severe cases. In many milder cases there is spontaneous recovery.

Emotionally determined immature articulation occurs quite frequently in children showing other evidence of delayed emotional maturation. There may be over-protection by the parents. Sometimes the child talks normally when away from the mother, relapsing into 'baby talk' when with her. The same process may occur when the young child is faced with severe stress causing regression in other spheres, as in regressive soiling. The diagnosis in these cases depends on a general assessment. If there is a clear history of normal, or at least better, articulation in certain circumstances, this supports the diagnosis. So also does the presence of emotional immaturity in other spheres, with overdependence on parents, or at least a need or wish for such overdependence. Some of these disorders are more appropriately categorised as adjustment reactions. Treatment is likely to involve some combination of psychotherapy with the child and help for the family (see Chapter 16). The outcome depends on the nature of the underlying psychiatric problem.

Specific Motor Retardation

Some children's motor development is specifically retarded, relative to their development in other spheres. This can take the form of severe clumsiness which may interfere with a child's school work, games or physical education. If unrecognised or unsympathetically handled it can lead to great unhappiness or to secondary emotional disturbance. This condition is sometimes known as 'developmental apraxia' (Walton *et al.*, 1962).

Characteristically these clumsy children are late in developing motor skills such as dressing, feeding and walking. They usually experience difficulty in writing and drawing, and even in copying. They perform badly at ball games, tend to break crockery and are poor at handicrafts. Sometimes there is also defective articulation. On the other hand, intelligence is normal, even above average, on verbal tests. In verbal work these children usually do well, but because of their inability to put what they know down in writing they may be regarded as dull, or even mentally handicapped. Sometimes they are regarded as lazy and the view is taken that they could do better if they tried.

Clumsy children do not usually show evidence of any abnormality in the motor pathways controlling voluntary movement. That is to say, they can carry out all normal movements but co-ordination of them to perform a particular task is defective. The condition is analogous to developmental reading disorder, in which the subject can see writing but cannot organise it into the meaning it represents.

Children with this condition may present at psychiatric departments, sometimes with secondary emotional disorders. Careful history-taking usually indicates the diagnosis which can be confirmed by asking the child to write and draw. Administration of the Wechsler Intelligence Scale for Children (see Chapter 14) usually reveals a much lower performance than verbal IQ. These children usually read better than they write. Similar clumsiness also occurs in children with severe mental handicap, but in these cases it is but part of generally retarded development and thus not a specific developmental disorder.

Treatment necessitates first the recognition of the disability and its explanation to child, family and teacher, and then the provision of special teaching and training. Modification of the school routine may be needed, especially along the lines of relieving these children of attempting games and other motor tasks which are clearly too difficult for them.

A full account of this syndrome, including two population surveys and information on the various neurological disorders which may cause clumsiness, is to be found in the book *The Clumsy Child* (Gubbay, 1975).

Mixed Developmental Disorders

Mixed developmental disorders consist simply of combinations of the various conditions described above. The coexistence of reading, spelling and language disorders is particularly common, but various other combinations also occur.

CHAPTER TEN

Psychosomatic Disorders

Psychosomatic disorders are physical conditions in which emotional factors play an important part. There is evidence that emotional factors play some part in most, perhaps all, disease processes, but in predominantly 'physical' conditions their part is relatively small. Even in such clearly organic disorders as pneumonia or appendicitis, however, the individual's emotional state and attitudes towards treatment and recovery can, it seems, affect progress. But these are not psychosomatic disorders as usually defined. Pinkerton (1974) has described psychosomatic disorders as those in which disordered physiology and psychopathology 'are so intimately interwoven that both components actively and concurrently contribute to the natural course of the disorder'. Examples are bronchial asthma, infantile eczema, ulcerative colitis, peptic ulcers, migraine, the periodic syndrome and obesity

Related to psychosomatic disorders, but somewhat different, are what Pinkerton (1974) calls 'pseudosomatic' disorders; these are disorders in which, although the condition presents as a physical problem, no organic disorder can be shown to be present. Examples include many cases of enuresis and soiling and various sleep and feeding disorders. *Anorexia nervosa* is also included in this group by Pinkerton, but is nevertheless considered in the present chapter.

A third group of conditions comprises those Pinkerton calls 'somatopsychic states', in other words disorders in which there is a basis of organic pathology which causes psychological consequences, so that psychiatric treatment may be needed. This is the case in many children with serious physical handicaps. Important examples include epilepsy (see Chapter 8), brain damage and its consequences

(Chapter 2), diabetes, cystic fibrosis, congenital heart conditions, some skin diseases, head injury and various forms of *spina bifida*.

A fuller discussion of psychosomatic medicine is to be found in the book *Childhood Disorder: A Psychosomatic Approach* (Pinkerton, 1974).

Causes

The effects of the emotions on bodily functions are familiar to all. Thus people can be 'scared stiff' or 'shaking with laughter'. When anxious or frightened they may lose their appetite or feel the urge to urinate or defecate: in extreme cases they may actually do these things. Some people's peptic ulcers get worse when they are worried or under stress. In psychosomatic disorders these factors combine with constitutional weakness, or an individual's tendency to react in a particular way, to produce the disorder.

The reasons for these constitutional weaknesses are not fully understood, but it appears that genetic factors play a part in at least some of these disorders. Thus bronchial asthma and eczema tend to run in families, though the exact mode of inheritance is not established. Migraine has been found to occur in the families of about three-quarters of the sufferers from the condition, and it is also said to be more frequent in the families of subjects with bronchial asthma than it is in the general population.

In particular disorders other factors, for example infective and allergic ones, play a part too. This is well illustrated in bronchial asthma.

Minuchin and his colleagues (1975) have proposed an explanation of psychosomatic disorders based on systems theory. They believe that certain types of family organisation favour the development and maintenance of children's psychosomatic symptoms, which in turn play a major role in maintaining family homeostasis. They consider that for a severe psychosomatic disorder to develop the child must be physiologically vulnerable, the family must show four characteristics in its transactional patterns – enmeshment, overprotectiveness, rigidity and lack of conflict resolution– and the sick child must play an important role in the family's pattern of conflict avoidance. These enmeshed families, in which everyone is deeply involved with and responsive to everyone else, show a high degree of protectiveness between all family members.

The rigidity of these families is shown in reluctance to change in response either to outside circumstances or to internal events, such as a child reaching adolescence. The enmeshment, overprotectiveness and rigidity combine to cause these families to have very low thresholds for conflict. These conflicts are not resolved. Instead each family has its own particular way of avoiding conflict; this is brought into action again and again and involves the continuation of the child's psychosomatic problem.

Minuchin and his co-workers (1975) report good results from treatment directed at these family difficulties in cases of intractable asthma, anorexia nervosa and 'superlabile diabetes' — that is diabetes which frequently gets out of control in association with emotional factors. The book *Psychosomatic Families* (Minuchin *et al.*, 1978) by this group, deals more fully with this work, and contains extensive descriptions of therapy in cases of anorexia nervosa.

Description

Psychosomatic disorders are best described by means of examples, and bronchial asthma is a good one. It consists of attacks in which there is constriction of muscles in the walls of the smaller air passages in the lungs. In addition to the contraction of the muscles, liquid secretions often accumulate in the air passages, and the walls of the passages swell. The secretions cannot be coughed up as they normally would be, and so cause further blockage. Breathing out is more difficult than breathing in, because the negative pressure created by the expansion of the chest wall during inspiration tends to dilate the air passages. The reverse happens on expiration. Thus the lungs tend to get over-filled with air and they and the whole chest are over-expanded.

The muscles of the air passage walls are supplied by nerves of the autonomic nervous system. This network of nerves, with connections in the brain, is responsible for the correct ordering of certain physiological functions, for example heart rate, blood pressure and the diameter of the air passages in the lungs. It is not under conscious control. As well as responding to the needs which arise in activities such as exercise (in which more blood supply to the muscles and more oxygen supply to the blood are required) the system is also sensitive to emotional changes. This is a relatively primitive physiological reaction. Thus the startled or frightened animal has to be ready for 'fight or flight'; and a quick physiological response to danger was probably important for survival in our ancestors, if not in man today. A means thus exists for changes in the lungs and blood vessels and other tissues to occur as a result of alterations in the emotional state of a person.

The diameter of the air passages can also be affected by at least two other factors. One of these is infection, whether by bacteria or viruses. The other is allergy. By an allergy is meant an adverse bodily reaction to a substance which may be present in the environment, and which is not normally harmful. Pollen and many other allergens can also irritate the air passages in the lungs, causing production of liquid secretions and thus their blockage. Infections have a similar effect.

There are therefore three possible precipitants of an attack of asthma: infection (which may start as a cold or bronchitis), exposure to an allergen, and emotional factors. A particular asthma patient may be more sensitive to one or other of these, but their effects tend to be cumulative. An attack of asthma becomes more likely with increasing severity of any of the precipitating conditions; if two or three operate at the same time it is more likely still, and will probably be more severe.

Asthma is often preceded by infantile eczema. This is a skin disease in which there is widespread eruption with inflammation and irritation, coming on during the first year of life. If severe, it is a serious condition with risk to the baby's life. It is often replaced, at least partially, by asthma after a year or two. Thus by the age of three or four the asthma may be the bigger problem, though the two often coexist and the 'asthma-eczema syndrome' is common in children. The onset so early in life is in itself suggestive of a constitutional weakness in the child. It seems that these patients are constitutionally vulnerable individuals who may react in at least two ways (eczema and asthma) to at least three types of stress.

Paula was referred for psychiatric opinion at the age of eight. She was the younger of two siblings, the other being a boy of thirteen, in good health. She had had eczema in infancy; she had been in hospital several times for this. The eczema and admissions to hospital had caused her family great anxiety. She still had some areas of relatively mild eczema but her skin condition had greatly improved.

Asthma had started in the second year of life. At first a diagnosis of 'bronchitis' was made, and it was not until the age of four that the condition was labelled asthma. This in itself caused the parents much concern as the maternal grandfather had been, so mother said, a lifelong asthmatic who died of the condition at the age of fifty-four.

Paula was referred by a paediatrician because of the increasing frequency of attacks which were causing her to miss a lot of school. At interview Paula appeared a bright, attractive girl of average intelligence. She talked freely, gave a good account of her life situation and acknowledged, but made light of, her asthma. Some patches of mild eczema were visible on her arms. She maintained that she liked school, but went on to say that very often her mother would not let her go because of her bad chest.

Paula's parents gave a slightly different account of things. They said that the asthma tended to be worse when Paula was supposed to be going to school. They felt unable to be firm with Paula over school attendance, and indeed over other things, too, for fear she might have an asthmatic attack and perhaps die, as her grandfather had done. Moreover, Paula had had some severe attacks of asthma at school time, requiring the presence of the family doctor and the administration of drugs to help terminate the attack. The school report indicated that Paula did quite well despite her frequent absence, but did not mix much with the other children.

It rapidly became clear that the parents', and especially mother's, anxiety and fear of Paula dying were important features. Paula had only to develop a mild cough to be kept off school. Mother over-indulged Paula, and was seldom firm with her lest she precipitate the asthma.

Paula's anxiety about her asthma, gradually emerged in psychotherapeutic interviews. She spoke of her dreams, the subjects of which (not identified as herself) died or nearly died, and then recovered or came back to life. She also played in an animated way with the family figures in the doll's house. The children were frequently being cared for in bed by the parents, but were also at times aggressively defiant towards the parents (which Paula never was in real life).

Paula, her mother and sometimes father, were seen weekly over a period of about three months, then less often. Paula played and talked out her fears and fantasies in individual sessions and gradually came to link them consciously with her asthma and its consequences. The parents were able to discuss their great anxiety and fear about Paula, indeed at first mother talked of little else. They gradually came to understand how anxiety and protectiveness increased Paula's anxiety. Supported by the therapist the parents became better able to be firm with Paula over things like bedtimes and her demands for toys and presents, as well as over going to school. To their surprise, Paula's cough and asthma became better, not worse. After about two months' treatment mother arrived one day and said, 'I've come to the conclusion she's been having me on a string all these years.'

Comment

There was clearly a constitutional predisposition to asthma, perhaps with a genetic basis, in Paula's case. Allergic factors were not prominent, but there was a history of exacerbations when she had minor colds which, as the parents said, 'went straight to her chest'. Hence the anxiety about her cough. Paula's ill-health had come to dominate the family, and Paula shared the parents' anxiety and fear of her dying. She also came unconsciously to use the asthma as a means of getting her way and avoiding things like going to bed or to school. She thus almost had a vested interest in it. Treatment of child and parents brought gratifying results, with a great reduction in asthmatic attacks in the next two years and only occasional absences from school, as compared with an absence rate of over fifty per cent previously.

Similar processes occur in other psychosomatic conditions. In *ulcerative colitis* there is apparently a constitutional weakness predisposing to inflammation and ulceration of the large intestine. Emotional factors seem more important in some cases than others, infection can play a part and so possibly can 'auto-immune reactions' (reactions thought to be due to normal substances present in certain tissues of the body). There is also evidence that the condition is more frequent in Jews than in other races, suggesting a genetic basis (though the racial incidence could be due to dietary habits). The condition usually presents with diarrhoea, abdominal pain, passage of blood with the faeces and other symptoms such as fever, loss of appetite and weight, nausea and malaise; there may also be depression, irritability and difficult behaviour. The interplay of emotional and other factors in this often serious, and even fatal condition, is complex and demands that psychiatric and other treatments are closely integrated.

Migraine consists of recurrent headache, usually unilateral, often preceded by visual disturbances and accompanied by vomiting (Bille, 1962). It is a common disorder (about one person in five has an attack at some time during his life), and again genetic, allergic, emotional and perhaps other factors combine to cause the symptoms. Onset is often during adolescence, but the condition occurs in children also.

The *periodic syndrome* occurs in the first decade of life. Attacks of headache may be accompanied by photophobia, abdominal pain, vomiting, and a miserable whimpering appearance in the child. Any one of these symptoms may predominate. No organic disease is found on investigation and the condition is probably a variant of migraine, having similar causes. One variety of it is called 'cyclical vomiting'. This seems often to be associated with emotional problems within the family (Davenport *et al.*, 1972).

Other psychosomatic conditions include *peptic ulcer* (commoner in adults than children), and possibly *deprivation dwarfism* (Silver and Finkelstein, 1967), in which growth failure is associated with environmental, especially family, stress — though in such cases undernutrition may often be a major factor (Whitten *et al.*, 1969).

It is also probably reasonable to regard *obesity* as a psychosomatic disorder, though its cause is complex, with genetic and environmental factors both playing their part (Grinker, 1981). It does seem, however, that emotional and social factors can, in predisposed children, play a part in causing obesity (Bruch, 1974). Certain individuals are said to have a high count of adipose cells. This may be genetically determined but there is evidence that it may also be caused by overnutrition in the early months of life. The deprived, unwanted child may eat excessively as a compensation for lack of affection. A mother who, perhaps unconsciously, feels guilty about her rejecting or aggressive attitude towards a child may over-feed the child in an attempt at compensation. Over-feeding may also be motivated, again unconsciously, by a parent's desire to keep the child in a close and dependent relationship. It may thus be but one aspect of a disturbed parent–child relationship, the child being used to fulfil the parent's own needs to have a mutually dependent relationship. Despite these points however it seems that obese children as a group are not seriously disturbed or deviant (Sallade, 1973).

Emotional problems can also result from obesity which may have endocrine, metabolic or other physical causes. The fat child may be teased and so come to feel self-conscious. It can be hard to get children to keep to a reducing diet when one has been prescribed. This can lead to tension and even strife between family members, though severe problems of this sort usually prove to result from pre-existing family relationship difficulties. In some instances it may be hard to discover whether obesity is the cause or the effect of the family problem, or whether it has simply become the focus of a problem which would have been centred around something else had the child not been obese.

Janice was referred at the age of eight. She was the youngest of three girls. The pregnancy had been unwanted, but mother gradually became reconciled to it in the hope that she would have a son. The father, a country postman, seemed to play little part in the family. Mother had apparently been critical of Janice from birth onwards. At the time of referral she complained of Janice's poor school progress and rather gross obesity. Investigation showed Janice to be of above average intelligence, and the teacher said she was doing well at school, if anything better than her sister. Mother said Janice would not keep to her diet, stealing biscuits from the kitchen and money from the house to buy sweets. There was a running battle between mother and daughter, and Janice if anything got fatter.

Janice attended weekly for psychotherapy. She proved a friendly girl with a talent for drawing, through which she gave various indications of her feelings of rejection by, and anger towards, her mother. Mother was seen weekly by a social worker, to whom she expressed her disappointment at having a third daughter and also a husband who, she felt, had contracted out of the family. Once mother was engaged in discussing these problems, a big improvement in the family emotional climate followed. Janice's school progress ceased to be a problem in mother's eyes and it was reported that Janice no longer ate food illicitly; she got only a little thinner, however.

Comment

The obesity was being used by child and mother as a focus for their mutually hostile feelings, based probably on mother's long-term rejection of Janice. Whether it was primarily caused by the psychological problem (its failure to disappear being due to incomplete resolution of the emotional problem), or whether it was due to other causes, and exacerbated by the emotional problem, was not clear. This case history is typical of children with psychosomatic disorders referred for psychiatric help in that there was a contribution the psychiatric clinic was able to make, but psychiatric help on its own did not solve the problem.

The *treatment* of psychosomatic disorders involves the removal, amelioration or prevention of any of the causative factors in a particular case. Thus infections and allergies are treated, or contact with the substances to which the child is allergic is avoided. Appropriate medical treatment is given; in asthma, for example drugs which dilate the air passages in the lungs are given, combined as necessary with antibiotics, oxygen or breathing exercises.

The extent to which psychiatric help is needed will vary with the relative importance of emotional factors in the particular case, but the emotional state of child and family must always be taken into account when the treatment plan is worked out. Some psychosomatic disorders, for example asthma and ulcerative colitis, can be life-threatening and may cause anxiety and fear in child and family, as well as being in part caused by emotional factors. Psychotherapy may be required by child, parents or the whole family. Increasingly the whole family is being taken as the unit for treatment, as these disorders come to be seen as playing a role in the maintenance of a dysfunctional family system. The various forms of treatment are discussed further in Chapter 16.

Outcome: It is difficult to generalise about the outcome in such a diverse group of disorders, varying as they do in their nature, causation and severity. In most cases, however, treatment leads to good results if a comprehensive formulation is made, and a similarly comprehensive treatment plan, taking in all aspects of the child's and family's problems, is carried out.

Anorexia Nervosa

In anorexia nervosa there is severe and prolonged refusal to eat with progressive loss of weight, but without evidence of physical disease. The disorder occurs mainly in adolescent girls.

Causes: In most instances, anorexia nervosa is a neurotic condition; less often there is depression of psychotic intensity, and occasionally the condition is an early manifestation of schizophrenia.

In the neurotic cases − over three-quarters of the total − there is usually complex psychopathology involving the family as well as the patient. The condition tends to occur in families in which there is much emphasis on food and eating. The latter is perceived by the patient as necessary for growing up and becoming sexually mature, and a major feature of the patient's psychopathology is usually a fear of growing up. The unconsciously intended purpose of the refusal to eat is to remain in a prepubertal state. As Crisp (1977) puts it, 'the search for security and self-esteem has proved incompatible with growth, which has therefore come to be stifled and avoided'. It is also generally agreed (Bruch, 1973; Liebman *et al.*, 1974; Crisp, 1977) that there are usually serious family problems. Many cases of anorexia are hysterical neurotic reactions to family stress.

Liebman and his colleagues believe that the parents deny their problems and avoid dealing with them by concentrating on the child patient's symptoms. The families have the characteristics described above – enmeshment, overprotectiveness, rigidity and lack of conflict resolution. Generational boundaries are weak and the parents are divided and ineffective, while individuals in the family are given little autonomy or privacy. These rigid systems cannot resolve conflicts, solve problems or deal effectively with stressful, frustrating situations.

Description: Anorexia nervosa is a disease of adolescence rather than of childhood. It is almost confined to girls but occasional cases occur in boys. It usually starts after menstruation begins, though sometimes there have been only one or two periods before the onset of the anorexia and it may occur before puberty. Menstruation ceases as the patient loses weight.

The condition often begins as 'normal' dieting arising from the patient's feeling that she is too fat, which is sometimes the case at the onset. The dieting, however, develops into a profound aversion to food with consequent severe and progressive weight loss. In many cases there develops a serious state of starvation with danger to life; it sometimes leads to death. Yet the subject typically shows a total lack of concern about her symptoms, as in hysterical illness generally. She is often abnormally active (this does not apply in the minority of depressed patients) and, at least in the early stages, adopts a superficially cheerful manner and enjoys feeding food to, or preparing it for, others. She will not eat it herself, however, and she may resort to all sorts of subterfuges to dispose of what she is supposed to eat.

In some cases the subject loses weight by means of self-induced vomiting (Russell, 1979), though how far those who do are a distinct group is unclear (Bhanji and Mattingly, 1981). DSM–III (American Psychiatric Association, 1980), however, has a separate coding for 'bulimia', the syndrome of episodic binge eating, with awareness that the eating pattern is abnormal, fear of being unable to stop eating voluntarily and self-deprecating thoughts. There is often subsequent induced vomiting.

There are often disturbances of body-image. As the condition progresses, the physical effects of starvation come to dominate the picture.

Once anorexia nervosa is established *treatment* is an urgent matter, for the condition can lead directly to a fatal outcome. It also differs from many other child psychiatric conditions in that toleration of the symptom while the underlying psychological problem is treated may not be possible.

In severe cases admission to hospital is required, preferably before there has been deterioration of the patient's physical health. Bed rest is often advised as an initial step until weight gain has started. Psychotherapy for the patient and the family is also necessary. A variety of psychotherapeutic regimes have been used. The team working at the Philadelphia Child Guidance Clinic and Children's Hospital claim particularly good results from their family therapy programme (Minuchin *et al.*, 1978). In addition various drug regimes have been suggested, involving particularly chlorpromazine and insulin; while these help patients gain weight during the acute stage they do not deal with the underlying psychopathology. Behaviour therapy programmes can also be useful, as is pointed out in a helpful review of the treatment of anorexia nervosa (Van Buskirk, 1977). Behaviour therapy principles are indeed used by the Philadelphia group in their programme.

Outcome: Anorexia nervosa is not an easy condition to treat successfully but in most cases recovery occurs, though sometimes only after long and difficult treatment. Unfortunately, relapse is quite common and sometimes there is recurring anorexia for years. This is probably due to incomplete resolution of the underlying emotional disorder. One 5- to 20-year follow-up of children treated when under the age of 16 suggested that outcome is closely related to personality type, 'hysterical-manipulative' patients, the biggest group, doing best, while those with obsessive personalities did less well and those with schizoid personalities did worst (Goetz *et al.*, 1977). Minuchin and his group (1978) report strikingly better results than have been found in most other follow-up studies. Rollins and Piazza (1981) report outcomes which fall between the gloomy statements of, for example, Russell (1977) and the optimistic ones of Minuchin and his colleagues.

CHAPTER ELEVEN

The Psychiatry of Infants and Young Children

The psychiatry of infancy and early childhood has received increasing attention in recent years. This has been reflected in the appearance of books on the subject (for example Osofsky, 1979; Howells, 1979), as well as increasing study of young children and their families by psychiatrists and their colleagues. A special section of the *Journal of the American Academy of Child Psychiatry* for Spring 1981 (volume 20, number 2) dealt with 'infant psychiatry' — the psychiatry of children aged up to age 2½. In one of the papers Minde and Minde (1981) review the concept of infant psychiatry and discuss especially the various treatment approaches available for use with infants.

As Minde and Minde point out, it has long been believed by many workers in our field that early experiences are of profound importance in human development. Yet psychiatrists, and many other child mental health professionals, have seemingly been reluctant to get involved directly in the study of very young children. Their attention has been largely confined to the more severe disorders, such as infantile autism and severe developmental delay, though it is now being turned to problems of bonding between parents and their infants as well as the variations in, and effects of, the different temperamental styles of infants. These issues are discussed in Chapters 1, 2 and 6. Other conditions which may affect infants and young children and which are discussed elsewhere in this book, include hyperactivity, encopresis and enuresis (Chapter 7) and disorders of speech, language and motor development (Chapter 9). This chapter will consider other issues concerning the development of infants and young children.

In pre-school children the family is particularly important as the child has relatively little contact with people outside it. Independent reports, for example from teachers, are not usually available and a self-report from the child is not as easy to obtain as it may be at a later age. The intimate involvement of child and family in this age period means that the child is particularly susceptible to tensions and problems in the family group, and that careful assessment may be necessary to determine whether the problem is essentially a disorder of the child's development or is primarily a manifestation of family dysfunction. These are not mutually exclusive, however, so that a careful assessment both of the child's level of development and emotional state, and of the family as a whole is necessary.

While the conditions to be described usually have their onset in the first years of life, and are mainly prevalent in that age group, many of them may persist into middle childhood.

Prevalence of Disorders

Richman and her colleagues (1975) reported a survey of 3-year-old children in a North London Borough. They found that 7 per cent had moderate or severe behaviour problems and a further 15 per cent had mild problems. There were no significant sex differences in overall prevalence rates, but overactivity and wetting and soiling problems were more frequent in boys, and fearfulness in girls. Children with delayed language development are not included in these figures, and the survey did not cover 'immigrant' families. As the authors point out, prevalence figures of this type can be misleading since young children are highly reactive to the environment, and considering them in isolation from their parents is artificial.

In later papers Earls and Richman (1980a, 1980b) compared the prevalence of behaviour problems in the children of West Indian-born parents living in London with those in children of British-born parents at age 3 and at follow-up 12—18 months later. Despite the fact that the former group lived in poorer housing and had experienced more separations, they did not show more behaviour problems; indeed in the follow-up survey they tended to show fewer and less severe behavioural problems.

The above prevalence rates are similar to those found in an earlier study in Newcastle-on-Tyne, in which 8 per cent of under-fives were considered to have behaviour problems (Miller et al., 1960). Further information about the behaviour and problems of pre-school children can be found in the book *Four Years Old in an Urban Community* (Newson and Newson, 1968).

Assessment of Infants and Young Children

The assessment of infants presents special problems. These have been reviewed by Gaensbauer and Harmon (1981), who suggest a systematic approach to the direct observation and assessment of infants — as distinct from simply obtaining an account from parents or other adults. These authors suggest the following method, which they believe is particularly useful in the age-range 9 to 21 months:

(1) A free play period with mother and infant, during which the infant can play either with toys or with the mother.
(2) Approaches to the infant by a stranger and by the mother. This was designed to discover the extent to which the mother is used as a source of security.
(3) Developmental testing using the Bayley Scales of Infant Development (see Chapter 14).
(4) A separation and reunion sequence involving the mother's departure and return three minutes later.

Gaensbauer and Harmon (1981) report differences in the responses to all four experiences in a group of 'abused/neglected' children when these were compared to a group of normal controls. While this work clearly requires further development it is an interesting attempt to assess more systematically the emotional state of infants.

Earls and colleagues (1982) discuss the measurement of 'behavioural adjustment' in pre-school children and describe the testing and validation of a twelve-item questionnaire designed for use in interviewing parents of 3-year-olds. This seems to be a useful instrument for screening populations of young children.

Common Problems

Temper tantrums are normal in toddlers (see Chapter 1) but may become a problem if they are severe and persistent. This is likely to happen if they are reinforced by attention and gratification. This may occur in unstable families in which other aspects of the care of the children are unsatisfactory. They are thus often part of a more widespread disturbance.

Since temper tantrums are an expression of rage at being frustrated, their escalation or cure depend upon how situations that are frustrating for the child are handled by the parents and other care-givers. Firm but kind limit-setting in an emotionally warm, accepting context will usually bring about a rapid improvement. Inconsistent or hostile attitudes, and especially the intermittent reinforcement of the tantrums by giving into them, will tend to cause them to worsen. A central issue, with this and with many other behaviours, is how secure the child's relationship with the parents is − one of the issues which Gaensbauer and Harmon's assessment procedure addresses. At the same time some children seem constitutionally more prone to tantrum behaviour than others, and children seem to differ in the ease with which tantrums can be extinguished.

Sleep Problems
Failure to sleep as and when expected by the parents may simply be due to unrealistic expectations by the parents, or a lack of knowledge of the amount of sleep needed by a child of the age in question. Moreover, the amount of sleep needed by different children seems to vary considerably. Failure to conform to a regular pattern of sleeping behaviour may occur in chaotic and disorganised homes where there is no regular bedtime and a bedtime routine is not adhered to, so that the child does not have the opportunity to learn a set pattern of sleeping and waking behaviour. Failure to sleep, with crying, is common in babies, but normally settles after a few months if feeding and the general care of the infant are satisfactory. Persistence of the trouble into the toddler years is quite common, however. There appears to be an association between waking at night and other behavioural and temperamental difficulties, particularly lack of malleability and rhythmicity (Richman, 1981a).

In many instances of sleep problems however, the child is in other ways mentally and physically healthy and the trouble is transient, clearing up after some weeks or months.

Night terrors can be alarming to parents who have not seen them before, but are common in perfectly healthy toddlers. These children wake up in a frightened, even terrified, condition. They are inaccessible and do not respond when spoken to, nor do they appear to see their surroundings. Instead they may appear auditorily or visually hallucinated, talking to and looking at people and things not actually there. They may be difficult to comfort at first, and the period of disturbed behaviour and altered consciousness may last up to fifteen minutes, occasionally even longer. Eventually the disturbance subsides with or without comfort from a parent, and the child goes back to sleep. There is usually no memory of the incident when the child wakes up in the morning.

Night terrors have been shown to occur on waking from 'stage 4' (deep) sleep. They persist into later childhood in 1–3 per cent of children (Keith, 1975). There is evidence that they are associated with dream content which touches on an area of intense emotional conflict for the subject; also that severity is related to the duration of stage 4 sleep (Fisher *et al.*, 1974).

Nightmares are unpleasant or frightening dreams. The child does not wake up, nor necessarily become overtly disturbed while having a nightmare. If woken up the child reacts normally and there is no period of altered consciousness or inaccessibility such as occurs in night terrors. Nightmares occur in 'REM' (that is 'rapid eye movement', or light) sleep.

Sleep-walking, or somnambulism, may accompany either nightmares or night terrors. Apparently the content of the dream or terror is acted out in a state of sleep or altered consciousness.

All forms of sleep disturbance are liable to be exacerbated by physical or emotional disorder. Nightmares and restless sleep are common in acute febrile illnesses. The possibility of nocturnal epilepsy must also be considered, since some epileptic children with major fits have their attacks only at night.

Very often no evidence is found of any other abnormality. The sleep disorder can then usually be regarded as a transient phase in development, and the parents reassured accordingly. It may indeed represent a reaction to the normal anxieties of the toddler period, during which the child has to meet and cope with many new experiences and situations. Sometimes, however, there is evidence of emotional disorder in the child or in the family group. In that case treatment for a neurotic disorder (see Chapter 5) or for the family as a whole may be needed. It has also been suggested that the drug diazepam (see Chapter 10) may be of value in the treatment of night terrors (Keith, 1975).

Sleep Apnoea

In 'sleep apnoea' there is frequent waking during the night, associated with periods of reduced or no breathing. Other features are loud snoring and excessive sleepiness during the day. The main importance of the syndrome to psychiatrists and their colleagues is that its diagnosis may be missed because it is mistaken for a psychogenic disorder. This is because associated symptoms include intellectual deterioration, depression (sometimes with suicidal thoughts), personality changes, sudden outbursts of irrational behaviour and suspiciousness. Morning headaches and hypnagogic hallucinations (those occurring as the subject goes to sleep) have also been reported. The cause may be mechanical obstruction to breathing or a failure of the neurological mechanism controlling breathing, or a mixture of the two. The condition occurs at all ages; it is not particularly a disorder of young children. It has been described by Guilleminault *et al.*, (1976) and a recent concise review is that of Martin and Lefebvre (1981) who also described the successful surgical treatment of a 13½-year-old boy with the condition. Recognition of the disorder is important since it can be fatal.

Young children's sleep disorders have been reviewed by Anders and Weinstein (1972) and Richman (1981b).

Feeding Problems

Feeding problems are common in young children, in whom they sometimes occur in the absence of other significant problems. Children may eat, or be thought by their parents to eat, too little or too much; they may be excessively particular over what they eat (or 'faddy'); or may eat items not normally regarded as edible (this is known as 'pica').

It has been mentioned in Chapter 7 that *food refusal* may be present in cases of soiling. It may also occur on its own. The psychopathology is often similar to that present in children who soil. The parent is attempting to control the child, perhaps in a rigid, obsessive way. The child reacts by refusing to eat what the parent considers an adequate diet. The parent may have an exaggerated idea of the importance of adequate nutrition, and perhaps unrealistic fears of what will happen if the child does not eat enough. The child is unconsciously or consciously aware of this and so chooses this particular symptom, while showing a total lack of concern about the 'problem'. Such children are usually perfectly satisfactorily nourished, and so have been receiving adequate diets, though it may not be very easy to persuade the parents of this.

The management needed resembles that used in case of negativistic soiling. The food refusal itself should be ignored. A lot of work may require to be done with the parents to enable them to understand and accept this. Where the parent (most often it is the mother) has very set, rigid ideas about feeding, the problem may have its roots in her own childhood.

Special food should not be prepared, and no attempt should be made to persuade the child to eat. An ordinary menu should be offered on a 'take-it-or-leave-it' basis. If this is done, children normally select a diet which provides adequate nourishment. (This does not of course apply in anorexia nervosa, a disorder of adolescents – see Chapter 10.)

The outcome is usually satisfactory. In many cases food refusal is simply a phase in development, particularly in toddlers who are trying to assert their individuality and are rebelling against constraints they find are placed on their behaviour. Where parental attitudes or the family environment are seriously disturbed, the outlook may be less good, but this is because of the background problems rather than the food refusal. In cases of this sort treatment by a family therapy approach may be helpful (Chapter 16).

Food fads often occur in children with food refusal. Many types of food are refused, which may cause anxiety to the parents. Nevertheless these children are usually well nourished and thus appear to be receiving an adequate diet. Relatively mild food fads are common in normal, healthy children. They are probably largely a means whereby children instinctively select a balanced diet suited to their present nutritional needs.

Pica is the eating of items not usually regarded as edible, for example paper, soil, paint, wood and cloth. Many other materials may be involved. The symptom has many causes, including adverse environmental factors and emotional distress; it is often associated with distorted developmental patterns, brain damage and mental retardation, but is sometimes seen in children of normal intelligence. The children often have relationship difficulties. The condition is frequently associated with iron deficiency anaemia (due to a generally poor diet) and lead poisoning, which itself can cause anaemia. Lead poisoning often results from ingesting old paint containing lead; it can lead to severe brain damage (Chapter 6).

Associated sleep and behaviour problems are common, and the families tend to be disorganised and poor. In severe cases treatment usually involves admission to hospital as well as intensive work with the family. Bicknell (1975) has provided an excellent review of the condition.

Breath-Holding Spells

Breath-holding spells occur commonly in pre-school children. They usually start before age 2, but seldom before 6 months. Livingstone (1972) reports a mean age of onset of 12 months and a peak frequency between ages 2 and 3. The spells usually die out by age 5 or 6.

Breath-holding spells are usually precipitated by some minor upset or frustration. This is followed by crying which increases in intensity until the child reaches a state of rage. Breathing then stops, usually in expiration, and cyanosis becomes manifest in blueness of the face, especially around the lips. Occasionally the period of breath-holding leads to a major epileptic fit, but in most cases the child starts to breathe again in half a minute or so and recovery quickly occurs. The three distinguishing factors are a precipitating factor, violent crying and cyanosis. The spells seem to be used by some children to alarm their parents, who may reinforce them by a show of concern and indulgence. They are better treated calmly and with as little fuss as possible. The outcome is usually good and there is no increased incidence of epilepsy in these children.

Thumb-Sucking and Nail-Biting

Both these behaviours are common in young children, though nail-biting also occurs frequently in older children, and in one population survey was found to reach a peak at 9 years in boys and 11 years in girls (Shepherd *et al.*, 1971). Thumb- and finger-sucking are normal in babies and gradually lessen during the second and subsequent years. Persistent thumb-sucking usually has little significance on its own but may be one feature in a pattern of regressive behaviour in a child who is anxious or under stress. It often requires no treatment, but if necessary can usually be stopped by simple reminders, rewards or even sanctions. Occasionally it becomes a severe, compulsive behaviour associated with rocking or masturbation, and more active treatment is required. Severe thumb-sucking can cause dental malocclusion in older children and may merit treatment for this reason.

Nail-biting is also usually a tension-reducing habit and tends to occur in anxious and tense children. Direct treatment is not usually needed, but the underlying condition may need treatment in its own right. Nail-biting often disappears at puberty if it has not done so previously.

Treatment

Minde and Minde (1981) divide treatment into direct and indirect approaches. While most psychoanalysts have refrained from analysing infants, a few have reported doing so. Behavioural approaches have also been used and mothers have been trained to act as therapists for their infants. Indirect treatments include counselling of parents and other caretakers by mental health professionals and paediatricians, and the provision of special 'early intervention' programmes for children at risk, in day care or pre-school settings or in the home. Another matter to which attention has been given is the care of small children who need to spend long periods in hospital. Minde and his colleagues (1980) report a study in which parents of very small premature infants were randomly allocated to self-help groups or to 'control' conditions – that is no group meetings – with apparent benefit to those in the self-help groups and their infants. The problems of infants and young children can also be looked at in the context of the family systems of which they are part, which may lead to treatment using family therapy approaches (Chapter 16).

CHAPTER TWELVE

Emotional Disorders in Mentally Handicapped Children

Mental Handicap

Mental handicap, or mental retardation, is usually defined in social terms, as well as according to the subject's level of intellectual function. Thus it is considered to be present when low intelligence is combined with failure to adapt to society. It is therefore a psycho-social concept. Definitions couched in psychosocial terms have been developed mainly to help in deciding which individuals require institutional care or special educational arrangements. For these purposes they have obvious value. But the division of children, for the purpose of providing them with psychiatric services, into those who are mentally handicapped and those who are not has disadvantages. There is much to be said for considering the psychiatry of all children as a part of the main stream of clinical child psychiatry. In the past the psychiatric care of duller children has tended to be provided in hospitals for the mentally handicapped, sometimes far away from the children's homes and families. Moves to reverse this trend have fortunately been under way for some years now (Kushlick, 1975).

Prevalence of Emotional Disorders

The Isle of Wight epidemiological study of 10- and 11-year-old children (Rutter, Tizard and Whitmore, 1970) showed that 'intellectually retarded' children (defined as those whose Wechsler Scale IQ − see Chapter 14 − was two standard deviations or more below the mean for 'control' children) had psychiatric disorders 3 to 4 times more often than children in the normal control group. Among severely retarded children not attending school, psychiatric disorder was found in 50 per cent of the children compared with 6.6 per cent of the general population. Among these severely disturbed children psychoses and the hyperkinetic syndrome were proportionately more common than in children of higher intelligence (Rutter, Graham and Yule, 1970).

As well as psychiatric disorders as defined in this book, a variety of forms of deviant behaviour are commoner in children of lower IQ than they are in more intellectually able children. Table 3, for example, illustrates this using some findings from the Isle of Wight survey.

TABLE 3: SYMPTOMS REPORTED IN 10- AND 11-YEAR-OLD GIRLS
(Isle of Wight survey)

	IQ 120 or more	*IQ 79 or less*
Poor concentration		
Parents' report	2·6%	26·4%
Teachers' report	9·1%	62·3%
Fighting		
Parents' report	1·3%	9·9%
Teachers' report	2·6%	11·0%

Causes and Clinical Associations

Some of the causes of mental retardation have been referred to in Chapters 2 and 6. As with other conditions, delayed intellectual development may be due to genetic factors (either specific or poly-genic); to brain damage occurring before, during or after birth; and to environmental factors — notably lack of stimulation, emotional and physical deprivation, and serious malnutrition which can stunt intellectual as well as physical growth.

The assessment and formulation of the psychiatric condition of mentally handicapped children follow the same lines as those set out in Chapter 3. The details and consequences of the child's intellectual limitations are likely to figure prominently in the formulation. These limitations tend to make it specially difficult for such children to adapt to social situations, as well as to cope with the various learning tasks of childhood, including school. How well they do cope depends on the environments they find themselves in, and the skills and dedication of their teachers.

For a more detailed discussion of the causes and types of mental retardation the reader should refer to a textbook such as Penrose (1972) or Kirman and Bicknell (1975).

Any of the forms of psychiatric disorder described elsewhere in this book may affect intellectually handicapped children, but there are established associations between low intelligence and infantile autism and other infantile psychoses, and between low intelligence and hyperactivity. Stereotyped repetitive movements are also commoner in dull children than in bright ones; so too are nail-biting, stuttering and some other behaviours.

The mechanisms responsible for the associations between intellectual handicap and psychiatric disorder are complex. The following points are relevant:

1. There is a relationship between IQ and deviant behaviour in children of normal intelligence as well as in dull children. Thus children who are intellectually above average show less deviant behaviour than those of average intelligence. This could mean that greater intellectual capacity makes social adaptation easier, and thus deviant behaviour less likely; indeed this is almost certainly an important factor.
2. There is little evidence that emotional disorders are the cause of a low IQ except in so far as they may impair a child's co-operation in intelligence testing.
3. Organic brain disease is commoner in dull children than in bright ones, and is virtually universal in children with IQs below 50 (Crome, 1960). In such children the organic condition often plays a part in causing the psychiatric disorder. In the Isle of Wight study (Rutter, Tizard and Whitmore, 1970), psychiatric disorder was found to be 3 to 4 times commoner in brain-damaged children than in the general child population. In children with chronic physical disorders which did not involve the brain, such as asthma and diabetes, it was found only slightly more often. Epileptic disturbances (see Chapter 8) are also associated with an increased incidence of psychiatric disorder (Eyman *et al.*, 1970). Moreover behaviour disturbance often lessens or even disappears

following hemispherectomy, an operation sometimes performed to remove half the cerebral cortex when this is badly damaged in children with infantile hemiplegia; similar improvement may also occur following the surgical removal of an epileptogenic focus from the temporal lobe. This suggests that the behaviour problems are due to malfunction of the brain in these cases.

4. Social factors may adversely affect both intellectual development and emotional stability. In particular, depriving, hostile and rejecting parental attitudes may have both effects. Studies have also shown that instability is commoner in the families of mentally handicapped children than in those of brighter ones, perhaps in part because there is a positive correlation between the intelligence levels of parents and those of their children. Retarded children may also be rejected by other children, to the detriment of their emotional development and mental health.

5. The developmental immaturity affecting retarded children means that their language and other social skills are less than those of their peers. These problems, combined with their delay in reaching motor and toilet training milestones, are additional handicaps which may be factors in bringing about the development of psychiatric disorder.

6. Educational failure is strongly associated with psychiatric disorder (another finding of the Isle of Wight study), and dull children inevitably progress more slowly than their brighter peers. In some retarded children, long-standing failure at school seems to be a major factor in causing emotional disorder.

7. Institutionalisation can adversely affect both intellectual development and emotional growth. The unsuitability of many institutions for children was clearly shown in the sociological investigations reported by King and his colleagues (1971).

The association between psychiatric disorder and intellectual handicap in children has been discussed helpfully, and more fully, by Rutter (1971a).

Treatment

The principles of treatment are discussed in Chapter 16. As in other cases, a comprehensive assessment of the child in the context of his or her family, school and neighbourhood is essential first; the formulation should pay special regard to the clinical associations discussed above. It is often found that social factors such as an unstable or depriving family background and educational failure are militating against the child's healthy emotional development, in addition to the various biological factors which may be operating. Both social and educational stress are in theory susceptible to modification, though the facilities available to achieve this are not always adequate.

In many developed countries there have been established centres and clinics devoted to the early detection and remediation of developmental delays and problems. Paediatricians, psychiatrists, psychologists, speech therapists, educationalists, social workers and professionals from other disciplines are available to investigate the nature of developmental problems, learning difficulties, perceptual deficits, emotional disorders and social background problems of children. Many of the problems of mentally handicapped children can be resolved or better still avoided, by adequate assessment of the children's needs, followed by the provision of the right kind of educational and living environment.

Institutional care is necessary for some children, including most of the very severely retarded. The need is usually determined by the degree of the intellectual retardation, together with the effects of any associated physical handicaps (and these are common in the severely retarded) or emotional disorder. The family is an important factor too, since the capacities of families to cope with handicapped children vary. Institutional care of mentally handicapped children, when it is necessary, should be in small, well-staffed units as near as possible to the children's families. Only a minority of the most severely handicapped require the full facilities of a hospital. In many instances hostels or group homes are better, as well as being less expensive to run and often nearer to the families. Unfortunately many children are still accommodated in large, ill-equipped and frequently under-staffed wards of antiquated hospitals and other institutions. This is not to be recommended.

Psychotherapy with mentally handicapped children presents special problems because of the poor verbal skills and limited concentration of these children. Where emotional problems exist in the child or family, family therapy is often easier to carry out and may be a more hopeful approach.

Behaviour therapy is widely used in treating mentally handicapped children (Yule and Carr, 1980). Forms of psychotherapy that involve verbal language skills are of limited value in these children, but operant conditioning can be very effective. Suitably constructed programmes can promote successful toilet training, the extinction of deviant behaviours like temper tantrums, rocking and head banging, the acquisition of motor and language skills and many other therapeutic aims. As well as the reduction or removal of specific symptoms, successful modification of problem behaviours can have helpful secondary effects on the child's emotional state.

Drug treatment can be of value in the treatment of psychiatric disorders in mentally handicapped children. Epilepsy, if present, should be controlled by the use of appropriate anticonvulsant drugs. Since motor hyperactivity sometimes responds well to such drugs as haloperidol, phenothiazines and methylphenidate, these substances can be helpful in treating the considerable number of retarded children who show this symptom. All these treatment methods are discussed further in Chapter 16.

In conclusion, some general points about helping intellectually handicapped children are worth stating. A middle course has to be steered between asking too much of a handicapped child and asking too little. Facing such a child with tasks in school which are quite beyond him or her can be damaging and lead to anxiety, even despair, and a needlessly poor self-image. On the other hand, asking too little, as may for instance happen to the inmate of a large hospital ward, means that the child's potential is not realised. Continuous assessment of these children and their progress, including their reactions to the education, treatment and other help they are getting, is essential. Assessment cannot be a once-for-all process. Continuity of care is important, too. Duller children find change more difficult to deal with. Finally, the needs of the family must always be considered. It is possible for the attention given to a handicapped child to affect adversely the care given to other children in the family. The presence of a severely retarded and disturbed child can also affect the parents and the stability of their marriage. All these factors must be taken into account in the management of these difficult problems.

Mental 'handicap' may be regarded as the extent to which intellectual retardation affects an individual's capacity to cope with life in the family and society in which he is living. It is thus as much a function of society as of the individual. Intellectual limitations are a greater problem in a technologically well-developed country than in a less well-developed one where most people are doing unskilled work. The extent to which the handicapped reach a satisfactory adjustment in any society will depend partly on such factors and also upon how society reacts to those who are handicapped.

CHAPTER THIRTEEN

Disorders in Adolescence

The principles underlying the assessment and treatment of psychiatric disorders in childhood apply also to disorders of adolescence, but there are some practical differences. The pattern of disorders prevalent in adolescence is also somewhat different from that seen in childhood. Adolescence is a time of rapid change — physical, emotional and social. The developmental tasks of this period have been outlined in Chapter 1; the main development is the gradual adoption of the adult role — social, vocational and sexual. During this process doubts, fears and feelings of inadequacy are common. These may cause anxiety which may not be openly expressed Instead the individual may become aggressive and defiant, or moody and unpredictable. Adolescents often make a show of rejecting adult standards, and of having interests and pursuits other than those of which their parents approve. The moods and attitudes of adolescents may vary strikingly over short periods of time.

Prevalence of Disorders in Adolescence

The prevalence of psychiatric disorders in adolescence differs considerably from that seen in childhood. This subject has been reviewed by Rutter (1980) in the book *Changing Youth in a Changing Society*, an important book reviewing many aspects of adolescence and its disorders. Extensive use of this book has been made in the preparation of this chapter.

Studies of adolescent populations have yielded prevalence rates of psychiatric disorder between 8 and 21 per cent, depending on the criteria used, the population and the sex of the subjects (Krupinski *et al.*, 1967; Henderson, 1971; Leslie, 1974; Rutter *et al.*, 1976; Latvik, 1977). Rates are generally twice as common, or more, in urban than in rural areas. There are also changes in the sex ratios found in adolescence, compared with those in childhood: whereas in childhood psychiatric disorders are much commoner in boys than girls, as adolescence proceeds the ratio becomes equal and it is reversed in adult life. This is mainly because of an increase in the prevalence of affective disorders, including depression, in girls.

Adolescent emotional disorders include:

1. Unresolved childhood disorders.
2. Disturbances related to the stresses of puberty and adolescence.
3. Insipient adult-type disorders.

Unresolved Childhood Disorders

Childhood emotional disorders which have neither resolved spontaneously nor been successfully treated will persist into adolescence. Much disturbed behaviour in middle childhood (but not that occurring in the pre-school years) does indeed persist into adolescence (McFarlane *et al.*, 1954).

Sometimes *neurotic disorders* improve at or around puberty. This may be due to the biological drives towards independence which become more active. The peer group, which tends to become a more important influence in adolescence, may also help. The change from primary to secondary school sometimes promotes emotional growth; if the child can face the challenge of an often larger school containing bigger children and requiring more responsibility and independence of decision on the part of its pupils, this can be a useful experience. All these factors may assist the emotionally immature child, who has been overdependent on his parents, to grow up, become more self-reliant and thus come to experience less anxiety in stressful situations. But sometimes they are insufficient. Faced with the challenges of adolescence some neurotic children cannot cope. Such drives towards independence as exist are not enough and the individuals fall back into the security and comfort of their families. Such children, realising unconsciously, if not consciously, their incapacity to fill age-appropriate roles, may become even more anxious, with a worsening of their condition.

School refusal in adolescence may be either a continuation or an exacerbation of a problem which existed before puberty, or a symptom appearing for the first time. Even if onset is during adolescence, however, the origins can usually be traced back to well before puberty. The pattern of school refusal in adolescence tends to be different from that seen in younger children. Adolescents who are anxious about going to school may hide when efforts are made to enforce attendance; others may stay at home and cling to their mothers. In many adolescents with school refusal, difficulties at school are more prominent than is usual in younger children. The 'problems' there, which often concern relationships with peer group or staff, would not be problems to children whose emotional development had been normal and whose family relationships were secure.

The difficulties which the parents of school-refusing children often have in expressing aggression in normal ways, and asserting independence, are usually present in the children too; but in adolescence they frequently become intensified. The adolescent's desire, conscious or unconscious, to be independent, and his awareness of parental 'smothering' and protectiveness which prevent this, can cause a buildup of intensely aggressive feelings. This may be expressed through violently aggressive outbursts, especially under stress, the child behaving at other times in a passive and dependent fashion. In these cases treatment of the whole family group is essential if the underlying problem is to be resolved. Sometimes the members of the family are not willing to enter into such treatment, or the situation proves insufficiently remediable if they do; there is then no alternative, in severe cases, to removing the adolescent from the family for treatment in a residential setting. It seems that school refusal in adolescents tends to be associated with more serious pathology in child and family than is usually the case in younger children (Coolidge *et al.*, 1970; Hersov, 1976b).

Conduct disorders are often exacerbated with the onset of puberty, as the individual's antisocial feelings are reinforced by the normal rebelliousness and rejection of adult standards seen at this age. In one study children who were most aggressive at age 8 to 10 were found to be especially likely to become violent delinquents (Farrington, 1978), though such an outcome is by no means inevitable. The adolescent who does not have a secure relationship with his parents, and lacks 'internal' behavioural controls based upon identification with the parents, is very much at risk. He is readily influenced by others of his age, from whom he may well get more acceptance and satisfaction than he receives at home. The nature of the peer group is partly a matter of chance, or at least of what is available in the neighbourhood, but the choosing of friends by adolescents is also influenced by their own attitudes and feelings. If the adolescent becomes part of a delinquent gang the conduct disorder will probably worsen, but some peer groups are beneficial in their effects. One of the aims of youth clubs and other youth organisations is to provide groups which will be constructive and useful to their members.

Psychotic disorders do not themselves usually get either better or worse at adolescence. If they have been improving the improvement often continues, but generally the handicaps of autistic and other psychotic children persist through adolescence (Rutter, 1970a). Similarly, a child who has been gradually adapting to a chronic neurological handicap may continue to do so. There may, however, be secondary emotional disorder due to the child's awareness of the increasing discrepancy between his or her own capabilities and those of the peer group. As these children get bigger, and should be getting more independent, their handicaps may show up more strikingly than hitherto. At this stage some psychotic and brain-damaged children who have previously been cared for at home may require admission to residential care or schooling.

Hyperactivity often lessens in adolescence. This applies both to hyperactive psychotic children and to the 'hyperkinetic syndrome' itself. The associated antisocial behaviour and learning problems often continue however (Mendelson *et al.*, 1971; Minde *et al.*, 1972). A follow-up study of young adults aged 17 to 24 showed that poor socialisation skills and poor sense of well-being were still present significantly more often than in control subjects. This applied also to scholastic skills and restlessness, but not to adjustment in work and living situations, nor to antisocial behaviour, non-medical use of drugs or serious psychiatric disturbances (Hechtman *et al.*, 1976).

Disturbances Related to Stresses of Puberty and Adolescence

Most of the disorders of the adolescents referred to clinics have started before puberty (Capes *et al.*, 1971), whereas just over half of those found in population studies have started during adolescence (Rutter *et al.*, 1976). This is probably because the disorders starting earlier tend to be more severe. Rutter (1980b) also points out that disorders starting in adolescence differ in several other respects from those starting before puberty: the ratio of boys to girls (1.3 to 1) is lower than that in disorders with earlier onset (2.3 to 1); specific reading retardation (Chapter 9) is less common, indeed no more common than in the general population, as opposed to being 3 or 4 times commoner in cases with earlier onset; and family difficulties are much less common.

The majority of the psychiatric disorders starting during adolescence are either neurotic (or 'emotional') or conduct disorders — as is true also of those starting before puberty. However, the excess of conduct disorders is no longer apparent, indicating that more neurotic and depressive than conduct disorders start during adolescence.

The decision where to draw the line between 'normal' rebelliousness and rejection of adult standards and conduct disorder; and also between the shyness, diffidence and lack of self-confidence with which some adolescents react when they experience difficulty adopting an adult role and neurotic disorder, is in some measure arbitrary. Similar considerations apply also to the much-discussed question of whether 'adolescent turmoil' is 'normal' or should be regarded as a psychiatric disorder (Rutter *et al.*, 1976). More important is the assessment of the nature, causes and seriousness of any problems present, leading to appropriate help. If a psychiatric label is to be attached it will sometimes be one of adjustment reaction.

During adolescence there is need for much give and take between parents and their children. If parents' attitudes are unduly rigid and inflexible, defiance may be provoked in their children. At the same time the adolescent, especially the early adolescent, still very much needs the security of home and family. It can be as unfortunate, even disastrous, for the parents to give too little support to, and take too little interest in, the adolescent, as for them to be excessively strict and rigid.

It is not always the parents who complain or feel worried. The adolescent too often feels anxious, tense or under strain during this period. There are several possible reasons for this.

(a) *The dependence–independence conflict.* The adolescent feels an innate urge to be more independent and to take decisions, and also perceives that this is socially expected of him or her, but may not be able adequately to play such a role. The alternative is to fall back on the family, and others, for support, but reluctantly. Thus help and support given by parents may be accepted in an off-hand and ungracious way.

(b) *Uncertainties about sexual role and sexual adequacy.* The onset of the physical and emotional changes of puberty can vary widely at least, between the ages of ten and seventeen. This can cause individuals to feel out of step with their peers, which may lead to anxiety. Fears of sexual inadequacy are common during this period.

During adolescence there is an upsurge of sexual activity, and relationships with the opposite sex become more prominent. During the transition there is often some confusion of feelings and difficulty in dealing with the new situation. The individual may wish to enter into relationships with the opposite sex, but shyness and lack of confidence may make this difficult and embarrassing. On the other hand, early sexual activity may, and in recent years increasingly has, led to unwanted teenage pregnancies (Schinke *et al.*, 1979). Pregnancy, whether it is carried to term or aborted, can also be a considerable stress to the adolescent girl.

(c) *Peer group influences.* As adolescents draw away from their parents, their peer groups become of greater importance. Adolescent groups are sometimes all of one sex, or they may include both boys and girls. One important purpose they serve is that of providing support for the anxious and insecure individual who feels unable to play an appropriate role unsupported. Members identify with the standards of the group as a whole, and with the support of the group can do things they would feel unable to tackle on their own. Adolescent groups may be as small as two or three but membership may run to ten, twenty or even more. Some are fairly constant, but usually they change, as members leave to form or join other groups, and others join. A particular adolescent may belong to several groups of different sizes or types at the same time.

Groups of this sort can be beneficial, helping their members to achieve normal behaviour and adjustment by providing support over a difficult period. The opposite can happen, however, as in the case of delinquent gangs.

Difficulties arising from group membership are mainly concerned with being, or feeling, different from the group. The problem may be one of appearance, race or religion. The groups usually demand a fair amount of conformity to their standards, and inability to meet these may cause the individual anxiety and even lead to rejection by the group.

Adolescent conduct or behaviour disorders, are characterised by antisocial behaviour, generally similar to that occurring in conduct disorders of younger children. They may present as an exaggeration of normal adolescent rebelliousness. The child may stay out later than the parents lay down, truant from school, be generally disobedient or steal. In more severe cases there may be frank delinquency with conflict with the law. The parents complain of things like the young person's mode of dress or hairstyle, and may consider him or her generally out of control. These disorders may be subdivided as described in Chapter 4.

These conditions are in part manifestations of breakdown in the relationships between young people and the adult world, particularly the parents. During adolescence the parent—child relationship has to undergo much change. Its soundness before puberty is an important factor in determining the extent to which the adolescent will rebel and 'test out' the parents. Another factor is the way the parents react to adolescent behaviour in their son or daughter. Great flexibility, tolerance and understanding, combined with the right amount of firmness and control, are needed. Sometimes abnormal rebelliousness and antisocial behaviour are unconsciously designed to get the parents to control the behaviour of a child who is insecure and afraid of his or her own aggressiveness. In other instances it is a protest against over-strict demands which the parents make. In yet others it is a reflection of rootlessness and aimlessness in children who have been, in varying degrees, deprived of love and security. Because of the poor quality of their relationships, conscience-formation has been defective and the conflicting pressures and anxieties of adolescence upset the delicate and uncertain balance which has hitherto resulted in reasonably conforming behaviour. In most cases the child's problems are but part of a wider family problem, and are more easily explicable when seen in this context. As well as being a useful treatment, family therapy can be a valuable way of learning how the adolescent's antisocial behaviour fits into the family's structure and functioning.

Many adolescent conduct disorders seem worse than they really are. The reported severity of the behavioural disturbance is on its own an inadequate criterion. Many adolescents emerge as mentally healthy individuals, adjusting satisfactorily to society, after going through a period of difficult behaviour. Factors to be considered in deciding how serious the problem really is include the child's adjustment before puberty, family stability and parental attitudes, and the individual's adjustment in circumstances where the parents are not directly involved. These include school, peer group and the interview situation with physician or other professional.

Running away from home is a common and apparently increasing problem in many societies. The term is applied to leaving or staying away from home, with the intention of staying away at least for some time, in circumstances in which the individual will be missed by those remaining at home. While it occurs at other ages also, it is particularly a problem of adolescents. About 1 in 10 of the youths aged 12 to 13 in the USA have run away from home at least once. About 300 000 run away for the first time each year (Justice and Duncan, 1976). These figures do not include institutionalised youths. The homes of runaways are characterised by much parent–child conflict and are broken by parental death, divorce or separation more often than in the population generally. Running away can be an escape from such conflicts or a means of avoiding defeat in the battle for independence from the parents.

Adolescent drug taking appears to have increased in the last few decades, although reliable prevalence figures are hard to obtain. Blumberg (1976) in an excellent review, quotes reported prevalence rates in American high school students as varying from 9 per cent to 42 per cent for marijuana use, 3 to 15 per cent for barbiturates, 2 to 7 per cent for LSD and 1 to 4 per cent for opiates. These figures are for students who had ever used the drug in question, even if only once, and are based on pre-1970 studies. Jalali and colleagues (1981) reported a survey of 2131 adolescents in five New Jersey schools. Their ages ranged from 12 to 18, with most in the age range 15 to 17. As in other studies, much the most commonly used drug was marijuana. Only 49 per cent of the subjects stated they had never used this drug Other drugs the adolescents had used included amphetamines (26.3 per cent), barbiturates (25.3 per cent), hallucinogens (21.1 per cent), cocaine (13.6 per cent), inhalants (13.2 per cent) and opiates (9.3 per cent). Onset of drug use was most often between 13 and 15, but earlier in the case of marijuana.

There were significant sex differences only in the case of marijuana: 70 per cent of the users of this drug were girls.

The same study also looked at alcohol use. Over 80 per cent of the subjects reported alcohol use from an early age – 34 per cent at 8 or younger. Alcohol was most commonly first obtained in the family, whereas other drugs were obtained from peers, usually at school. Only about a quarter of the subjects used drugs at home, whereas nearly half of them used alcohol in the family setting. In this population at least, drug use seemed to arise largely from contacts at school, or with peers in other situations, while alcohol use was more a family activity. Alcohol use among adolescents is closely associated with its use, and especially its abuse, by parents.

It is useful to divide drug users into experimental, situational (or recreational) and compulsive groups. Most adolescents probably experiment, at least with marijuana, at some stage. A smaller number use it at parties and in other social situations, while an even smaller group become dependent on a drug or drugs. In most cases, therefore, social pressures and causes are major factors. Availability is of course also important; this is probably why alcohol, tobacco and (in many communities) marijuana are the most widely used substances. Socio-economic factors play a part too: drug use, especially of marijuana, has been found in many USA studies to be commoner among whites than blacks, which is probably in part a consequence of their better economic status, providing them with the money with which to buy drugs.

Gibbs (1982) studied a particularly troubled group of adolescents, namely 48 delinquent girls, and has also provided a concise review of some of the relevant literature. Among this group she identified four personality patterns: 'borderline' (7 girls), 'antisocial' (14), 'neurotic' (18) and 'socialised delinquent' (9). Ninety per cent of these girls had used at least one drug, most often marijuana, but there was a long list of other drugs that had been used by the group. The average age of initial use was 12.5 years. Seventy-nine per cent of the girls had used alcohol at least once, a rate not much different from that found in some school populations, but five of the girls (10.5 per cent) claimed to have serious drinking problems. The girls with antisocial personalities had the highest mean drug and alcohol abuse scores, while the socialised delinquents (roughly the same group as the socialised conduct disorder group described in Chapter 4) had the lowest. The other two groups occupied intermediate positions.

There is a significant correlation between drug and alcohol abuse and both delinquency and failure at school. Other factors which have been found associated are social isolation, low self-esteem, poor relationships with parents, depression and unconventional beliefs and values concerning drug use (Gibbs, 1982). It seems that individuals seek to have their felt needs for affiliation, satisfaction of curiosity, altered state of consciousness, recreation, anxiety reduction and general drive reduction met by drug use (Blumberg, 1976).

A study of young adolescents by Hundelby *et al.* (1982) has shown a very significant correlation between drug use and 'sexual behaviour' (heavy petting, dating, sexual intercourse, long telephone conversations with opposite sex). There were also lesser but significant correlations between drug use and both 'general delinquency' and 'school misbehaviour', though the latter seemed to be largely independent of each other.

Drug use can also be seen as a learnt habit if the subject finds it rewarding. If some felt need is met, use of the drug is likely to be reinforced. Thus what starts as experimentation as a result of group pressure may be continued for other reasons.

Among adolescent drug users there is a small proportion who have serious personality problems which usually pre-date the drug use. Drug *abusers* tend to show evidence of psychopathology, while the simpler drug *user* appears, from most research studies, to be more like the general run of young people of similar age (Amini *et al.*, 1976). The psychopathology may be predominantly depressive, rather than a personality disorder. Some drug abusers have a history of early deprivation.

There is apparently a stepwise progression in drug use. This starts with beer or wine, going on to, successively, cigarettes and hard liquor, marijuana and then other illegal drugs such as heroin, cocaine and LSD. Not all adolescents who start on this sequence complete it of course, and indeed the proportion who reach the final stage is quite small (Hamburg *et al.*, 1975; Kandel and Faust, 1975).

Progression to 'hard drugs', such as heroin, is serious since these often produce major problems of addiction. The taking of drugs by injection, for example, amphetamine drugs ('speed'), barbiturates and heroin is also a bad sign. Complications due to dirty or contaminated injections (infection or hepatitis), and overdosage are ever-present risks.

Drugs used by adolescents include the following:

(a) Alcohol — This is a serious problem in society at large, and its use by adolescents reflects this. It is a drug of dependence, it causes serious health risks (notably liver damage) and it is an important contributing cause of road traffic accidents. There is some reason to believe its use among teenagers has been increasing, though it is hard to be sure about this (O'Connor, 1977).

(b) Tobacco — Cigarette smoking is powerfully addictive and shares with alochol use the problem of being widely abused by society. Tobacco products, like alcoholic drinks, are widely advertised, often to appeal to young people. Smoking predisposes to lung cancer, heart disease, arterial disease and other health hazards.

(c) Marijuana — (cannabis, hashish, 'pot') is an intoxicant which produces a euphoric state similar to that produced by alcohol. It is illegal in most western countries, though in many, penalties for its use have been lightened in recent years. It does not cause physical dependence, though users may become psychologically dependent on it. Long-term effects of its use are not certainly established, but in the short term it can cause mental confusion and can make a person as dangerous at the wheel of a car as can alcohol.

(d) Amphetamines ('speed') — are used to produce a state of euphoria; their use can lead to physical dependence and to a psychotic state. Intravenous use can have particularly serious effects.

(e) Hallucinogens — the best known of which is lysergic acid diethyl-amide ('LSD' or 'acid') are used often to provide an altered state of consciousness and unusual subjective, including hallucinatory, experiences.

(f) Barbiturates are used both orally and intravenously, and can lead to marked states of dependency. There is real danger of overdose, and suicide by barbiturates is quite frequent.

(g) Other tranquillisers and sedatives ('downers') are frequently used to produce altered states of consciousness by adolescents.

(h) Solvents such as glues used for model-making, nail-polish remover and typewriter correction solutions are quite often used by young people. They are inhaled, often from inside a plastic bag in which the vapour is concentrated. The process is usually known as 'glue-sniffing'. A euphoric state can be produced, leading to mental disorientation and even unconsciousness. The habit seems to be

increasing. It carries a significant risk of causing brain damage,
liver damage, kidney failure and blood and other disorders
(O'Connor, 1979).

(i) Heroin, cocaine and other major addictive drugs are used relatively
infrequently by young people, but their use is serious since
dependence readily develops, and the long-term prognosis for
those who are addicted is generally poor.

Neurotic disorders arising *de novo* in adolescents are often expressions of anxiety arising out of difficulty in coping with the
developmental tasks of adolescence. Many individuals who develop
neurotic symptoms have previously shown evidence of emotional
immaturity. Clinical pictures similar to those described in Chapter 5
are seen. Anxiety states and depressive disorders are commonest;
obsessive–compulsive, hysterical and phobic conditions are considerably less common. Sometimes adolescent neurosis presents as school
refusal occurring for the first time.

Anorexia nervosa, a condition affecting mainly adolescents is
discussed in Chapter 10.

Adult-type Mental Disorders Arising in Adolescence

Schizophrenia and affective psychoses become increasingly common
once puberty is past. Both are still fairly rare during the first year or
two after puberty, though depressive illness may be difficult to
recognise at this time. During middle and late adolescence the
frequency of the conditions increases considerably. The late teens
and early twenties are the commonest time for schizophrenia to
commence.

The main features of *schizophrenia* have been described in Chapter
6. The diagnosis can be difficult to make in this age period since shyness, diffidence and vagueness of expression are common in anxious
adolescents who are feeling unsure of themselves but are not psychotic.
It is important not to make a diagnosis of schizophrenia lightly, and
without positive evidence such as is set out in Chapter 6. Nevertheless, the condition's onset can be insidious and it may be necessary
to await developments while bearing the possibility of schizophrenia
in mind. Sometimes a period of observation in a hospital psychiatric
unit is helpful in making the distinction.

The commonest form of *affective disorder* is depression, which may be atypical in adolescence. Many adolescents with depressed mood are reacting in a way which can be understood in the light of stress which they face. Depression of psychotic intensity (that is with delusions or other disordered contact with reality) also occurs. The onset may be acute, in a boy or girl who has previously been well, and who may or may not be faced with any special family stress or other obvious difficulty; or it may be insidious. The presenting symptoms may not include obvious depression of mood; there may rather be anxiety (perhaps about going to school), panic attacks or somatic symptoms such as headaches or abdominal pain. Slowness of movement or thought may be evident. The presence of depression of mood may only emerge during conversation, in the course of which the adolescent may reveal that he has been or has felt like weeping, has wished he were dead, can get little or no pleasure out of life and may even have contemplated suicide or, perhaps, running away.

There may also be tiredness, irritability, poor concentration, difficulty in coping with school work which the subject could previously manage, sleep disturbance and poor appetite. Some of these symptoms may be confirmed by the parents who may describe the contrast between the patient's present listless, apathetic and unhappy self, and his normal more active, energetic and cheerful personality.

Manic-depressive, or bipolar affective, disorders are rare in early adolescence but become less so in late adolescence. Many cases are now on record with onset before age 16. Hassanyeh and Davison (1980) report 10 such cases, 5 boys and 5 girls, as well as reviewing earlier reports. They found that mania was easier to diagnose than depression, which was sometimes diagnosed retrospectively, though mild degrees of mania can easily be mistaken for manifestations of conduct disorder. This is especially so when restlessness, hostility and verbal abuse predominate. In addition to euphoria, irritability, hyperactivity, pressure of speech, flight of ideas, grandiosity, sleep disturbance and distractibility, the manic adolescent often hurled verbal abuse at parents and denied that anything was amiss, even in the face of wildly disturbed behaviour. In girls, sexually provocative behaviour, including wandering about the house naked, was common. The manic patients' hospital rooms were in a state of total disorder, which Hassanyeh and Davison termed the 'bomb-in-the-room' syndrome.

In their depressed phases these patients showed depressed mood, self-depreciation, agitation, sleep disturbance, diminished school performance, diminished socialisation, changed attitudes towards school, somatic complaints, lack of energy, loss of appetite and/or weight, suicidal ideation and psychomotor retardation. The first two items in each list had to be present, together with at least three (for mania) and two (for depression) of the others, for the relevant diagnosis to be made. Two of the depressed subjects presented in stupor and others showed severe psychomotor retardation — that is a slowing of thought processes and movements.

Suicidal Behaviour in Adolescence

Suicide rates in the 10- to 14-year age rates are low. In the USA in 1978 one child in 123 000 in this age bracket committed suicide, a rate of 0.81 per 100 000. Boys outnumbered girls by more than three to one and most of the deaths were in the 12–14 age range. The suicide rate in the 15- to 19-year age range was much higher at 7.64 per 100 000, representing a total of 1686 suicides. Boys outnumbered girls by more than four to one (Shaffer and Fisher, 1981).

The incidence of suicidal attempts is very much higher than that of completed suicides, but it is also much more difficult to estimate accurately. What is clear is that the sex ratio is reversed. 'Deliberate self-poisoning' has been found to be as much as nine times commoner in adolescent girls as in boys (Hawton et al., 1982). Of course, not all self-poisonings represent attempts at suicide: some are ways of expressing distress or of attempting to stimulate concern in adults or to achieve other changes in the environment. Despite this they may occasionally have a fatal outcome. The sex differences in adolescent suicidal behaviour, and other aspects of such behaviour, are discussed by Rosenthal (1981) whose paper appears in a volume of Adolescent Psychiatry (volume 9, 1981) which contains an interesting collection of articles on 'adolescent suicidology'.

The possibility of suicide should always be borne in mind when an adolescent presents with depressive symptoms. The risk is greater when the situation is the culmination of a period of depression, but it also varies with the severity of the depression. Suicidal behaviour is more likely the less communication there is with others; the isolated depressed child is very much at risk, especially when communication channels have recently broken down. Any previous history of attempted suicide is important in assessing a suicidal adolescent. A long history of self-destructive behaviour is particularly serious; and the more serious any previous attempts have been, the more the subject may now be at risk. Also important is how far an attempt at suicide has been intended as a means of communication and whether the communication has been heeded by those to whom it was directed. If there has been little impact on the environment, the risk of recurrence is greater. Most serious of all are attempts at suicide in isolation, especially when accompanied by a strong desire to die.

Treatment of Adolescents

Treatment is generally along lines similar to those used at other ages, but psychotherapy with adolescents can present special problems. In particular the tendency for adolescents to regard the adult generation in a hostile light, and to resent those in authority, can make establishing a working relationship difficult. It may indeed prevent the adolescent coming for treatment at all.

Treatment can be particularly difficult when the relationship between the adolescent and the parents is disturbed. Adolescents may give a totally different picture of their family situation, and of their relationships with their parents, from that given by the parents. They may deny that any problems exist, while the parents have a long list of complaints about them. In such instances family therapy can be helpful. The point of view of each party in any disagreements can then be stated while all are present, as a first step to examining the problem and trying to resolve it. Family therapy is valuable in a wide range of non-psychotic disorders of adolescence. Its value in psychotic conditions is less clear, despite its having been originally introduced in the USA for this purpose.

Haley (1980) has looked especially at the therapy of families containing adolescents who are attempting to become more independent of their families but are having difficulty with the processes. In the case of some of the more severely delinquent adolescents from highly disturbed families, residential treatment of the adolescent may be necessary before the whole family can be usefully engaged in therapy (Burquest, 1979).

Particularly difficult to treat are adolescents who have suffered prolonged and severe deprivation. Many of them have profound difficulty establishing trusting and intimate relationships with people; this limits the effectiveness of psychotherapy, and involvement in a living situation in which the subject can have the opportunity gradually to learn interpersonal skills may offer the best chance of overcoming the problem. This need may be met in a family receiving family therapy, or in a therapeutic group – often the living group in a residential treatment setting. Even then treatment is usually long, difficult and often unsuccessful. Some of these young people abuse drugs which can come to replace human relationships in their lives (Wieder and Kaplan, 1969).

Schizophrenia is a serious condition requiring specialist treatment, often initially in hospital. Phenothiazine drugs may be of benefit.

Depression also requires energetic and prompt treatment, but not necessarily in hospital unless there appears to be a danger of suicide. Antidepressant drugs are often effective. They should be combined with such other measures as the formulation of the case suggests are needed, for example psychotherapeutic support, and alleviation, where possible, of any reality stresses the patient faces, whether at home, school or elsewhere.

Manic-depressive disorders often respond well to treatment by lithium carbonate (Hassanyeh and Davison, 1980). This and other treatments are discussed further in Chapter 16.

Threats and attempts at suicide in adolescents should always be taken seriously. In many cases the suicidal adolescent is found to be isolated and to have problems of communication. The therapist must at once set about establishing communication with the subject (which can be difficult) while showing appropriate interest and concern. This approach should be combined with attempts to open up communication between the adolescent and the family and other significant people, as well as alleviation of any other stress which the subject faces.

Outcome

There is a strong association between antisocial behaviour in adolescence – and also in childhood – and similar behaviour in adult life. While most antisocial adults have shown antisocial behaviour earlier in life, the converse is not true, that is most antisocial young people do not become antisocial adults (Robins, 1978). In the case of neurotic disorders the outlook seems to be better. Most conditions in childhood and adolescence do not presage adult psychiatric disorder; severity seems to be a factor which determines whether they do. Much the same applies to depressive disorders; these often appear in adulthood for the first time (Rutter, 1980b). Psychotic conditions tend to persist into adult life.

In summary, much disturbed behaviour in adolescence does not persist into adult life. Much can usually be done to help, especially when the family as a whole actively seeks treatment. On the other hand, a disinterested family is a bad prognostic sign.

CHAPTER FOURTEEN

Psychological Tests

Psychological tests can add to the knowledge obtained at interview about children and their families. The results can help in assessing children's development and evaluating the results of treatment. The administration and interpretation of psychological tests is a part, though a small one, of the work of clinical and educational psychologists; but all who use the information obtained should know something about the tests and what they measure. The tests used with children include:

(a) Intelligence tests.
(b) Tests of educational attainment.
(c) Personality tests.
(d) Tests of specific psychological functions.

Intelligence Tests

Intelligence tests are designed to place children in order according to their ability to perform various tasks. They give an idea of the general ability of each child in relation to the whole population of the same age, and also provide information about how a child functions on particular types of task.

The *Wechsler Intelligence Scale for Children, Revised* (WISC-R) is probably the intelligence test most widely used for children in the clinical setting. It has separate verbal and performance sections, with sub-test scales as follows:

Verbal	Performance
General information	Picture completion
General comprehension	Picture arrangement
Arithmetic	Block design
Similarities	Object assembly
Vocabulary	Coding
(Digit span)	(Mazes)

The items in brackets are alternative tests, not usually used and correlating less well with the rest of the scale than the other sub-tests. While the names of the sub-tests give a general idea of the items concerned, the student should examine the actual test materials to discover precisely what their content is.

The test has been standardised on large populations of children so that the mean verbal, performance or full scale IQ at any age is 100. All the ten sub-tests have a mean (scaled) score of 10, though often there is a good deal of 'scatter', a child doing relatively better at one sub-test than another. The standard IQ deviation is 15, which means that about 66 per cent of children will have an IQ between 85 and 115. Two standard deviations (IQ 70–130) will cover about 95 per cent of the population, and three (55–145) will cover over 99 per cent.

The verbal and performance scores give an indication of the child's relative abilities in these two sorts of task and are often clinically more useful than the full scale IQ. The pattern of the sub-test scores can also give useful information, and the WISC-R is nowadays often used more as a diagnostic tool than as just an intelligence test. The child's responses can give the experienced clinician valuable information about thinking disorders, problems with impulsivity and learning difficulties.

The WISC-R is designed for use in the age range six to sixteen. Another scale, the *Wechsler Pre-School and Primary School Intelligence Scale* is used for children in the age range four to six-and-a-half. It is designed on principles similar to those used in the WISC-R.

Another widely used intelligence test is the *Stanford-Binet Intelligence Scale*. The latest (1960) version, known as form L-M, derives ultimately from the test devised by a Frenchman, Binet, in 1905. It covers the age range from two up to adult life. It includes a wide variety of tasks, but these vary at different ages and tend to be verbal rather than non-verbal. The result thus depends largely on the linguistic ability of the child, and for this reason the test is useful in relation to educational achievement and potential. It gives a 'mental age' as well as an IQ but the test gives less diagnostic information concerning the pattern of the child's abilities than does the WISC, and IQs at different ages are not strictly comparable.

The concept of mental age is used less than it was, but a child's IQ was originally conceived by Binet as the ratio between his mental age and his chronological age, expressed as a percentage. Thus an eight-year-old of exactly average ability would have an IQ of 100. If he functioned like an average seven-year-old, he would have an IQ of $7/8 \times 100$, that is about 88. If he had a mental age of nine-and-a-half his IQ would be $9.5/8 \times 100$, that is 119.

Raven's Progressive Matrices consist of a series of patterns or 'matrices', from each of which a part is missing. This test can be used for the age range six to thirteen. The child being tested is presented with a series of shapes and has to decide which one will complete the matrix. An advantage of this test is that the material is non-verbal; and the task can be demonstrated to deaf or aphasic children, and to non-English speaking children. It is also easily and quickly administered and scored. Although it is quite unlike either the WISC-R or the Stanford-Binet scale, its results correlate reasonably well with the results of these tests. It is a useful non-verbal reasoning test and is thought to reflect innate ability (rather than learned skills) better than most other tests. The test results are expressed as centile scores which can be divided into grades.

The *Peabody Picture Vocabulary Test* is widely used as an easily-administered test of verbal skills.

Several other tests for younger children exist. The *Merrill—Palmer Scale* covers the age range from eighteen months to six years. Allowance can be made, in scoring the test, for items refused or omitted and the test can be scored without the verbal items. The result can be expressed as a mental age, as a centile rank or as a standard score. The test is useful for obtaining a general estimate of a young child's abilities.

The *Griffiths Mental Development Scale* is designed for children in the first two years of life. It has five sections: locomotor, personal-social, hearing and speech, eye and hand, and performance. A mental age can be derived from the five sub-test scores. There is an extension available for use in the age range two to eight.

The *Bayley Infant Scales of Mental and Motor Development* were developed in America, and have also been standardised on British children. The test has separate scales for 'motor' and for 'mental' development, and gives a score for each.

The *Gesell Developmental Schedule* can be used to assess the development of pre-school normal children and of older mentally handicapped children. Four aspects of development are covered: motor, language, adaptive behaviour and personal-social. A developmental age is obtained and a developmental quotient (DQ) can be derived by using the formula:

$$DQ = \frac{\text{developmental age}}{\text{chronological age}} \times 100$$

The DQ is not equivalent to an IQ as obtained on tests like the WISC, since the nature and construction of the test is quite different. These tests are of value in giving a general estimate of the child's level of development, and of areas in which he is lagging or is developing precociously. The precise developmental ages, or DQs, are not of much significance, however, and correlations with IQs on tests for higher ages are low.

The Interpretation and Value of Intelligence Test Results
The IQ is sometimes misunderstood and over-rated. An IQ may get attached to a child as a sort of permanent label, and is quoted as part of his description. This is an abuse of the whole concept of intelligence testing. One is only entitled to say that on a certain date the child's IQ on a particular test was such and such. The psychologist's comments on the results should also be taken into account. These will usually say whether or not the child was disturbed or co-operative during testing and how reliable the results seem to be. Because of the misuse of IQ figures, psychologists nowadays tend not to quote numerical IQs, but either quote a range or give a verbal description (e.g. 'upper end of average range'). The child's approach to cognitive tasks of various kinds is generally considered more important than the test scores.

The question as to what intelligence tests measure is difficult to answer. Strictly speaking, they cannot be said to measure anything other than the ability to do the tasks of which the tests consist. Their practical value results from the correspondence between test ability and performance and the capacity to learn in school and to cope with verbal and manual tasks generally.

Tests of Educational Attainment

While intelligence tests indicate a child's general level of ability and expected achievement at school, they do not measure actual attainments. For this purpose a number of educational tests have been devised. The most important are those which test reading. Tests of arithmetic and spelling also exist.

Attainment tests consist of a series of tasks — word or sentence reading, or arithmetical tasks — of increasing difficulty. The tests are standardised on the general child population, just as are intelligence tests, and the child's performance can be compared with that of an average child of the same age. The results are usually expressed as reading, arithmetic or spelling ages. Quotients can then be obtained, if desired, by comparing, say, the child's reading age with the chronological age, just as an IQ can be obtained from a mental age (see previous section).

It is important to know, in interpreting attainment test results, the population on which the test has been standardised, and how much it differs from the population from which the child tested has come. Levels of attainment vary in different countries, and even in different parts of the same ones. They also differ from decade to decade.

Many different educational tests are available, and only a few examples will be mentioned. In Britain one of the most widely used reading tests is the *Neale Analysis of Reading Ability*. This consists of tests covering word recognition and comprehension, as well as various diagnostic measures, including sound production, auditory discrimination and syllable recognition. In North America the *Wide Range Achievement Test* is much used. As well as testing word recognition, it also assesses achievement in mathematics and spelling. It extends from the 4-year-old level to adult life. Other educational tests are the *Gates-MacGinitie Reading Tests*, which extend from the reading readiness level up to the level expected at about age 14, and the *Canadian Tests of Basic Skills*.

Arithmetic tests are less used nowadays because of the varied and changing methods of teaching arithmetic. Now that schools place less emphasis on mechanical arithmetic and use a more interesting approach to numbers and their relationships, it is usually better to obtain from the teacher a report on the child's progress. There is less emphasis, too, on spelling, and the use of spelling tests has declined accordingly.

Personality Tests

The assessment of personality is more difficult than the estimation of intelligence or educational attainment, and the extent to which tests are used for the purpose varies greatly from clinic to clinic and centre to centre. Many tests have been devised, and undoubtedly a child's response to them is related in some way to his personality characteristics and emotional state. The difficulty lies in interpreting and scoring the results and comparing them with the normal. It is easier to define average reading attainment or average intelligence than to define an average personality. Despite these problems, the results of personality tests can contribute significantly to clinical diagnosis.

Projective tests. The oldest and best known of these is the *Rorschach Test*. In this test the child (or adult) is asked to look at a number of printed shapes, originally derived from ink blots, and to say what they seem to resemble. The blots in themselves have no designed meaning, so any response the child produces must be a projection. Interpretation is difficult and special training and experience are considered necessary first. In Britain there are relatively few workers who are fully trained in the Rorschach test, and it is used more extensively in North America. The value of the test, even in the hands of those fully trained in its use, is disputed by many psychologists and psychiatrists, but equally its proponents consider it a useful diagnostic tool. The *Children's Apperception Test* (CAT) is probably more commonly used than the Rorschach. It consists of a number of somewhat ambiguous pictures about which the child is asked to tell a story.

The *Thematic Apperception Test* (TAT), although designed for adults, is used instead of, or as well as, the CAT by many clinicians. The TAT has more realistic pictures and also offers a wider variety of pictures and situations.

Two other widely used tests are the *Draw-a-Person Test* and the

House—Tree—Person Test. In each case the child is asked to draw the items mentioned in the name of the test. The results can be analysed qualitatively and quantitatively to give information about the child's personality and emotional state.

These tests, and similar ones, are not scientific instruments, and do not give scores as valid and reliable as, for example, those of educational attainment. Nevertheless, they can be useful ways of supplementing the clinical interview even if not scored, and may reveal information about the child, and his view of the family and the world generally, which may not emerge during an interview. The Rorschach and CAT, in particular, resemble techniques used by psychiatrists who may ask the child to make up a story, comment on a picture he or she has drawn, give three wishes, make up a dream and so on.

Two tests of 'social adjustment' are quite widely used. The *Vineland Social Maturity Scale* consists of a series of questions which are put to the child's mother, or to someone with a good knowledge of the child. It is concerned with such abilities as dressing, feeding oneself, walking and talking and is a useful and quick way of assessing the level of social development of infants and young children. The various sub-test scores (self-help generally, self-help dressing, self-help eating, self-direction, occupation, communication and locomotion) give a sort of clinical shorthand summary of the child's development. This test can also be used for older children, but for them a combination of clinical interview, IQ and attainment tests is often more useful.

The *Bristol Social Adjustment Guides* consist of questionnaires designed to examine the adjustment of children in school, in residential care and in the family. There are questionnaires for teachers, residential child care staff and social workers, and there are boy and girl versions. Examination of the completed questionnaires often reveals interesting and useful information about the subjects, but the value in clinical practice (as opposed to research, for which the guides have been much used) of the various scores which can be derived from the tests, is uncertain.

The *Bene—Anthony Family Relations Test* consists of a number of figures, representing the various members of the family and one representing 'nobody', each with a little box attached. The child is then asked to 'post' cards with various statements on into whichever box he considers appropriate. If the statement applies to no one in his family it goes into the 'nobody' box. The test is intended to give a picture of the child's view of emotional relationships in the family.

The *Children's Personality Questionnaire of Catell* is an example of a questionnaire-type test. The parent or other adult familiar with the child answers a series of questions. From the responses an estimate of the child's personality and emotional state is made. This test is not widely used.

Tests of Specific Psychological Functions

There are various tests which aim at measuring specific aspects of functioning, other than those which have been mentioned. A few of the more important ones only will be mentioned.

The *Illinois Test of Psycholinguistic Abilities* (ITPA) is a test of various aspects of language development, and it also gives a total language score. It aims to measure 'decoding', the capacity to decipher auditory and visual stimuli (that is, things heard and seen), and 'encoding', the transfer of ideas into speech and into motor functions. There are also tests of visual and auditory memory, of auditory—vocal and visual—motor association, and of auditory and visual closure. The 'closure' tests are designed to investigate the child's capacity to identify and select different auditory and visual stimuli as appropriate.

This test is a useful clinical and research tool for the investigation of disorders of language development. In cases of delayed development it gives an indication of the nature of the defect, and thus of the sort of treatment needed. It gives a test age for each of the sub-tests, as well as a total language age. The results can be expressed on the test form as a graph or profile which gives a pictorial impression of the child's language capacities and of how much variation there is among them. The test covers the range 2 years 4 months to 10 years 3 months.

The *Reynell Developmental Language Scales* comprise two scales measuring verbal comprehension and one measuring expressive language. The verbal comprehension test 'B' is intended to be parallel to test 'A' but requires minimal responses from the child and so is useful for cerebral palsied or very shy children. The test has been standardised on a large population of English children. There are separate norms for each sex, and an incidental point is that girls develop language (as assessed by this test) more quickly than boys. These scales are valuable clinical tools in the assessment of children with delayed language development.

The *Lincoln—Oseretsky Motor Development Scale* is a test of the motor ability of children. Some of the items involve hand and arm movements and others large body movements, for example jumping and balancing tasks. Norms are available and the test enables motor development to be assessed in relation to age and compared with intellectual development. The test is useful in investigating 'clumsy' children (see Chapter 9), and some children with brain disorder.

The *Bender Visual Motor Gestalt Test* involves the copying of a series of designs. The child's copies are then scored in a particular way. It has been suggested that the test can help establish a diagnosis of brain damage, but its practical value for this purpose is very limited. It merely provides a brief sample of the child's visual—motor abilities.

The *Berry Visual Motor Test* also involves copying figures, but has been better standardised on normal populations than the Bender Test, in place of which it is often used.

The *Frostig Test of Developmental Perception* is designed for use with children aged about four to ten years. It is a useful screening test for children suspected of needing special perceptual training. It deals with five important areas, namely eye—hand coordination, figure—ground perception, the ability to perceive 'constancy in shape' and 'position in space', and spatial relationships; it is linked to a series of training programmes. Both the tests and the training programmes can be administered individually or in a group setting.

General Points

This survey is far from complete but gives an idea of the range of behaviour which psychological tests try to measure. Tests should always be administered and interpreted by someone trained and experienced in their use, normally a clinical or educational psychologist, and their limitations, as well as their considerable usefulness, must always be borne in mind. This applies, perhaps with even greater force, to 'group tests'. These are often used in schools to measure educational attainment and 'intelligence'. A group of children, large or small, write answers to various questions and/or instructions on a form. The tests are often constructed on multiple choice lines, the subject being given a number of answers from which to choose. While these tests have obvious practical value, the results are less reliable than those of individual tests, and it is harder to detect the child who for one reason or another (perhaps illness, fatigue or hostility) is not co-operating. The results of group 'intelligence tests' sometimes differ greatly from those of individual tests; they also tend to be predominantly verbal tests, and so reflect the child's level of academic attainment. They are considered to have practical value in schools, however.

For further information on tests, various reference books are available (Johnson and Bommarito, 1971; Anastasi, 1976) and the test materials themselves may be examined.

CHAPTER FIFTEEN

Legal Aspects of Child Psychiatry and Problems of Child Abuse

All developed countries have found it necessary to have a framework of law to deal with children who offend against society in various ways, or who are neglected, inadequately cared for or physically abused by their parents or others. Psychiatrists and other professionals working in the mental health field are sometimes asked for help in such cases by courts and other statutory bodies, for example the 'children's hearings' established in Scotland, and also by social agencies concerned with child welfare. In Great Britain these include the social services departments of local authorities and various voluntary agencies. In North America this function is often carried out by state-funded child welfare agencies called Children's Aid Societies, Family Service Agencies and such like. Many children and adolescents referred for psychiatric assessment or treatment are already in the care of statutory agencies either because they have committed offences or because they have been inadequately cared for or have been abused.

It is necessary for professionals working in this field to have a sound knowledge of the relevant legislation. This varies according to the country, state or province concerned and there are so many differences that it is impossible even to summarise them in an intro-ductory book such as this. Moreover, changes are often made in child welfare legislation.

Two important aspects of the practice of child psychiatry and related disciplines are the writing of reports for use by courts and the assessment and treatment of families in which there has been, or may have been, abuse of a child by the parents or others. Expert advice and help is also sometimes sought in cases where there are disputes between separated or divorced parents about custody of or access to the children of the marriage. Referrals of this nature appear to be getting more frequent, probably because of rising divorce and family breakdown rates.

Writing Reports for Courts

While the form and content of court reports will differ according to local practice, the type of court concerned and the circumstances of the case, certain general principles are widely applicable. The assessment of these children and their families should be done in the same way as in other cases (see Chapter 3). It is important that the parents as well as the child are seen; this can present difficulties if the child is in custody, but it is important to have at least one face-to-face interview with everyone concerned. However good a report is, it can never be a substitute for an in-person meeting.

A school report is often available; if not, one should be obtained. It may be important to interview, either in person or by telephone, the child's teacher, or one of them. Reports should also be obtained from any other agencies that have been involved.

In writing the report the following general points are important:

1. Write in plain, readily understood English, without the use of jargon. Always remember that judges, magistrates and lawyers may not understand medical or psychological terms.
2. Bear in mind that your report may be read out in court or shown to the defence, so that the subject or the family may learn of its contents. If the report includes essential information which must not be disclosed in court (which is not, for example, the best place for a child to learn that he was born illegitimately or was adopted), this should be plainly marked 'confidential'.
3. Avoid referring to questions of guilt or innocence. These are for the court to decide.
4. Do not quote information given by the child, the family or others as if it were fact. It is better to use phrases like 'He said that . . .' or 'They described . . .'
5. Do not repeat information given in other reports, unless you have a special reason for doing so.
6. Make sure that your meaning is expressed plainly and unambiguously, avoiding vague terms and phrases like 'immature' or 'border-

line intelligence', both of which, if used at all, would require further definition. Rather than saying, 'He is immature' say, 'In his relationships with his parents and other family members he behaves more like a child five years younger'. Do not quote IQ figures; instead explain your view of the child's level of intellectual function and its significance in the particular case.

The precise form of the report is less important than ensuring that all the relevant information is included. A useful way of setting out reports is as in the following numbered paragraphs, each of which can be the subject of a paragraph or, in a long report, a section with its own sub-heading.

1. State the sources of information which you have used, including any reports (from school, social worker, etc.) you have read, as well as when, where and whom you interviewed.
2. Draw the court's attention to what you consider are the important points of the history you obtained and that presented in other reports.
3. Outline the results of your examination of the child, avoiding technical terms, but explaining in language a lay person will understand the nature and consequences of any psychiatric disorder which you found to be present.
4. Formulate the case in lay terms, so as to explain how, in your opinion, the behaviour or circumstances leading to the child's appearance in court have arisen. The formulation should take into account all relevant emotional, biological, social, educational and other factors.
5. Conclude with any recommendations for treatment, or other suggestions which you think may be helpful to the court in taking the best course of action.

Word the report in moderate terms. Avoid apportioning blame. Remember you are giving guidance to the court, not telling it what to do. Use short sentences and words as far as possible.

Most children seen for juvenile or family courts prove not to have any major psychiatric condition such as a psychotic illness. The psychiatrist's report, while useful to the court in ruling out such a condition, may mainly be of value in the understanding which it gives of the case as a whole.

The following specimen report illustrates one form which a report to a court may take.

Child Psychiatry Clinic
Endhampton District Hospital
Farr Road
Endhampton

Special Psychiatric Report on Andrew Barry Charles, born 1.1.70 [Address].
Charged with theft of bicycles, house-breaking.

I saw this boy on 31 December 1982. He was accompanied to the clinic by his parents and by Miss Harris, the social worker concerned with his case. I interviewed Andrew first, then saw his parents, following which I saw all three together for a short time; I then had a discussion with Miss Harris. In addition, I have read Miss Harris' social report dated 29 December 1982, the report prepared by Mr James, Andrew's school principal dated 20 December and that of the educational psychologist, Dr Keen, dated 18 December.

History
Miss Harris' report covers the points about Andrew's development and the family situation. I think the following matters are specially relevant.

1.   Andrew was born with a harelip and cleft palate, which caused feeding difficulties and repeated admissions to hospital during his first two years of life. Although these deformities were in due course surgically repaired, the Court will notice that there is still some slight disfigurement.
2.   Andrew's relationship to his mother seems never to have been a close one. The parents told me they feel this was due to his frequent admissions to hospital early in life, and they say he was never a 'cuddly' baby like their older son, Luke.
3.   There were difficulties of adjustment when Andrew first went to school, and he was late learning to read. His educational progress has always been poor and I note that the psychologist finds Andrew's reading to be about two-and-a-half years retarded, despite average intelligence.
4.   Adjustment in the secondary school at which Andrew started at the beginning of last term has been particularly poor. Andrew is said to have played truant repeatedly and the offences for which he is appearing in court were committed while truanting and in company with another child who was also playing truant.
5.   Andrew has been a life-long bedwetter.
6.   There have been difficulties in the relationship between the parents. Mr Charles left Mrs Charles 18 months ago to live with another woman, but returned 6 months later. Although Mr and Mrs Charles were able to

tell me about this, and say that the relationship between them has now improved, they also indicated that considerable tensions persist. Mrs Charles seems bitter about having been 'deserted for 6 months', as she puts it.

7.   Miss Harris reports that the neighbourhood in which Andrew lives is one in which there is a high level of delinquency.

Examination

I found Andrew to be a friendly, co-operative, pleasant boy. He was well dressed and seemed well cared for. I noted the scar and slight facial deformity mentioned above. He spoke freely and answered questions readily. Once he had settled down in the interview he gave a full and apparently frank account of his life, including his situation at school and at home. I detected no abnormality of his thought processes, nor was there any evidence of any abnormal mental processes (such as delusions or hallucinations). His mood was appropriate to the situation.

Andrew told me that he has never liked school, and in particular dislikes his present school which is 'too big' and where he feels he has been bullied and teased a lot. He denies, however, that he is teased about his facial appearance. He said he finds most subjects difficult, but enjoys woodwork and games. According to Andrew another boy he met on the way to school suggested that they stay off school, and it was also this boy's idea that they should steal the bicycles, which are the subject of one of the charges against Andrew. He was prepared to talk freely about the incidents which led to his appearance in court.

Andrew was also able to talk about the tensions in the home. He told me that he feels his parents favour his brother who has been more successful at school and has never got into any trouble with the police. Andrew is also sensitive about his bedwetting, a problem his brother does not have. He spoke about the period when his parents were separated and I got the impression that he would like to think of that as in the past, but is not completely confident that he can.

I found no abnormality on physical examination, except for the facial deformity I have mentioned.

Opinion

In my opinion Andrew is not suffering from a major psychiatric disorder, but there are psychological factors which may have contributed to his recent delinquent acts. He appears to be a boy with a poor self-image, not adequately secure in his family relationships and not getting much satisfaction from school. Family relationships generally do not seem to be warm, and Andrew appears to be the less favoured of the two children. He is seen by his parents as a less attractive child, and his congenital deformity, the subsequent periods in hospital, the difficulty in feeding him (his mother says he was always a sickly child) and his bedwetting have all probably militated against the development of a warm relationship between Andrew and his parents, especially his mother. In addition, there are tensions in the marital relationship, and the parents were separated for a time. A further problem is that Andrew has never settled well into school, nor obtained much personal satisfaction from it. Lacking fulfilment both at home and at school, it is not surprising that he has drifted into delinquent activities with other children with whom, perhaps, he can achieve more status.

Recommendations

The family as a whole need continuing help of the type Miss Harris has recently started to provide. Andrew's problems should be dealt with in the context of his home and family. I do not believe he would benefit from removal from the family at present, but I think a supervision order would be helpful. Miss Harris could then continue working with the family, as she tells me she would like to do. She could also, in consultation with the psychologist and school staff, look into how Andrew might be helped at school. If he can achieve greater success there it is likely to help his self-image.

I do not think that Andrew requires psychiatric treatment, but the family might benefit from family therapy. This would involve a series of treatment sessions involving the whole family. Miss Harris might like to consider this and discuss it with the family. If, in due course, the family wish to participate in a series of such interviews I should be glad to co-operate with the social worker in trying to arrange the treatment at this clinic. In any event Andrew will inevitably remain 'at risk' of getting into further trouble for some months after treatment starts.

A report should be no longer than is necessary to convey the information the court needs, but opinions and conclusions unsupported by an indication of the information on which they are based carry less weight than those which are so supported. The report should help the court to a better understanding of child and family as well as, if possible, offering advice on treatment or placement. It should be interesting and readable. An over-long report may be skimmed through, not read. Sometimes it is helpful, in discussing recommendations, to list various possible courses of action and then discuss the relative merits and disadvantages of each, perhaps without coming down firmly in favour of any particular one.

Further guidance on preparing reports for courts is to be found in a paper by Gibbens (1974).

Child Abuse

Child abuse is being recognised with increasing frequency. This is reflected in the more frequent referral of children, parents and families in which abuse is suspected to psychiatrists and their colleagues. Historical accounts suggest that child abuse has occurred for as long as records exist but it seems to have increased in frequency and severity with the onset of the industrial revolution. It is only fairly recently, however, that the frequency of violence towards children within families became appreciated. In 1946 Caffey, a radiologist, described cases of multiple fractures of the long bones in association with subdural haematoma in children. He suggested that the fractures were due to trauma, and it has subsequently become established that physically abused children often show X-ray evidence of old fractures.

In 1962 the term 'battered child syndrome' was coined (Kempe *et al*. 1962). Other terms used include 'child abuse' and 'non-accidental injury in children' (Scott, 1977). Kempe (1971) suggested that in the USA 6 children per 1000 suffer non-accidental injury annually, a total of 40 000 known cases, though rates certainly vary in different places.

A good epidemiological study was that of Baldwin and Oliver (1975). These authors investigated the extent of severe child abuse involving children aged under 5, in north-east Wiltshire, England, during a seven-year period. The last 1½ years of the period were studied prospectively, the rest retrospectively. Strict criteria for 'severe abuse' were used. A much higher rate of abuse – nearly 1 per thousand in the first three years of life – was found in the prospective study. This was 2.6 times the rate in the retrospective study. There were four deaths in the retrospective study and two in the prospective. Both studies probably underestimated the true incidence, and aimed only to cover severe cases. Overall, 225 separate incidents of abuse were recorded in 38 children, a mean of 5.9 per child, with a range of 1 to 23. Many injuries would of course have healed and so must have gone undetected. This valuable paper contains much other useful information on these children and their families.

The *causation* of child abuse is complex. Factors in the parents, factors in the child and social factors all play their parts. Many abusing parents are judged to have personality disorders; they often appear immature and many have been abused themselves in childhood. They frequently seem to have a poor 'internal model' of how to rear children and make quite excessive demands on their children in terms of the behaviour they expect at any particular age. Some abusing parents are depressed or otherwise mentally ill.

Factors in the child undoubtedly contribute too. Children's temperamental differences have been mentioned in Chapter 1. A child who cries a lot, is very active and has low biological rhythmicity and negative mood quality is likely to be more at risk for abuse than a child with easier temperamental attributes.

The quality of the parents' marriage, if there is one, is likely to be important too. The more mutually satisfying the relationship between husband and wife the less likely is the occurrence of child abuse. The wider social context is important too. Young inexperienced mothers are sometimes left to bring up children in states of social isolation, often in multistorey buildings with difficult or no access to play facilities, and cut off from the extended family. It is also usually possible to see these as dysfunctional families and to make a diagnosis in family system terms.

Gil (1975) suggests that there are three levels at which child abuse occurs. The first is the home, where the abusers are usually parents or permanent or temporary parent substitutes. The second is that of the institutional level: day care centres, schools, courts, child care agencies, welfare departments and correctional and other residential settings may abuse children by failing to provide them with the circumstances needed for their healthy development. The third level is that of society at large, which allows 'millions of children in our society' to live in poverty and to be denied adequate nutrition, health care, education, housing and neighbourhood conditions generally. This, however, is to take a wider view of child abuse than simply the physical injury of children.

Clinical features: Cases of child abuse present in many ways, but seldom do families come asking for help with the problem. Physically abused children are often brought to hospital emergency departments with a story that they have fallen downstairs or out of bed or against an item of furniture or household appliance. The tales told by parents can be detailed and imaginative, but they are usually inconsistent and nearly always incompatible with the child's injuries. Moreover, a full and careful examination of the child usually reveals evidence of previous injury and X-rays of the long bones and skull may show evidence of old fractures in various stages of healing. Cases of child abuse are sometimes reported to child welfare agencies by neighbours or relatives, who perhaps hear the child screaming or observe the injuries. Other cases come to notice at school, in day care centres or during routine physical examinations. The injuries may consist of bruising of any degree of severity, fractures, injury to internal organs, perhaps with internal bleeding, intracranial haemorrhage with consequent damage to the brain or loss of vision due to ocular injuries. Death occurs in from about 1 to 23 per cent of cases in various surveys reported (Scott, 1977).

In addition to the physical injuries, many abused children show evidence of being under-fed and otherwise neglected and ill-cared for. Medical attention may not be sought when needed. These factors can adversely affect development. On the other hand, some children who have been physically injured appear in other ways well cared for. It seems that in these cases satisfactory general physical care is interrupted by episodes of rage on the part of parent or other adult, during which injury is inflicted on the child.

Sometimes an off-hand, uncaring parental attitude, a failure to relate normally to the child and a lack of concern about the child's condition on the part of the parent are present. The parents may be reluctant to have the child admitted or investigated and may have been to many hospitals on different occasions. There are often other family and marital problems and alcohol or drug abuse. The parents may give a history of abuse or neglect when they were children.

Abused children tend to show difficulty in enjoying themselves, behavioural problems, low self-esteem, withdrawal, oppositional behaviour, hypervigilance, compulsive behaviour, a pseudo-adult manner and learning problems at school (Martin and Beezley, 1977). They may appear fearful towards their parents, for example getting upset when father is heard returning home, and they may show 'reversed caring' by anxiously looking out for the parent's needs, offering mother one of her cigarettes and so on. In severe cases of neglect the child may be obviously ill-cared for, dirty, under-nourished or dehydrated. Child abuse occurs in all socio-economic groups.

Assessment and *treatment* present great difficulties and require mature clinical judgement, extensive experience and a patient, painstaking and empathic approach to the families concerned. Thorough clinical and X-ray examination of the child is essential in any suspected case. Sexual molestation sometimes occurs as a feature of child abuse and the examination should include inspection of the genitals and anus (Sgroi, 1975).

Treatment is inevitably a multidisciplinary process, once child abuse is established. The relevant child welfare agency is responsible for the immediate welfare of the child and must decide whether to remove the child from the care of parents or guardians. Admission to hospital may be necessary, and paediatric or surgical treatment may be needed. Meanwhile investigation of the family is carried out, usually by a social worker from the child welfare agency. Psychiatric help is often sought at this stage, either for parents, for the child or for the whole family group. These families must be approached in a sympathetic, non-punitive way. It is best to tell the parent(s) about the child's injuries, making it clear that they are not compatible with the story given, but not demanding an admission or confession. The interview can then often proceed on the basis of an unspoken under-standing of the parents' part in the problem. It is unhelpful to get angry with people who abuse children; this militates against forming a therapeutic relationship and the therapist must control the feelings of outrage which most of us sometimes feel when dealing with these cases. It is also important not to get over-involved. Many child abusers are plausible, attractive, even charming people; or the therapist may come to feel sorry for them because of their hard or deprived lives. They may be expert at manipulating social agencies and auth-ority figures, for example by suggesting that their behaviour and attitudes are changing, and so flattering the therapist, when there has been no real change in the situation. The naive therapist can easily be deceived.

Long and difficult treatment is usually necessary. The treatment and management of the child must be integrated with help for the family. The return of the child to the family requires careful consider-ation, full assessment of the current situation, close supervision and detailed follow-up.

Since these are essentially family problems, treatment by family therapy has been suggested. While this is indeed helpful in some cases, the reported results, generally 'offer little optimism', as Kinard (1982) points out. This author favours the provision of psychiatric help for the parents, placement of abused children outside the home and psychiatric evaluation and treatment of the children – depending of course on the details of this case. He advances the view that separation of child and parents need not be harmful, depending on the child's environment following separation.

Some abused children have to be removed permanently from their families; others require prolonged treatment or substitute care to repair the emotional damage done prior to treatment.

The *outcome* of child abuse is grim. Scott's (1977) review indicated that permanent mental handicap, blindness and cerebral palsy may occur in surviving seriously injured children. Between 2 and 4 per cent of children in hospitals for the subnormal in Britain are said to be brain-damaged through assaults by parents. Lynch (1978) has also reviewed the prognosis of child abuse and lists as *sequelae* death, subsequent injury, permanent physical damage, growth failure, intellectual retardation and personality and behaviour problems. She emphasises the importance of comprehensive, thorough treatment of these children, not just 'crisis intervention'.

Prevention of child abuse is obviously much to be preferred to treatment. There is reason to believe that a preventive health service for young children and their families, with more frequent visits of nurse or other workers to such families is helpful (Wynn, 1974).

Vigilance by all professionals concerned with families containing children is essential. In all jurisdictions there are provisions for the compulsory reporting of suspected child abuse to the relevant authorities, and those with such suspicions should not hesitate to report them. In addition, the wider social problems of which gross child abuse is but an extreme example need to be tackled. Approaches to this are discussed in Chapter 17.

Many areas maintain a register of cases, or suspected cases, of child abuse. This can be helpful as these families often move frequently and consult a succession of hospitals, agencies and doctors.

Sexual Abuse and Incest

Sexual abuse is a special form of child abuse which merits separate consideration. It includes, but is not limited to, certain forms of incest, which is usually defined as sexual intercourse between persons so closely related that a legal marriage would not be possible. Thus it may occur between adults, between adults and children, and between children — indeed the commonest form is said to be between children. The most commonly reported variety is father (or stepfather)—daughter incest.

Child sexual abuse includes activities which fall short of intercourse by related persons and also the sexual exploitation of children by unrelated persons. It thus includes everything from forcible rape to such activities as fondling the breasts or genitals. While sexual abuse may be accompanied by physical violence, in many cases it is not.

The incidence of sexual offences against children is hard to assess but appears to be high. Sarafino (1979) estimated that there might be 74 725 reported cases in a one-year period in the USA. Clearly many cases go unreported, but how far the total nationwide estimate of 336 200 cases is accurate it is hard to know.

Parent—child incest usually occurs in very troubled families. There tend to be serious problems, including sexual ones, in the marital relationship, as well as personality disorders in the parents — especially those involved in the incestuous activities. Father—daughter incest often occurs when father and daughter feel abandoned by the mother. This may occur following childbirth or when the mother turns to another person (perhaps the grandmother or another man) or develops another interest. As the mother grows older and becomes less attractive as well as less involved, the father may turn to the young, sexually developing daughter who reminds him of the young, attractive wife he once married. The lonely and fearful daughter accepts the father's sexual advances as expressions of the affection she feels she needs, while the mother, by her non-involvement and lack of interest in what is going on, tacitly encourages the process.

Not all father—daughter incest cases follow this pattern. Sometimes incest is but one part of a pattern of gross family disorganisation. The term 'character-disordered family' has been applied to this type of family by Anderson and Shafer (1979). In such families there are also chemical dependency problems and a tendency to the use of physical violence. The term 'multiproblem family' is also used, but is perhaps too vague and general to be of much value.

Treatment in these cases should include both therapy for the family group and treatment of the individuals concerned. Hard data on the results of treatment are largely lacking, but the various approaches to the treatment of child victims — individual, group and family therapy — are discussed by Boatman et al. (1981).

Extra-familial child sexual abuse is a different issue. There is usually severe psychopathology in those committing such acts, highlighted in the occasional widely reported cases of individuals who sexually assault and murder whole series of children.

An excellent source of further information on incest is Meiselman's

(1978) book *Incest*. A briefer review has been provided by Rist (1979). It seems to be generally agreed that brother—sister incest is the least damaging variety. It often goes undetected and unreported and may have few or no adverse *sequelae*. Parent—child incest has more serious consequences, adversely affecting the psychosexual development of the children concerned. Sex is given a different meaning to girl victims (there are much less data on boys), much guilt and distress may result and the incest taboo may be subtly broken in succeeding generations. Cooper and Lormier (1982) have pointed out that incest may be intergenerationally transmitted.

Custody and Access Disputes

Psychiatrists and other mental health workers are sometimes asked for help in cases in which parents are in dispute about who should have custody of children, or about access to children in the custody of, usually, the other parent (Chamberlain and Awad, 1979). This situation may arise in relation to divorce proceedings, or simply when there is a separation, legal or otherwise. Sometimes disputes of this sort continue long after a divorce and seem to be a vicarious way in which the parents continue their relationship.

The assessment of these children and their families follows the same principles as apply in other cases (see Chapter 3), and reports can be written along the same general lines as described earlier. There are, however, some special problems. The psychiatrist or other professional is often retained and paid by one or other side. This can lead to a situation in which two expert witnesses, each having access to only one side of the story, make conflicting recommendations. This is not usually in the best interests of the children.

A better plan is for the psychiatrist or other professional to be retained by both parties, each of which contributes to the fee. Irving (1981) has described the process of 'family mediation', which consists of negotiation in an atmosphere of support and trust. The process starts with the establishment of an agreement among all concerned, including the lawyers for both parties, as to the terms of the mediation process. Irving describes three phases of the process: 'understanding through exploration', 'problem solving' and 'resolution'. The mediator must provide emotional support to all concerned, assist the parties in identifying the problem or problems, elicit enough factual information to find a solution to the problem, help develop and identify all possible alternative solutions, assist the parties in selecting one of the alternatives, develop an agreement on what steps are needed to ensure that the selected alternative is successful and, finally, follow up or monitor the implementation of the agreement.

The agreement made is put into writing and the lawyers use it as the basis for a settlement in court. This process is not possible, of course, if the parties are not willing to participate and it is not always successful. It often is, however, and it represents a way psychiatrists and their colleagues can be of help in such cases.

CHAPTER SIXTEEN

Treatment of Child Psychiatric Disorders

Since child psychiatric disorders are multifactorial in origin, a variety of treatment approaches may need to be used. These include:

Individual psychotherapy.
Help for the parents.
Family therapy.
Group therapy for children or parents.
Behaviour therapy.
Drug treatment.
Inpatient treatment.
Daypatient treatment.
Alternative families.
Educational measures.
Speech therapy.
Other measures, including removal from parental care.

Individual Psychotherapy

Many models of psychotherapy exist. An essential element of all is the relationship between the patient (or client) and therapist. Every contact between child and therapist is of emotional significance, and may be either of psychotherapeutic value or, if it is an unsatisfactory contact, antitherapeutic. Certain principles, therefore, need to be borne in mind when dealing with any emotionally disturbed child, whether or not psychotherapy is the specific treatment which is being employed.

1. Never criticise the child. Children must be accepted as they are. If a child's symptoms are the expression of repressed anxiety or hostility, disapproving attitudes in the therapist are likely to make the anxiety or hostility, and thus the symptoms, worse. Acceptance of children, however, does not imply approval of all they do. Indeed child and therapist will often agree on aspects of the child's behaviour that require to be changed.
2. Bear in mind that most children do not come for treatment of their own accord. They are brought by others, usually their parents, who are worried about them or angry with them. They may thus come for treatment with the expectation that they will meet someone who is also going to be anxious about or angry with them. Indeed some parents have, before coming for help, told the child to expect 'a good talking to'. In such cases the therapist often has to work hard to gain the child's confidence and it may take several interviews to do so.
3. Do not plunge straight into a discussion of the symptoms, unless these are raised by the child.
4. Instead, try to understand the child's feelings and point of view. It is only when there is this sort of understanding between child and therapist that free communication, such as is essential to successful treatment, becomes possible. The child should come to see the therapist as someone who is concerned to help. This will not prevent the expression of angry feelings, in fact when the child has strong aggressive feelings which need expression it will help this process.
5. Remember that limits have to be set, in a psychotherapeutic interview as in other situations. While the free expression of feelings is to be encouraged, there are naturally things the child cannot be permitted to do. These will include physically hurting the therapist and dangerous activities like playing in a hazardous way with live electrical fittings. There are also limits which must be set to the damage permitted to the fabric of the building, or its equipment. Limits should be imposed on the basis of 'I can't allow you to do that', but with an understanding of the child's desire to do it and explanation of the dangers of what is desired or the reasons why it cannot be allowed.

The techniques and application of psychotherapy can be learned only by working with disturbed children, and carrying out treatment, under supervision. Before embarking on psychotherapy it is necessary to have a clear aim, and to know what the treatment is intended to achieve. This aim should have been stated in the initial diagnostic formulation. *Supportive therapy* is aimed at helping the child to cope more easily with any current stress. The stress may be an acute one likely to subside in course of time, for example the illness or admission to hospital of a parent, or the grief reaction following a bereavement. Alternatively, the stress may be a continuing one which cannot easily be removed. The child may thus need long-term help in dealing with a difficult reality situation, for example a family disturbed in one way or another.

Quite different is *psychoanalysis*, which aims at achieving a radical change in the child's emotional state and reactions. Between supportive therapy and full psychoanalysis there is a range of intermediate possibilities, designed to achieve more limited goals than analysis, or to deal with particular facets of the child's emotional life. Psychoanalysis is a highly specialised treatment for which long and expert training is needed. It usually involves hour-long treatment sessions up to five days a week over a period of months or even years, so that even in clinics where trained psychoanalysts are available the number of children they can treat is strictly limited. The object of the treatment is to explore fully the child's unconscious life and fantasies, and deal with any problems found, in the context of the relationship between child and therapist. Anna Freud (1966, 1972) and Melanie Klein (1932) were pioneers in the field of child analysis.

Psychotherapy with children usually has more limited aims than those of psychoanalysis, which is perhaps more a research tool, and a means of developing theoretical understanding of emotional disorders, than a widely applicable treatment. Psychoanalysis has, however, contributed greatly to the practice of psychotherapy generally.

There are wide variations in technique, depending on the theoretical orientation of the therapist, the treatment goals and the patient's age. Some therapists make extensive use of verbal interpretation of the child's statements and play; others make little or even no use of interpretation. Some therapists take a more active and directive role than others.

As a rule, the younger the child, the more contact has to be made through the medium of play, but some children even as young as three or four do talk freely. How freely they communicate verbally depends on their intelligence, language development and emotional state. Common to all psychotherapy are, first, the development of a working relationship with the child; secondly, an appraisal of the feelings and ideas the child expresses in the context of the relationship; and thirdly the use of the relationship to help resolve the child's problems.

How does the treatment help the child? At the first level there is the simple process of acceptance of the child's feelings. We all know that we often feel better after we have spoken to an accepting and understanding person about things that are worrying us or which we are angry over or ashamed of. This applies also to the feelings of disturbed children. It accounts for the considerable improvement which sometimes follows a single interview, even one intended primarily as diagnostic. For some children it is a new experience to be listened to and given the full attention of an accepting adult; and when such children find that their revelations do not shock, worry or cause the therapist to feel outraged, this may reduce the intensity of their emotions.

Very often it is not sufficient for children simply to express their feelings and have them accepted by an adult with interest in and concern for their point of view. There also has to be emotional interchange with the child over a period of time. In these emotional transactions children often manifest behaviour and attitudes similar to those they manifest towards their parents, or other key figures. They can thus play or talk about their difficulties with the therapist, rather as young children work out things in fantasy play. This too may sometimes be sufficient to enable them to overcome their problems.

At the next level 'interpretation' is added to the emotional interchange with the child. This aims to put the problems or conflicts into words and thus help the child to understand them. Interpretations are generally withheld until the meaning of a child's play or talk is clear. Speculative interpretations which are incorrect may be harmful, though they are often ignored or rejected by the child.

The above methods of therapy are based principally on a 'psychodynamic' view of psychiatric disorders. With the possible exception of purely 'supportive' therapy, they all aim to resolve the child's problems, which are understood as being due to repressed conflicts (see Chapter 1), in the context of the child/therapist relationship. This is the essence of the methods of such therapists as Allen (1942) and Adams (1974). In recent years, however, a number of 'strategic' therapies have come into use. These can be used with individuals, groups and families.

Strategic therapies aim to change the subject's behaviour by other and various means. Cade (1980) has described the strategic approach as 'essentially pragmatic' and based on the belief that problems are maintained through the operation of repetitive behavioural sequences. Strategic methods include 'reframing', changing the sequences of behaviours, giving paradoxical directives and using therapeutic metaphors.

The term 'reframing' is given different meanings by different therapists, but in essence it refers to the process of giving a symptom, or a repetitive pattern of behaviour, a different meaning. Closely related is 'positive connotation'; by which a behaviour regarded by the subject, or by others related to or having contact with the subject, as problematic is labelled as a strength or as serving a useful purpose. Such re-labelling can often lead to the modification or abandonment of the behaviour (Barker, 1981a, 1981b).

A pioneer of the use of paradox was Frankl (1960), who used the term 'paradoxical intention' for his approach to problems which worsened as the patient struggled to counter the behaviour or feelings. He encouraged his patients to bring on or increase their symptoms, but often in a humorous context and always in a way which enabled the patient to distance himself or herself from the symptom. Remarkably rapid relief of symptoms can follow the use of such methods, which are discussed elsewhere (Barker, 1981b).

Therapeutic metaphors are stories related in some way to the subject's situation, leading to one or more suggested solutions or different ways of looking at the problems which have led to therapy. They are particularly suited for use with children who are generally receptive to fairy tales and other stories. The construction and use of therapeutic metaphors has been discussed by Gordon (1978).

Milton Erickson, a psychiatrist and hypnotist who employed many creative approaches in therapy, was a master of strategic therapy – though he did not so call it. His work has been described by Haley (1973). It has also been studied, along with that of other outstandingly effective therapists, by Bandler and Grinder (1979; Grinder and Bandler, 1981), who have developed 'neuro-linguistic programming' (NLP), a method of communicating with others designed to bring about change as effectively and economically as possible. The body of techniques and approaches to communication and therapy which makes up NLP offers the therapist many easily learnt ways of bringing about change in children and adults alike.

While space does not permit detailed discussion of any of the many therapy methods available, including the use of hypnosis, it is important to know that they exist. They are discussed further in the references mentioned, and training courses and supervision are also available and are necessary for the competent use of these methods.

Help for the Parents

Psychotherapy with the child is sometimes combined with help for the family. It is usually the parents who most need help, but there may be other family members – grandparents, uncles, aunts or siblings – who also require to be involved. Sometimes it is satisfactory for the same person to see both the parents (or other family members) and the child, but it is sometimes considered advantageous to have two different therapists involved.

Sussenwein (1976) has reviewed the methods used by social workers in working with families. She has identified the following: the provision of advice and material aid, the use of interaction in the interview, techniques designed to modify behaviour and the promotion of environmental changes.

These four methods of intervention cover the main needs which the parents of disturbed children may have. Some lack factual information about how to handle or bring up their children, and benefit from direct advice. Some also lack the knowledge, means or initiative to obtain material things required and can be helped to do this. Interviews provide opportunities for the release of feelings, for the clarification of issues in the client's mind, for encouragement and for promotion of increased understanding of the self. The relationship which develops between social worker and client can also provide a secure base in the client's emotional life and it can be a social and emotional learning experience.

Sometimes social workers and others who work with parents, use techniques based on learning theory. The essence of this approach is to identify the circumstances which precede or follow behaviour which is to be modified. Once this has been analysed the behaviour may be modified by altering these circumstances (see below).

The environmental changes which social workers promote may include mobilising community resources (play groups, day-care centres, youth groups and the like) and community workers (youth leaders, school counsellors, credit counsellors and so forth) to help the family as appropriate. Sometimes the environmental change may involve the family's relationship with neighbours or the extended family. Isolation of the nuclear family can be a very real problem.

These measures are not necessarily combined with the provision of psychotherapy for the child. They may be used along with any other form of treatment given to the identified disturbed child, or they may be the main or the only intervention in a particular case.

Family Therapy

The family therapist looks at the symptoms reported in the 'identified patient' as but one aspect of the functioning of the family as a whole. This is not to deny that individual children have their own problems for which they may require special help, but it aims to provide this help in the context of the family as a whole. (Of course if the sole problem is, for example, a child's reading difficulty, and in other respects the family is functioning well, no question arises of psychotherapy of any sort.) It is uncertain how often family therapy is the best approach, but some centres nowadays use it as their principal treatment method. It may be that these centres differentially attract referrals suitable for family therapy, other children being sent elsewhere. It is also the case that many children have no functional families and are in the care of child welfare agencies; but even in such instances a 'family' approach to problems may be possible, the child's substitute parents or family being involved in place of the natural family. Indeed a better name for family therapy is probably 'systems therapy', since the treatment may be applied to systems other than families. A brief account of systems theory appears in Chapter 2 and an outline of how to assess family groups is to be found in Chapter 3. Both topics are discussed more fully in the companion volume *Basic Family Therapy* (Barker, 1981a), which also discusses the different schools of family therapy and the wide range of therapeutic techniques used by family therapists.

Among the many family therapy approaches available, the 'structural' approach of Minuchin (1974; also Minuchin and Fishman, 1981) is a good one which is widely used. It starts with a 'structural' assessment of the family. The basic idea is that within a family unit members relate according to certain arrangements, which govern the transactions between them. These arrangements, which are not usually explicitly stated or even recognised, form a whole – the structure of the family. The family structure cannot be immediately assessed by the therapist, who can only discover it by joining the family.

'Joining' the family implies participating in its conversation and in its non-verbal communications. But first what Minuchin calls 'accommodation' is necessary. Accommodation consists of the adjustments the therapist must make in order to join the family. Initially the therapist accepts the family's organisation and way of doing things. Processes used in accommodation include 'maintenance', the deliberate supporting of the family's structure as when the dominant mother is treated as the leader or the subsystem pattern is accepted or even encouraged; 'tracking', the following by the therapist of the family's communications and behaviour which are encouraged to continue; and 'mimesis', the adoption by the therapist of some aspects of the family members' behaviour, for example their speed or style of speaking, or the sharing with them of some common experience.

Having joined the family the therapist becomes a participant-observer and can form a working hypothesis, or family diagnosis. This leads to a plan of intervention which tests the hypothesis. If the hypothesis is correct, and the interventions are well planned, change comes about. If not then it probably doesn't, and another hypothesis or intervention must be formulated. Change occurs as a result of the therapist's behaviour, including the directives and tasks given the family. The process can only be learnt on the job. It is best taught using one-way observation screens, closed circuit television and videotape. The learner can thus observe other therapists at work, as well as participating in and carrying out treatment under the supervision of a more experienced therapist. Particularly valuable are the opportunities videotapes provide for therapists to examine and discuss with others their recorded treatment sessions.

The following case history is quoted to illustrate, not teach, the process. Family therapy is discussed much more fully in *Basic Family Therapy*, in which can be found references to the extensive literature on the subject. All methods, however, involve altering the family's 'homeostasis', or fixed patterns of functioning, preferably in a way that will promote growth.

The Y family consisted of Mr Y, aged 49, Mrs Y, aged 44 and three children, Karen (15), Bruce (12) and Pamela (6). Pamela was referred because she was very 'insecure' (as her mother put it) and afraid of being alone and of the dark. She would not go to bed, or to the toilet, on her own. She was sleeping with her parents and she was a 'whining' child who, when she wanted something, usually persisted till she got it. Karen was reported by the parents to be rebellious and difficult, and to communicate little with her parents, while Bruce was well behaved and presented no problems. Mr Y was much preoccupied with the 'illness' for which he had been treated by two psychiatrists, and had had a period of inpatient care. His symptoms consisted of depression, feelings of inadequacy and severe obsessive– compulsive symptoms of three years' duration. He had troublesome check- ing rituals which made it difficult for him to carry out his job in a bank.

At the first family interview Mr Y spoke of how depressed and useless he felt. He said he had lost interest in life and was no longer part of the family. Mrs Y agreed and said she felt like a widow, depending for what support she got upon the two older children. She spoke in a calm, smiling, condescending way. Karen complained that she and Bruce were not allowed to settle differences and have a relationship between themselves, because of interference by the parents. Mrs Y said she felt she had to intervene because otherwise Karen would 'kill' Bruce. Bruce, a big boy for his age, said he thought Karen and he could settle their differences on their own, but he didn't seem too concerned about the matter. Karen went on to complain of many restrictions the parents placed on her activities and of the way the family is 'ruled by the clock'. She said she was very unhappy, wanted to leave the family to live on her own as soon as she could and felt Bruce was favoured at her expense. Bruce agreed about the latter point. Pamela said little, and soon left the family circle to play on her own else- where in the room.

All members of the family saw Mr Y as useless and ineffectual, but Mrs Y and Karen were particularly forthright in saying this, and Karen asked why her father couldn't 'make an effort' as she had done recently when she returned to school after having influenza.

At the second session Karen complained bitterly of feeling left out of things in the family. She resented the fact that Bruce, as she saw it, was treated as more grown up than she was and she described Pamela as a 'menace' who always got her way either by making a nuisance of herself or by 'sucking up' to mother.

At this time the family structure seemed to be as follows:

Mr Y was on his own, far apart from the rest of the family.

Mrs Y was close to, and related warmly with, Bruce and Pamela (though she was irritated by Pamela's behaviour).

Karen was closer to her mother than to her father, but all her relationships in the family were characterised by much hostility.

Mr and Mrs Y did not operate as a parental couple, each independently stating his or her opinion on whatever was discussed, but never talking to each other or coming to a mutual agreement.

The aim of treatment at this stage was to establish the parents as an effective couple caring for the children in a united and appropriate fashion.

The closeness of Mrs Y and Bruce became increasingly obvious and it soon transpired that Mrs Y washed the hair and cleaned the shoes of this pubertal 12-year-old. She also turned to him for help in the house, for example to do odd jobs. Mr Y was considered by all to be 'too ill' to do these, and there had accumulated a long list of tasks too big for Bruce which, to Mrs Y's ire, had simply not been done. The therapist initiated a discussion of these jobs, asking Mr Y what they consisted of, how long each would take and which were the most urgent. With Mrs Y participating, an agreement was reached that Mr Y would carry out one of them (the repair of a kitchen shelf) by the next session. At the same session the question of whether Bruce could wash his own hair and brush his own shoes was discussed. Both parents, and indeed the whole family including Bruce, agreed that he could and should. Thus both parents had tasks to perform by the time of the next session, father to do a minor household repair, mother to allow her 12-year-old to do more for himself.

Having joined the family group and formed an opinion about the family structure, the therapist was trying to restructure the family through his interventions. He did not accept the father's uselessness. He looked for the positive aspects in all members' roles in the family, reinforcing and supporting them. Through his interventions he was able to help the family demonstrate, for example, that Mr Y could still repair shelves; Mrs Y did not have to wash Bruce's hair since Bruce was well able to do this himself; Karen was capable of going to watch an evening football match involving the team she supported without any harm coming to her (which the parents had not believed); and Pamela (who had been subjected to little discipline and much indulgence) could do as she was told. Moreover, as such demands were made on Pamela it became easier to get her to bed at night.

Throughout the twelve sessions of treatment with this family, the therapist tried to treat Mr and Mrs Y as a parental couple when discussing any matters concerning the children. If one expressed a view about any of the children (and initially it was usually the mother), the opinion of the other was sought. On many occasions the parents were encouraged to discuss matters together there and then, or occasionally between interviews, so that they could bring their joint decision to the next session, and an agreement was reached. The children too were encouraged to discuss things together, and by this means the many differences between Karen and Bruce were reduced. In fact Karen and Bruce proved to have a warmer relationship than had at first been apparent, and the ease with which many of their differences were settled surprised everyone.

As is almost invariable in such treatment, the family tended to resist change. In the early stages Mr Y complained of the 'tension' he felt and at the end of most sessions he asked for tranquillisers. During one two-week break between sessions he even consulted another psychiatrist (who agreed, in discussion with the therapist, not to offer treatment). Thus many of the changes in the family were followed by a tendency to resort to former transactional patterns. The therapist's response was to emphasise the positive aspects of the family's functioning and to maintain an optimistic, good-humoured attitude. It even became clear that Mr Y's role in the family had not been quite as negative as the whole family had indicated: for example, he had always helped Pamela with her schoolwork when she needed this.

Comment

The above is but an outline of the sort of thing that may happen in family therapy. The main point is that it was the family that was taken as the unit for treatment, which was concerned with the 'here-and-now' functioning of the family. Therapy aimed to alter the family functioning rather than to look at, or treat, any member of the family as an individual. Although the family came with Pamela as the presenting problem, they were quickly able to see that her symptoms were but part of a wider family problem. (Not every family is able to see this so readily, even when it is clear to the therapist.) In the course of twelve family therapy sessions, considerable changes in family functioning occurred, with a more equal relationship developing between husband and wife, and a happier one between the parental couple on the one hand, and the children on the other. There were still stresses in the marital relationship, however, and Mr Y's obsessive–compulsive disorder, while less troublesome, was still evident. The children's symptoms had greatly improved and all three seemed a good deal more content than they had been before.

Group Therapy

Children, adolescents or parents may be treated in groups (Ginott,

1961; Yalom, 1975). As with individual therapy, there are a variety of approaches to group therapy, but the basic idea is that members of the group help each other through their interaction and the modelling they can provide for each other. Thus the active, outgoing child can act as a model for the quiet, inhibited one, and vice versa. Group therapy may be particularly valuable for children who have difficulty with peer relationships.

Group therapy with younger children usually involves primarily the use of play, while with adolescents discussion is more usual, with the problems of the individual group members often being dealt with directly. In all forms of group therapy the therapist leading the group has an important role in facilitating constructive and helpful interchange between group members.

Parent groups can sometimes achieve many of the aims of individual casework with parents, both more effectively and more economically. The focus of the group is usually on matters concerned with problem children and their management. Variable amounts of instruction may be given by the leader, but an important part of the process is the interaction between the parents, and their group problem-solving. It can also be helpful to a parent to know that he or she is not the only one with a difficult child or with problems in child management. Philipp (1979) has provided an excellent account of the conduct of parent training groups. The emphasis is on finding solutions, rather than apportioning blame or elucidating causes, and social learning theory principles and behaviour modification techniques can be useful in this (see below).

Behaviour Therapy

Behaviour therapy seeks to use learning theory as the basis for altering children's behaviour and modifying or removing symptoms. It aims to achieve precise therapeutic goals, either the elimination of symptoms (for instance bedwetting, temper tantrums or obsessive—compulsive symptoms) or the development of behaviour regarded as desirable (such as attendance at school in the child who has difficulty in going, or various social skills). Behaviour therapists do not seek to interpret the behaviour they modify, nor to promote insight into the dynamics of the problem. Indeed, many behaviour therapists question both the value of interpretation, and the psychodynamic view of children's disorders. They take the view that problem behaviours are learned and can be eliminated and replaced by other behaviours through the provision of new learning experiences. Regardless of what theories are accepted, however, it is clear that behaviour modification is of value in certain conditions. It is perhaps not surprising that more models than one are applicable to the understanding and treatment of the wide range of psychiatric disorders of children.

Behaviour therapy can either alter the circumstances leading up to a behaviour or the circumstances following it. The first approach is known as 'respondent conditioning'. The second as 'operant conditioning'. In either case individual or group treatment may be used. An example of respondent conditioning is 'systematic desensitisation'.

Quentin was seen at the age of twelve. When he was seven he had seen the film *Born Free* and became frightened, and nearly fainted, when a snake was shown on the screen. But the fear of snakes seemed to have developed slowly before that, and had been evident during earlier visits to a zoo.

When seen, Quentin was handicapped in that he could not go to a zoo, into a pet shop (in case there was a snake there) or a toy shop (where there might be a rubber snake), watch animal programmes on television (lest a snake was shown) or go near the biology laboratory at school (in case there was a snake in it). All pictures of snakes had had to be removed from his biology books. There was also some fear of large worms, eels, frogs and lizards, probably generalised from his fear of snakes. Otherwise Quentin and his family appeared emotionally stable and there were no other problems.

Quentin was treated by systematic desensitisation. After training in relaxation he was asked to imagine snakes, then later shown black-and-white pictures, all in a controlled, graded fashion, in the context of relaxation exercises. Eventually he progressed to a large model of a snake and finally a visit to a zoo where he was able to enter the reptile house and view each snake for a satisfactory period of time. By the end of treatment he had become an expert on snakes, and showed eagerness to read magazine articles on them. At follow-up 2½ years after the end of treatment Quentin remained symptom-free.

In this treatment the child is first taught to relax muscle tension, prior to presentation of the phobic stimulus. After relaxation has been achieved the phobic object is presented in mild form, perhaps as a small, uncoloured picture, or even by asking the child to imagine it. There is then a gradual, planned increase in the intensity of the stimulus, the rate of increase being such as to enable the child to maintain his relaxed state. This treatment is usually successful for specific phobias, but results are less good when there is generalised anxiety.

Operant conditioning is the planned modification of behaviour through manipulation of the consequences which are seen to control the behaviour. If every time a boy touches something hot he receives a painful burn he will soon stop that behaviour; and if every time he has a temper tantrum he is given what he wants by his parents he will soon be using tantrums as a means of getting things. The behaviour of all of us is affected in this way; if every time we pass a door we try it and find it locked, we will soon stop trying the door. In behaviour therapists' terms the behaviour has been 'extinguished' by 'non-reinforcement'.

Operant methods include the planned positive reinforcement of desired behaviour, negative reinforcement of undesired behaviour and extinction of behaviour by providing no response to it. Positive reinforcers may be material items (e.g. candies), or they may be social (words of praise and a smile). In some settings token economy systems have been found useful. The children acquire tokens for certain behaviours, and in some systems lose them for others, and the tokens are later redeemable for material rewards such as money or for privileges or status. This sort of programme is used in some residential and day treatment centres, and has also been used successfully in schools, group homes and other settings. This method, like many of the forms of behaviour therapy, lends itself very well to the treatment of groups of children (Wagner and Breitmeyer, 1975; Hoefler and Bornstein, 1975).

Behaviour therapy, usually using operant methods, has been used for obsessive—compulsive behaviour, anorexia nervosa, temper tantrums, aggressive behaviour, delinquent behaviour, language disorders, enuresis and many other problems. In the treatment of obsessive—compulsive rituals (see Chapter 5) 'response prevention', the active restriction of the rituals, seems to be the most satisfactory method. If the rituals are consistently prevented, the urge to carry them out has been found to disappear (Stanley, 1980). The use of the pad and buzzer in enuresis is described in Chapter 7. Behaviour therapy techniques now have an assured place in child psychiatry. They continue to be developed and there appears to be a trend towards locating treatment in the child's environment (home, school, hospital ward,

—

treatment centre), rather than in the therapist's office. Many more detailed accounts of this treatment approach are available (Patterson, 1975; O'Leary and O'Leary, 1977).

Drug Treatment

Drugs have only limited usefulness in child psychiatry. The main indications for their use are in the control of epilepsy, and in the treatment of hyperactive children, certain depressed children and, possibly, some neurotically anxious children and children with particular behaviour problems.

Anticonvulsant drugs should always be prescribed for children having epileptic fits, and they are normally continued at least until the child has been free of fits for two years. While phenobarbitone is often effective in controlling fits, especially major ones, it can make behaviour disorders worse, or may even create them (in the form of aggressiveness, overactivity, poor concentration and generally difficult behaviour) where they did not previously exist. It is therefore best avoided where there is any question of associated psychiatric or behaviour disorder. Many other effective anticonvulsant drugs are available nowadays. For details, dosage and side-effects the reader should consult a text book of paediatrics or paediatric neurology.

In the treatment of hyperkinetic children, epilepsy, if present should first be controlled. This may be followed by a reduction of the hyperactivity. In most cases, however, there is no evidence of epilepsy and the choice of drugs lies between a stimulant drug, a phenothiazine such as chlorpromazine, and haloperidol. There is evidence that all these drugs are effective in reducing hyperactivity (Cantwell, 1977). The stimulant drug mainly used at present is melthylphenidate, but the chemically related amphetamine drugs are also effective. Methylphenidate has an unusually short half-life (the time taken for the blood level of the drug to be reduced by half) of two to three hours (Gualtieri et al., 1982). This means that doses have to be given every two to three hours to maintain therapeutic effect. When the drug is used for children whose hyperactivity is causing problems in school doses half-an-hour or so before starting school, and again at about mid-day usually prove the most effective regimen. The drug need not be given on days when the child is not attending school, unless there is a need to control the hyperactivity in other situations. Although these drugs are stimulants in adults, they have a paradoxical effect in children. Many phenothiazines have been used, particularly chlorpromazine and thioridazine, but it is generally agreed that they adversely affect learning and cognitive functioning. Haloperidol is of value particularly with certain target symptoms — excess motor activity, restlessness and aggressive and impulsive behaviour (Barker, 1975). These drugs may be given along with anticonvulsants in epileptic children whose behaviour remains hyperactive even after control of the epilepsy is achieved.

In other behaviour disorders, including some of those associated with brain damage, drug treatment may help, but only as a part of a wider treatment programme which takes into account the child's motor, perceptual, social and educational status. Phenothiazine drugs such as chlorpromazine, fluphenazine, perphenazine or thioridazine may help reduce symptoms, especially on a short-term basis; so also may haloperidol (see Table 4).

Drugs are of limited value in neurotic disorders, but temporary relief from acute and severe anxiety may be provided by such 'anxiolytics' as diazepam, chlordiazepoxide and perphenazine. Drugs should not be a substitute for a psychotherapeutic approach designed to help children in the context of their families and wider life situations. They may, however, occasionally help by controlling anxiety in the short term while other measures are being instituted.

Table 4 shows the doses and main side-effects of the various drugs which have been mentioned above. In all cases dosage should be adjusted individually with the aim of obtaining the response sought without serious side-effects. Children generally require higher weight-related doses than adults. Children below about age 4 (though these seldom require the drugs under discussion) tend to need 1.25 to 1.5 times those required by older children, though response is very variable. The estimation of blood levels is therefore helpful and is increasingly becoming available in clinical practice.

The question of the use of tricylic antidepressants such as imipramine and amitriptyline has been discussed in Chapter 6. Since depression in children is often reactive to severe environmental stress, a main therapeutic aim should be to reduce the stress, or to support the child in coping with it. Despite an increasing number of research studies which have been carried out in recent years (Puig-Antich, 1980), precisely when antidepressent drugs should be used remains uncertain. The view is gaining ground, however, that they should be

TABLE 4: DRUG DOSES AND SIDE-EFFECTS

Drug	Dose	Adverse effects
Phenothiazine drugs		
chlorpromazine thioridazine	1−3 mg/kg/24 h (night sedative dose up to 3 mg/kg/24 h)	Drowsiness Muscular rigidity and spasms Tremor Jaundice Precipitation of epilepsy Blood dyscrasias
fluphenazine	0.5−0.25 mg/kg/24 h	Urinary retention and incon- tinence
perphenazine	0.15−0.30 mg/kg/24 h	Skin rashes (chlorpromzaine may cause photosensitive skin rash)
Haloperidol	0.025−0.5 mg/kg/24 h	Painful muscle spasms Muscular rigidity and tremor Drowsiness Depression
Other drugs for hyperkinetic children		
dexamphetamine	0.25−0.5 mg/kg/24 h	Excitement Sleeplessness Loss of appetite Failure to gain weight and height Palpitations
methylphenidate	0.2−0.7 mg/kg/24 h	Headache Abdominal cramps Drug dependence (not usually a problem in hyperactive children)
Benzodiazepine compounds (dosage for over-fives)		
chlordiazepoxide	5−10 mg two or three times daily	Drowsiness Skin rashes
diazepam	2−5 mg two or three times daily	Muscle tenderness or weak- ness

Note: The muscle spasms and tremor which may be caused by phenothiazines and haloperidol can be prevented by simultaneous administration of an anti-Parkinsonian drug, e.g. benzhexol 1−5 mg twice daily.

seriously considered in the presence of 'major depressive disorder' as defined in DSM−III. This is especially true in the case of adolescents.

Table 5 indicates the doses of tricyclic antidepressants which may be useful in the age range five to twelve. Over about twelve, adult doses may be given. Doses at the lower end of the ranges mentioned should be given at first, with subsequent gradual increases every three days or so until a satisfactory response is obtained, adverse effects appear or the maximum recommended dose is reached.

Because of the danger of adverse cardiac reactions great caution should be exercised in using tricyclic drugs in children. Blood levels can vary widely with the same weight-related dose. Treatment should therefore be monitored by regular electrocardiographs and, probably, the estimation of plasma levels of the drug, which can now be measured in many centres. It seems that a plasma level of imipramine and desmethylimipramine (an active metabolite of imipramine) between 150 and 250 ng/litre should be sought. The subject is discussed further by Puig-Antich (1980, 1981).

The prescription of tricyclic drugs requires special caution also because of the danger of overdoses, either accidental or with suicidal intent. It is unwise to prescribe it for disorganised families or when there may be access to the tablets by someone presenting a suicidal risk.

TABLE 5: DOSES AND SIDE-EFFECTS OF TRICYCLIC DRUGS

Drug	Dose	Adverse effects
Imipramine Amitriptyline	1.5 to 5 mg/kg/day in 3 doses	Arrhythmias, blood pressure variations and other cardiac disorders Dry mouth Difficulty with visual accommodation
In enuresis		Tremor
Imipramine Amitriptyline	10–50 mg at bedtime	Precipitation of fits (in epileptics) Jaundice and blood disorders (both rare) Psychosis Amitriptyline may cause drowsiness

In nocturnal enuresis the administration of imipramine or amitriptyline at bedtime has been shown in controlled trials to reduce the frequency of wetting, but the effect tends to be short-lived, subsequent relapse being common.

In manic-depressive, or bipolar affective disorders lithium carbonate is often valuable. Given in a dosage which maintains a serum level of 0.8–1.2 milliequivalents/litre, it leads to a reduction or cessation of the attacks of mania and depression in many cases – perhaps about 80 per cent (Hassanyeh and Davison, 1980; Youngerman and Canino, 1978). The dose required may vary from 600 to 1200 mg or more per day, and is determined on the basis of frequent estimations of the serum lithium level. Adverse effects include tremor, confusion, drowsiness, abnormalities of cardiac function, nausea, vomiting and diarrhoea. Careful monitoring of the functioning of the heart, kidneys and thyroid is advisable, especially in children and adolescents.

Drugs do not appear to alter the course of infantile psychosis, but are sometimes useful in dealing with specific symptoms like hyperkinetic behaviour or sleeplessness. Older children with psychotic conditions resembling adult-type schizophrenia may be helped by phenothiazine drugs such as those listed in Table 4. Long-term maintenance therapy may lead to prolonged remission of symptoms, but on the whole children with late-onset psychosis of childhood seem to respond less well than adults with schizophrenia. Here again, however, there is a lack of satisfactory evidence from properly controlled trials.

TABLE 6: HYPNOTIC DRUGS: DOSES AND SIDE-EFFECTS

Drug	Dose	Adverse effects
Chloral Dichloralphenazone Triclofos	20–50 mg/kg/24 h Maximum dose 1 g	Nausea Vomiting
Promethazine	15–30 mg (in age range five–twelve)	Dizziness Lack of co-ordination Blurred vision Blood disorders (rare)

Sleeplessness may occasionally merit treatment with drugs, though toddlers who do not sleep can be difficult to sedate effectively. Table 6 shows the dose ranges for some hypnotics which may be used to induce sleep in children. Chloral and the following two compounds are closely related substances with very similar effects. If they are proved ineffective, chlorpromazine or thioridazine (see Table 4) can be useful, especially in young children, or promethazine may be tried.

Recent years have seen the development of a large, and sometimes confusing, literature on drug treatment in child psychiatry. Good recent reviews are those of Wiener (1977) and Werry (1982).

Inpatient Treatment

Children are admitted for residential treatment either because of behaviour so severely disturbed as to make treatment or even care elsewhere difficult or impossible, or because it is thought that removal of the child for a limited period from the home environment to one designed to provide a more helpful living and treatment situation will be beneficial. With increased emphasis on the role of the family and the use of family therapy, it seems that inpatient treatment is tending to be used in a more focussed and briefer way, with specific therapeutic aims; it is more often an episode in a wider and longer-term plan of treatment (Barker, 1983).

Examples of severe disturbance necessitating admission are extremely aggressive or hyperactive behaviour, serious depression with perhaps suicidal ideas, very bizarre and withdrawn psychotic behaviour and severe anorexia nervosa. Admission can also be of benefit in some neurotic disorders, for example severe school refusal.

Adverse environmental circumstances which may make it desirable to admit children for treatment include unstable homes with much marital disharmony, severe parental rejection of the child, gross overprotection and certain conditions of emotional deprivation. (These circumstances are often faced also by children admitted because of the severity of their disturbance.) Admission is indicated where it seems likely, or at least possible, that more can be done to alter the adverse environment while the child is having treatment in hospital than would be the case if he or she stayed at home for treatment. It is sometimes easier to help the family, and change the parents' attitudes for the better, while they are relieved of the constant irritant of the child's disturbed behaviour. The child who has received residential treatment at the same time may in due course be reintroduced to the family in a less disturbed state. Treatment may then continue on a daypatient or outpatient basis.

Admission must always be considered in the light of the family situation or the situation in the group home, foster home or wherever the child is living. Requests for admission are sometimes disguised attempts by parents or others to get rid of an unwanted child. Sometimes the request is a symptom of the 'scapegoating' of a child, and the right course is to treat the family as a group, to try and understand why this is and help the family to change. In such circumstances it may strengthen the family's disturbed way of functioning to collude with it by admitting the child.

An essential feature of the treatment provided for children in psychiatric inpatient units is the general emotional environment in which the children live. This may be supplemented by, and indeed is in part made up of, such other treatments as recreational and occupational therapy, educational help, administration of drugs and behaviour therapy. While all these things can be provided on an outpatient basis, inpatient care also provides for the child a living environment which can be altered to suit his particular psychological needs.

Most inpatient units are staffed by nurses and/or child care workers. These 'front line' staff are usually part of a larger treatment team including other professionals – psychiatrists, psychologists, social workers, perhaps occupational therapists and non-medical psychotherapists. An emotionally warm, relaxed atmosphere is needed; however disturbed and difficult the child's behaviour it should not be met by angry or rejecting attitudes on the part of the staff. Yet, as in individual psychotherapy, limits have to be set. The point is that the child's present clinical state and behaviour are accepted, while work proceeds to bring about the required changes in behaviour. It is to help achieve this that the staff are working with not against the child.

One approach to change, apparently useful in residential treatment as well as in other therapeutic situations, is 'positive peer culture' (Vorrath and Brendthro, 1976). This seeks to help individuals by creating a culture in which they help others. The emphasis is thus not on what is being done to the subject, but on what members of the group, or the group as a whole, can do for others.

The treatment needs of the different children in a hospital unit vary. The psychotic child who tends to withdraw must be brought into contact with people by any means available. Immature, over-dependent neurotic children must be given progressively more scope and encouragement to stand on their own emotionally, and cope with relationships with others without constantly requiring support from parents or the staff. Such children will need a steadily decreasing amount of non-anxious support as they improve. Children with severe conduct disorders require calm, consistent, accepting limit-setting. Such children often behave conformingly for the first few days, or even weeks. Once they begin to feel more sure of themselves in their new situation their aggressiveness, destructiveness and negativism emerge. Unconsciously they expect this to be met by hostility and rejection such as they have probably experienced at home and elsewhere. Indeed, their admission may be seen by them as a manifestation of rejection. Such children benefit from firm limit-setting (which may involve physically restraining them from damaging other people or property), while they themselves are nevertheless subject to warm attitudes of acceptance.

Inpatient units have a useful diagnostic function. In cases of particular difficulty, a period of observation while the child is resident may clarify the diagnosis. The assessment of psychotic children is sometimes made easier by inpatient observation; so also is the estimation of the relative importance of an adverse home environment in various other conditions.

Admission to a psychiatric unit is usually best avoided if the child has no home or a home so grossly disturbed or unsatisfactory as to be quite unsuitable. Such children, if admitted, tend to become over-dependent upon, and attached to, the unit with consequent emotional trauma and feelings of rejection when they are discharged. Children without homes in which they can live should first be found substitute homes, usually in conjunction with the appropriate child welfare agency. In such cases close co-operation with the child welfare agency is necessary, and some treatment centres have set up arrangements whereby specially selected, trained and supported foster parents provide homes for children during, and often following, inpatient treatment (Barker *et al.*, 1978).

Residential treatment is discussed more fully in the books *The Residential Psychiatric Treatment of Children* (Barker, 1974) and *Caring for Troubled Children* (Whittaker, 1979).

Day Treatment

Day treatment (Chazen, 1969; Gold and Reisman, 1970; Linnihan, 1977) can provide many of the benefits of inpatient treatment without totally removing the child from home, and at less expense. Children can spend a substantial part of their waking hours in a therapeutic milieu, yet continue to live with their families, who are, however, relieved of much of the stress of coping with their disturbed behaviour. Day treatment does not carry the risk, ever present in inpatient care, of child and parents losing contact with each other and of the problem coming to be denied on one or both sides. It can often be helpfully combined with family therapy or therapy with the parents.

Day treatment can also be useful when a child's behavioural problems are selectively manifest at school, adjustment at home being satisfactory. Since most day treatment units have teachers on their staff, the educational needs of these children can often be met during a period of attendance at such a unit.

Day treatment usually involves attendance from about 9 a.m. until 4 or 5 p.m., 5 days a week, but hours may vary and attendance may be for fewer than 5 days weekly or may be confined to mornings, afternoons or evenings.

Alternative Families

In recent years use has been made, in some centres, of families in the community as places where children can receive 'residential' treatment. Examples are the 'parent–therapist' programme in Hamilton, Ontario (Levin *et al.*, 1976), the Alberta Parent Counsellors (Larson *et al.*, 1978), and the Kent Family Placement Project in England (Hazel, 1977). In these programmes families are specially selected, trained and paid, and then take into their homes disturbed children needing treatment away from their own homes. The alternative families receive continuing help in this work, a main feature of this being regular group meetings under the leadership of a professional worker. Meanwhile work is done as indicated with the natural families, as it would be during inpatient treatment. These schemes appear to be of real value and can provide a good alternative to inpatient treatment. They are also less costly.

A somewhat similar scheme, the 'family care programme' in Toronto, provides alternative families for children receiving inpatient treatment, in cases where the child has no family that can provide a suitable home (Barker *et al.*, 1978). As well as visiting their child in the treatment centre, the 'foster care workers' provide, as necessary, a weekend home and, often, later a home for the child to live in upon discharge. In the rather frequent cases where the child's family has broken up or rejected the child, this appears greatly to facilitate and shorten residential treatment and prevent subsequent relapse.

Educational Measures

Where educational problems are present, as they often are in disturbed children, treatment must include appropriate educational measures. These may include remedial teaching for the child, a change of educational methods or transfer to a different class or school. Advice from educational psychologists is helpful on these matters.

In many countries special schools and classes exist for disturbed children, either as part of the general school system or as private establishments. In Great Britain local education authorities have a statutory duty to provide special education for 'maladjusted' children requiring it, and for this reason many run special schools for maladjusted children. There are also a number of privately run schools. There are both day and residential schools for maladjusted children; some take both day and residential pupils. In North America the arrangements for the education of disturbed children are more varied. Many of the schools that specialise in this area are privately run, but many boards of education run special classes. There are also a number of special schools attached to residential and day treatment centres. Children with chronically unstable, adverse family environments can often benefit greatly from attending these schools or special classes. Skilled, accepting care is combined with special educational help in small classes. The residential schools are often small (up to about 80 pupils, but normally nearer 40) and have a higher staff:pupil ratio than ordinary schools. While at school the children are often able to develop relationships with the staff which are more satisfying and constructive than those they have with their parents, with whom they live during school holidays, half-term breaks and perhaps weekends. Very often their adjustment at home improves as their educational problems begin to resolve as a result of their treatment in school. Many of these schools also have social workers on their staffs who can help families with their problems while the child is away at the school. The development of schools for maladjusted children has been well described by Bridgland (1971).

While special schools and classes are valuable for some children, most disturbed children are educated in ordinary schools and classes.

Many more minor educational problems can be dealt with in such settings, often with some additional help from educational psychologists or remedial teachers. A helpful recent review of the education of disturbed children is that of Laslett (1977).

Speech and Language Therapy

Most centres treating disturbed children have one or more speech therapists on their staff. Since speech and language disorders are often associated with emotional disturbance, it is important that expert assessment and treatment by a speech therapist should be available. Speech therapists have an important role in the assessment and treatment of children with developmental language disorders (see Chapter 9).

Removal from Parental Care

Some children do not have families with which they can live. This may be because of the death or desertion of one or both parents, but provision is also needed for the care of children who do not receive an adequate standard of care within their families. In all developed countries there are child welfare agencies, often run by the state, but sometimes by private organisations, to deal with these children.

Where a child has a family with which it would be possible to live if the care available in it was adequate, efforts should naturally first be made to improve the standard of care the family gives. This is one important function of the social workers who staff child welfare agencies. If these efforts fail, or when there is no family with which the child can live, alternative care is necessary. This can often be done with the consent of the parents, or next of kin, but it is sometimes necessary for the child to be taken into care against the wishes of the next of kin (see Chapter 15).

Many children who have had to be removed from their families have experienced unstable, rejecting and perhaps depriving conditions prior to being taken into care, so that their emotional development has been retarded and abnormal. They may show various behavioural problems and commonly have conduct disorders, developmental disorders, educational problems or other difficulties, often in various combinations. The child welfare agencies concerned have the often very difficult task of meeting these children's needs, and psychiatric help may be sought in the course of their efforts to do so.

The substitute environment provided for these children usually consists of either a group home or a foster home. The large and often rather impersonal 'children's homes', or 'orphanages', of the past have now been mostly replaced by much smaller homes, usually consisting of ordinary houses in which the children are cared for in the same way as in other families. Unfortunately, however, many mentally handicapped children are still cared for in large, impersonal and understaffed institutions, the drawbacks of which were well described by King and colleagues (1971). Happily there is a trend towards caring for these children also in smaller units, such as hostels or group homes.

Today substitute homes – often called 'group homes' – do not usually contain more than about ten to twelve children, and ideally should probably have rather fewer. An increasing number take the form of 'family group homes' in which a married couple, perhaps assisted by one or two other staff, look after the children, the husband going out to work at a job as would the father in an ordinary family. Foster care consists of placing the child in an ordinary family, the foster parents being selected from people who have volunteered for the work. They are paid a sum for the child's keep and care is provided in their own home.

Substitute care of some sort is the main need of some emotionally disturbed children. After removal from the disturbed family, their disorders often gradually settle in the more stable environment in which they are placed. As well as requiring skilled and patient management, however, they may also require some of the other treatment measures which have been described in this chapter. It is for this reason that child welfare agencies often seek help from psychiatrists and psychologists, as well as employing social workers. Inter-disciplinary assessment can be helpful in deciding the nature of a deprived child's problems and in planning placement and management.

Many western countries also have 'training' or 'correctional' schools for delinquent children, and especially adolescents. Their value has been questioned, and the environment and help they offer their clients vary greatly. In some, however, progressive and humane therapeutic programmes exist, whereas others are primarily custodial and/or punitive. In some jurisdictions these establishments have been abolished or greatly reduced in numbers. In Great Britain they were formerly called 'approved schools' and were under the jurisdiction of the Home Office, which also runs prisons for adults. They are now renamed 'community homes' and are run by social services departments, which are also responsible for other child welfare services.

CHAPTER SEVENTEEN

Prevention of Child Psychiatric Disorders

It is obviously better to prevent child psychiatric disorders than to treat them once they are established. Less attention has, nevertheless, in the past been given to prevention than to treatment services. It is important, however, since treatment methods are by no means uniformly effective and in any case are unavailable to many children and families who need them.

Types of Prevention

Prevention has been divided into primary, secondary and tertiary types (Caplan, 1964).

Primary prevention in the field of child mental health consists of planned programmes designed to reduce the incidence of specific pathological conditions, whether psychiatric illness or mental handicap, in a population of children not currently suffering from such conditions.

Secondary prevention aims at early diagnosis and case finding, followed by intervention to bring the disorder rapidly under control, so that there is minimal impact on the subject.

Tertiary prevention consists of measures taken once a disorder is established. It aims to limit the effects of the disorder, to prevent it getting worse and to give support to the afflicted individual or family.

This chapter will deal principally with primary prevention. The *prevalence* of a disorder is the number of cases at a given time in a specified population. It is a function of two independent variables —

incidence and *duration*. Incidence is a measure of the number of new cases occurring during a specified time period; duration is the length of time a disorder persists, that is, the time from onset until either recovery or death. An increase in either incidence or duration will thus cause a greater prevalence. It will be clear from the definitions of the different types of prevention mentioned above that primary prevention aims to reduce prevalence by lowering the incidence of disorders, while secondary prevention aims to do it by shortening the duration of disorders.

Primary Prevention

The publication of Caplan's (1964) book *Principles of Preventive Psychiatry* was an important step in the development of preventive psychiatry. More recently the same author has provided a valuable, concise account of methods of primary prevention which are currently available for use in child psychiatry (Caplan, 1980). The subject is discussed more fully in the reports of the Vermont conferences on primary prevention held in 1975, 1976 and 1977 (Albee and Joffe, 1977; Forgays, 1978; Kent and Rolfe, 1978).

Epidemiology is a basic tool in the development of programmes of primary prevention. It is concerned with the incidence, prevalence and distribution of disorders in communities. By means of epidemiological studies it is possible both to determine a baseline so that the effectiveness of a preventive programme can be judged, and also to identify *risk factors* which make the development of particular disorders more likely. Primary prevention is then based on this information and also on knowledge about *intervening variables*, those factors which determine whether individuals at risk do or do not develop the disorders in question. No risk factor is 100 per cent effective, and in any epidemic some individuals will escape. Primary prevention aims to alter the environment so that more escape.

Risk Factors Relevant in Primary Prevention

The following factors are known to be of significance for primary prevention:

(a)   Genetic factors. Reference has been made in Chapter 2 to genetic factors in the causation of child psychiatric disorder. It has proved possible, for example, to reduce the incidence of mental handicap due to phenylketonuria by the routine testing of the urine of newborn infants and the provision of an appropriate diet to those who show evidence of the condition. The provision of genetic counselling services can also reduce the incidence of certain genetic disorders. It is often combined with amniocentesis, in genetically 'at risk' pregnant mothers. Amniocentesis is the prenatal examination of the amniotic fluid, which enables a number of foetal abnormalities to be detected early in pregnancy. Pregnancy can then be terminated.

(b) Pregnancy risk factors. These include toxaemia of pregnancy, various infections of the mother (rubella, syphilis, toxoplasmosis) and other factors such as smoking and alcholism. Programmes designed to reduce these risk factors have met with great success. Congenital syphilis and the mental retardation and other results of maternal rubella in early pregnancy are now very rare where good antenatal care is practised.

(c) Birth trauma. It has long been known that birth trauma can cause damage to the brain, as well as to other parts of the foetus. Good obstetric care reduces this and is thus an important element in primary prevention.

(d) Prematurity and neonatal medical disorders. Apart from their direct effects, these may have indirect ones as a result of prolonged separation of infant and mother. Treatment in a special care unit may disrupt mother–infant bonding.

(e) Accidents in and outside the home. These are common causes of neurological and other injuries, which may lead to psychiatric disorder or mental handicap.

(f) Poisons. The most important is lead (see Chapter 6).

(g) Physical illnesses, especially of the central nervous system. The risks are particularly great when illnesses are prolonged and lead to repeated admissions to hospital.

(h) Cultural deprivation. Many studies have shown higher prevalence rates of psychiatric disorders, as well as of mental handicap and learning failure at school, in culturally deprived homes than in better endowed homes.

(i) Family disharmony and disruption. Children from such families generally have higher rates of emotional and behavioural disorders.

(j)   Parental mental illness. This is a particularly serious risk factor when both parents suffer mental illness, and also when the disorder is severe and prolonged.
(k)   Early school failure. This is often associated with specific learning disorders, hyperkinesis and neurological problems.
(l)   Experience of being in the care of a child welfare agency. This is discussed further below.
(m)   Large family size. This has been shown to be associated with an increased incidence of juvenile delinquency.

The above list of risk factors is not exhaustive, but in the case of all those mentioned there is some evidence to support the listing. Many other risk factors certainly exist. In some cases there is suspicion of their role but no proof; others are no doubt as yet unsuspected.

Protective factors may be contrasted with risk factors. They are factors which make the development of a disorder less likely. The World Health Organisation publication *Child Mental Health and Psychosocial Development* (1977b) lists the following possible protective factors.

(a)   Sex. For little understood reasons girls seem to be less susceptible to psychosocial stress in childhood.
(b)   Temperament. An adaptable temperament seems to protect against the effects of deprivation and disadvantage.
(c)   Isolated nature of stress. Even chronic stresses, if isolated, tend to cause little damage, but multiple stresses interact to potentiate the adverse results.
(d)   Coping skills. There is evidence that children can acquire the skills to cope with various stresses. For example it has been shown that children who are used to brief, happy separation experiences, such as short stays with friends or relatives, cope better with the stress of hospital admission.
(e)   A good relationship with one parent. Such a relationship helps protect against the adverse effects which result when a child is brought up in a discordant, unhappy home.
(f)   Success or good experiences outside the home. Good schooling can apparently help mitigate the effects of a bad home environment.
(g)   Improved family circumstances. Later years spent in a harmonious family setting seem to lessen the effects of earlier adverse family circumstances.

Rutter (1979) has provided a valuable review of factors relating to 'invulnerability' — the ability of some children to survive gross deprivation and psychosocial stress without developing psychiatric disorders. While affirming that genetic factors are important causes contributing to children's psychiatric problems, he also cites evidence that one way in which genetic factors operate is through their influence on the responsiveness of individuals to environmental stresses. This suggests that if the latter are reduced, the genetic predisposition may be countered.

Preventive Measures

Epidemiological data, combined with evidence concerning risk factors, intervening variables and protective factors, enable rational plans to be made for programmes of primary prevention. It has already been pointed out that the provision of genetic counselling services and of facilities for amniocentesis can reduce the incidence of cases of some forms of mental retardation. Our knowledge of risk factors also suggests that the provision of good antenatal and obstetric services will be of value.

Accident prevention, which can be achieved by making roads, vehicles and homes safer, is likely to have some primary preventive value. The removal of lead from paint and the safe disposal of lead-containing waste can be expected to reduce the incidence of cases of lead poisoning. Measures which control infectious diseases, especially those affecting the central nervous system, are relevant.

Factors such as cultural deprivation, family disharmony and parental mental illness present difficult challenges. It has been established, however, that social change which can lead to lessening of the psychiatric morbidity in communities can be brought about by specific interventions. A classical study is that of Leighton (1965), who described changes in a rural community over a 10-year period. At the start of the period the community was impoverished materially, culturally, educationally and socially, with a high prevalence of broken marriages, interparental strife and child neglect. As a result of a number of changes in the community, notably group action and the emergence of local leadership, there were great improvements in all these areas over a 10-year period. Factors that contributed to the change were activities of the official responsible for adult education in the area and those of the local teacher. Some external factors, such as electrification of the village, helped but for the most part the changes in the community came from within. Outside people and agencies did, however, act as catalysts. The role of the 'consolidated school', in a town several miles away, appeared to be important. The village children started going to this school during the course of the study. The influence of this school, through the ideas, concepts, values and standards of behaviour brought home by the children, seemed important and helpful. (More recent research has confirmed that the influence of the school, as a social institution, on the psycho-social development of its students is of great significance (Rutter *et al.*, 1979).) The changes described by Leighton are reported to have been accompanied by a great lowering of the prevalence of psychiatric disorder over the 10-year period of the study. This con-trasted with other communities that in 1952, when the study started, were equally disintegrated but remained so in 1962. These communi-ties showed no comparable decline in the prevalence of psychiatric disorder.

In most western societies rural poverty and disintegration is today less prominent as a problem than are various urban problems. A similar model for change can, however, be used. It is set out in a paper by Cordoza and colleagues (1975), though the example they use concerns not children, but the elderly. The essence of the approach is that 'conditions stressful to individuals frequently derive from the social characteristics of communities'. Communities may be regarded as systems containing various subsystems. These systems have two dimensions. One is the 'structure' of the community — its social stratification, kinship networks and leadership hierarchy. The other dimension consists of 'shared feelings, attitudes, values and opinions' which make up the structures and can be called shared sentiments. Structure and sentiment interact to make up the community's functioning, which may or may not promote good mental health in particular families and individuals. Cordoza and his colleagues describe the 'Sommerville' project, which seemed to show that the intervention of a 'catalyst', in this case a member of a mental health team, could change the structure of the community. The worker operated by 'weaving networks of communication between resources and people who knew about them'. The authors acknowledge that the study, like other similar ones, lacked a 'control' group. That is to say it is impossible to be absolutely sure that the beneficial changes did not come about by chance. Nevertheless, evidence that these measures are effective is increasing.

In Britain the term 'intermediate treatment' has been used for interventions of a similar kind. This approach involves the use of various social work techniques, but especially 'community work'; this seeks to involve 'the participation of the parents and adults of the neighbourhood in the planning of services to children and youth, while fostering the involvement of the youngsters in the life of their community'. In other words, the idea is to enable communities to function better as communities. The book *Intermediate Treatment* (Leissner *et al.*, 1977), from which the above quotation is taken, describes pilot schemes in seven 'areas of deprivation' in England. While results are difficult to evaluate, schemes of this sort seem to offer real hope of being of value in both primary and secondary prevention.

An important 'high risk' group of children consists of those who have been in the care of child welfare agencies at some time in their life. Such children show psychiatric disorder later in childhood much more often than children who have not experienced a period of agency care (Wolkind and Rutter, 1973). While the reasons for this are complex, and are probably related more to the instability of these families and their relative lack of supporting social networks than to the fact of the children having been in care, it is clear that this is a vulnerable group. The provision of excellent alternative care for children deprived of normal, stable, secure family life is likely to be of great preventive value. The question of the provision of services to such children, and how their results might be evaluated, is discussed further in the book *Care Can Prevent* (Barker, 1973).

The known association between large family size and juvenile delinquency (West and Farrington, 1973) suggests that measures which make birth control more readily available may be of value.

Caplan (1980) suggests that in addition to reducing risk factors, it is also helpful to take positive steps to improve the capacity of children to cope with crises, for example admission to hospital. He suggests two ways of doing this: 'anticipatory guidance' and 'preventive intervention'. The former consists of explaining and discussing the upcoming 'crisis' and the likely feelings and experiences the subject will encounter. The process is best done in groups. Tours of hospitals and the use of films are helpful additional tools. 'Preventive intervention' consists of guidance given to children and their families.

This is focussed on the here-and-now. The subjects are helped and supported in understanding what is happening, in finding solutions to problems, in countering blame of self or others, in maintaining hope and in finding outside help — from extended families, friends and professional care-givers — where appropriate. By these means children's 'coping skills' can be improved and what might have been an emotionally damaging experience can become a growth-promoting one.

Also helpful in both primary and secondary prevention are support and self-help groups. As Caplan (1980) points out, convening a support group for a person in need can have great preventive value. The people in need may be recent immigrants to a country, they may have a dying relative or they may face a natural or man-made disaster or one of a myriad of other stresses. A supportive group or network can help greatly in reducing the stress the subject experiences.

Many 'self-help groups' have grown up to provide support to their members. They range from associations for the families of children with cystic fibrosis or diabetes to 'Toughlove' (York and York, 1980), a network of groups for the parents of troublesome teenagers.

Secondary Prevention

This involves early diagnosis and case finding, followed by intervention to bring the disorder under control as rapidly as possible. The screening of populations to detect disorders at an early stage is of value here. In most school systems children are tested and assessed regularly to detect early evidence of both emotional disorders and learning disabilities. Many children in whom evidence of disorder is detected in this way come from troubled families. In these cases treatment often involves the whole family group, and what is secondary prevention for one child may be primary prevention for other, as yet undisturbed, children.

Many screening devices are available for detecting early signs of disorder in children. These include Rutter's scales for use by teachers and by parents (Rutter, 1967b, 1970b) and the Bristol Social Adjustment Guide (Stott, 1960).

The treatment methods required in dealing with early cases detected by secondary prevention programmes are similar to those required for established disorders, as described in the earlier chapters of this book. Many schools have special psychological and remedial services for children with learning problems.

Most communities have services which both provide support and help for families raising young children and are available to detect early signs of problems in the children. In Britain the principal service is that provided by *health visitors*, specialised nurses who have the statutory duty to visit the families of all children soon after birth and at intervals thereafter. In North America similar functions are performed by *public health nurses.*

Tertiary Prevention

This consists of measures taken once a disorder is established. It aims to limit the effect of the disorder, to prevent its getting worse and to give support to the affected individual or family. It requires active involvement and usually a lot of work by those doing the prevention but it may be essential, for example with families in which there has been serious abuse or neglect of children. Generally, however, primary and secondary prevention are preferable and more economic uses of scarce professional time. Various agencies and services run intensive programmes for families containing children at high risk. *Family service units*, for example, aim to give intensive help, if necessary over a long period of time, to families which are functioning especially badly. The staff are prepared if need be to spend substantial periods of time in the home, supporting the families; helping them with their emotional and social handicaps; demonstrating, if necessary, basic techniques of home management and the care of children, and gradually enabling the family to function better on its own. Despite their great value, such units are few in relation to the number of families they could help.

Other Points Concerning Prevention

One of the problems in discussing primary prevention is that, as Kessler and Albee (1977) have pointed out, 'practically every effort aimed at improved child rearing, increasing effective communication, building inner control and self-esteem, reducing stress and pollution, and such like — in short everything aimed at improving the human condition – may be considered to be part of primary prevention of mental or emotional disturbance'. It is, therefore, important that professionals in the field, when they recommend preventive pro-grammes, do so on the basis of data which at least suggest that the programme will be effective – and also cost-effective. Means of evaluating new programmes should be built into the plans.

This sort of approach is important because whether preventive measures are taken to deal with particular problems often depends on community attitudes, and especially those of community leaders. Wild claims, programme failures and extravagantly expensive schemes do not endear professionals to the communities they serve. Moreover in many instances it is the collective motivation of communities that determines whether or not preventive programmes are implemented. For example finances allocated to education authorities and child welfare agencies usually depend on delicate political considerations.

The widespread dissemination of information on the stresses which society places on its members, and on how such stresses may be alleviated is very important. In this connection the National Children's Bureau (8 Wakley Street, London EC1V 7QE) has published a series of brief reviews or 'highlights'. These summarise current knowledge about various groups of children that are at risk. They quote relevant references and are a useful guide to the literature.

At the level of society as a whole, the view is expressed by many people that modern, western society fails to provide an appropriate environment for the raising of emotionally healthy children. These people point to the rising crime, delinquency, family break-up and divorce rates as evidence of this. Writing from an ecological point of view Goldsmith (1977) sees modern urban society as undermining the essential functions of the family, which in turn is undermined as the basis of our social system. He believes that the educative, econ-omic, welfare and social control functions of the family have all largely been taken away by the modern industrial state. At the same time, increasing numbers of poor, dispossessed, alienated people struggle to bring up children in deteriorating inner city areas. Econ-omic and social problems make this increasingly difficult. Goldsmith's solution is 'de-urbanisation' – the settlement of people in smaller, ecologically balanced societies. But Goldsmith et al. (1972) and others like him believe that even more radical changes in society, such as those suggested in the 'Blueprint for Survival', are required if modern civilisation is to be set on the right tracks.

Writing from a mental health point of view Bronfenbrenner (1977) also points out that, 'in recent decades the American family has been falling apart'. He believes that children's needs are being met less and less effectively and he too sees this as due to changing social standards. How is it, he asks, that we can deliver men and survival systems to the moon, but not health care to the neighbourhood? Bronfenbrenner believes that it is the self-centredness of members of today's society, and the failure of people to contribute adequately to the community in which they live, which is at the root of the problem. His solutions are seemingly less radical than Goldsmith's, but nevertheless require drastic changes in society.

The decline in religion is probably related to the other changes in society. The great religions of the world offer sound codes by which human beings may live together. Many western nations have largely abandoned their former Christian heritage, with its obligation to love and help others, and to put God and other people before self. Instead a self-seeking materialism seems to be preferred in which, as Bronfenbrenner puts it, 'doing your own thing (is) our undoing'. Material possessions are the main aim of many in today's society. These have their limitations as a background for family life and the rearing of children.

These matters are of course political, social and moral issues rather than clinical ones. They concern all of society, not just mental health professionals. Nevertheless, those involved in the mental health field should be especially aware of such issues and bring them constantly to the notice of the wider society of which they are part.

References

Adams, P.L. (1973). *Obsessive Children*. London: Butterworth; New York: Brunner/Mazel.

Adams, P.L. (1974). *A Primer of Child Psychotherapy*. Boston: Little Brown.

Albee, G.W. and Joffe, J.M. (eds) (1977). *Primary Prevention of Psychopathology. Volume 1: The Issues*. Hanover, New Hampshire: University Press of New England.

Allen, F.H. (1942). *Psychotherapy with Children*. New York: Norton.

American Psychiatric Association (1980). *Diagnostic and Statistical Manual III*. Washington, DC: APA.

Amini, F., Salasnek, S. and Burke, E.L. (1976). 'Adolescent drug abuse: etiological and treatment considerations'. *Adolescence*, 11, 281–299.

Anastasi, A. (1976). *Psychological Testing*, 4th ed. New York: Macmillan.

Anders, T.F. and Weinstein, P. (1972). 'Sleep and its disorders in infants and children'. *Pediatrics*, 50, 312–324.

Anderson, L.M. and Shafer, G. (1979). 'The character-disordered family: a community treatment model for family sexual abuse'. *American Journal of Orthopsychiatry*, 49, 436–445.

Andrews, G. and Harris, M. (1964). *The Syndrome of Stuttering*. London: Heinemann.

Anthony, E.J. (1957). 'An experimental approach to the psychopathology of childhood: encopresis'. *British Journal of Medical Psychology*, 30, 146–175.

APA (1980). *See* American Psychiatric Association.

Asperger, H. (1944). 'Die autistichen psychopathen in kindersalter'. *Archiv fur Psychiatrie und Nervankrankheiten (Berlin)*, 117, 76–137.

Bagley, C. (1971). *The Social Psychology of the Child with Epilepsy*. London: Routledge and Kegan Paul.

Bakwin, H. (1971). 'Enuresis in twins'. *American Journal of Diseases of Children*, 121, 222–225.

Balbernie, I. (1974). 'Unintegration, integration and level of ego functioning as the determinants of planned "cover therapy", of unit task and of placement'. *Journal of the Association of Workers for Maladjusted Children*, 2, 6–46.

Baldwin, J.A. and Oliver, J.E. (1975). 'Epidemiology and family characteristics of severely abused children'. *British Journal of Preventive and Social Medicine*, **29**, 205–221.

Bandler, R. and Grinder, J. (1979). *Frogs into Princes*. Moab, Utah: Real People Press.

Barker, P. (1968). 'The inpatient treatment of school refusal'. *British Journal of Medical Psychology*, **41**, 381–387.

Barker, P. (1973). *Care Can Prevent: Child Care or Child Psychiatry?* London: National Children's Home.

Barker, P. (1974). *The Residential Psychiatric Treatment of Children*, ed. P. Barker. London: Crosby Lockwood Staples.

Barker, P. (1975). 'Haloperidol'. *Journal of Child Psychology and Psychiatry*, **16**, 169–172.

Barker, P. (1981a). *Basic Family Therapy*, St. Albans: Granada and Baltimore: University Park Press.

Barker, P. (1981b). 'Paradoxical techniques in psychotherapy'. In *Treating Families with Special needs*, eds D. S. Freeman and B. Trute. Ottawa: Canadian Association of Social Workers.

Barker, P. (1983). 'Residential treatment for disturbed children: its place in the "80s" '. *Canadian Journal of Psychiatry*, in press.

Barker, P., Buffe, C. and Zaretsky, R. (1978). 'Providing a family alternative for the disturbed child'. *Child Welfare*, **57**, 373–379.

Barker, P. and Swinson, R. (1980). 'Classification of psychiatric disorders'. *Canadian Medical Association Journal*, **122**, 748–750.

Barnhill, L.H. and Longo, D. (1978). 'Fixation and regression in the family life cycle'. *Family Process*, **17**, 469–478.

Bartak, L., Rutter, M. and Cox, A. (1975). 'A comparative study of infantile autism and specific developmental receptive language disorder'. *British Journal of Psychiatry*, **126**, 127–145.

Beard, R.M. (1969). *An Outline of Piaget's Developmental Psychology*. London: Routledge and Kegan Paul.

Bellman, M. (1966). 'Studies on encopresis'. *Acta Paediatrica Scandinavica*, Supplement 170.

Bender, L. and Schilder, P. (1940). 'Impulsions: a specific disorder of the behaviour of children'. *Archives of Neurology and Psychiatry*, **44**, 990–1008.

Berecz, J.M. (1968). 'Phobias in childhood: aetiology and treatment'. *Psychological Bulletin*, **70**, 694–720.

Berg, I. (1979). 'Day wetting in children'. *Journal of Child Psychology and Psychiatry*, **20**, 167–173.

Berger, M., Yule, W. and Rutter, M. (1975). 'Attainment and adjustment in two geographical areas'. *British Journal of Psychiatry*, **126**, 510–519.

Berney, T. *et al.* (1981). 'School phobia: a therapeutic trial with clomipramine and short-term outcome, *British Journal of Psychiatry*, **138**, 110–118.

Bever, T.G. (1970). 'The cognitive bases of linguistic structures'. In *Cognition and the Development of Language*, ed. T.R. Hayes. New York: Wiley.

Bhanji, S. and Mattingly, D. (1981). 'Anorexia nervosa: some observations on "dieters" and "vomiters," cholesterol and carotene'. *British Journal of Psychiatry*, **139**, 238–241.

Bicknell, J. (1975). *Pica: A Childhood Symptom*. London: Butterworth.

Bille, B. (1962). 'Migraine in school children'. *Acta Paediatrica*, **51**, Supplement 163.

Biller, H.B. (1970). 'Father absence and the personality development of the male child'. *Developmental Psychology*, **2**, 181–201.

Blumberg, H. (1976). 'Drug taking'. In *Child Psychiatry: Modern Approaches*, eds M. Rutter and L. Hersov. Oxford: Blackwell.

Boatman, B., Borkan, E.L. and Schetky, D.H. (1981). 'Treatment of child victims of incest'. *American Journal of Family Therapy*, **9**, 43–51.

Bowlby, J. (1961). 'Childhood mourning and its implications for psychiatry'. *American Journal of Psychiatry*, **118**, 481–498.

Bowlby, J. (1969). *Attachment*. London: Hogarth and New York: Basic Books.

Bowlby, J. (1977). 'The making and breaking of emotional bonds'. *British Journal of Psychiatry*, **130**, 201–210 and 421–431.

Bowlby, J. (1979). *The Making and Breaking of Affectional Bonds*. London: Tavistock.

Bradley, S. and Sloman, L. (1975) 'Elective mutism in immigrant families'. *Journal of the American Academy of Child Psychiatry*, **14**, 510–514.

Bridgland, M. (1971). *Pioneer Work with Maladjusted Children*. London: Crosby Lockwood Staples.

British Medical Journal (1977). 'Enuresis' (editorial). **1**, 4.

Broderick, C.B. and Rowe, P. (1968). 'A scale of pre-adolescent heterosexual development'. *Journal of Marriage and the Family*, **30**, 97–101.

Bronfenbrenner, V. (1977). 'Doing your own thing our undoing'. *Child Psychiatry and Human Development*, **8**, 3–10.

Brown, B., Fuller, J. and Gericke, C. (1975a). 'Elective mutism: a review and a report of an unsuccessfully treated case'. *Journal of the Association of Workers for Maladjusted Children*, **3**, 27–37.

Brown, B. and Lloyd, H. (1975). 'A controlled study of children not speaking at school'. *Journal of the Association of Workers for Maladjusted Children*, **3**, 49–63.

Brown, G.W., NiBrochelchain, M. and Harris, T.O. (1975b). 'Social class and psychiatric disturbance among women in an urban population'. *Sociology*, **9**, 225–254.

Brown, S.L. (1972). 'Family group therapy'. In *Manual of Child Psychopathology*, ed. B.B. Wolman. New York: McGraw-Hill.

Bruch, E. (1973). *Eating Disorders*. New York: Basic Books.

Bruch, H. (1974). 'Obesity' (part II). In *Eating Disorders, Obesity, Anorexia Nervosa and the Person Within*. London: Routledge and Kegan Paul.

Burquest, B. (1979). 'Severe female delinquency: when to involve the family in treatment'. In *Adolescent Psychiatry*, Vol. 7, eds S.C. Feinstein and P.L. Giovacchini. University of Chicago Press.

Busch, F., Nagero, H., McKnight, J. and Pezzarossi, G. (1973). 'Primary transitional objects'. *Journal of the American Academy of Child Psychiatry*, **12**, 193–214.

Cade, B. (1980). 'Strategic therapy'. *Journal of Family Therapy*, **2**, 89–99.

Caffey, J. (1946). 'Multiple fractures in the long bones of infants suffering from chronic subdural haematoma'. *American Journal of Roentgenology*, **56**, 163–173.

Cameron, J.R. (1977). 'Parental treatment, children's temperament and the risk of childhood behavioural problems'. *American Journal of Orthopsychiatry*, **47**, 568–576.

Cantwell, D. (1977). 'Psychopharmacologic treatment of the minimal brain dysfunction syndrome'. In *Psychopharmacology in Childhood and Adolescence*, ed. J.M. Wiener. New York: Basic Books.

Capes, M., Gould, E. and Townsend, M. (1971). *Stress in Youth*. London: Oxford University Press for the Nuffield Provincial Hospitals Trust.

Caplan, G. (1964). *Principles of Preventive Psychiatry*. New York: Basic Books.

Caplan, G. (1980). 'An approach to preventive intervention in child psychiatry'. *Canadian Journal of Psychiatry*, **25**, 671–682.

Caplan, H.L. (1970). M. Phil. Dissertation, University of London. (Findings summarised in Hersov, L. in *The Residential Psychiatric Treatment of Children* (pages 118–119), ed. P. Barker. London: Crosby Lockwood Staples.

Carter, E.A. and McGoldrick, M. (1980). *The Family Life Cycle*. New York: Gardner.

Chamberlain, C. and Awad, G. (1979). 'Clinical consultation in custody and access disputes'. In *New Directions in Children's Mental Health*, ed. S.J. Shamsie. New York: SP Medical and Scientific Books.

Chazen, R. (1969). 'Day treatment of emotionally disturbed children' *Child Welfare*, **48**, 212–218.

Chess, S. (1977). 'Follow-up report on autism in congenital rubella'. *Journal of Autism and Childhood Schizophrenia*, **7**, 69–81.

Cohen, D.J. (1980). 'The pathology of the self in primary childhood autism and Gilles de la Tourette syndrome'. *Psychiatric Clinics of North America*, **3**, 383–402.

Cohen, D.J. *et al.* (1979). 'Central biogenic amine metabolism in children with the syndrome of chronic multiple tics of Gilles de la Tourette'. *Journal of the American Academy of Child Psychiatry*, **18**, 320–341.

Cohen, I.L. *et al.* (1980). 'Behavioural effects of haloperidol in young autistic children'. *Journal of the American Academy of Child Psychiatry*, **19**, 665–677.

Connell, P.H. (1971). 'Suicidal attempts in childhood and adolescence'. In *Modern Perspectives in Child Psychiatry*, ed. J.G. Howells. New York: Brunner/Mazel.

Coolidge, J.C., Willer, M.L., Tessman, E. and Waldfogel, S. (1970). 'School phobia in adolescence; a manifestation of severe character disturbance'. *American Journal of Orthopsychiatry*, **30**, 599–607.

Cooper, I. and Lormier, B.M. (1982). 'Intergenerational transmission of incest'. *Canadian Journal of Psychiatry*, **27**, 231–235.

Corbett, J., Harris, R., Taylor, E. and Trimble, M. (1977). 'Progressive disintegrative psychosis of childhood'. *Journal of Child Psychology and Psychiatry*, **18**, 211–219.

Corbett, J.A., Matthews, A.M., Connell, P.H. and Shapiro, D.A. (1969). 'Tics and Gilles de la Tourette's syndrome: a follow-up study and critical review'. *British Journal of Psychiatry*, **115**, 122–141.

Cordoza, V.G., Ackerly, W.C. and Leighton, A.H. (1975). 'Improving mental health through community action'. *Community Mental Health Journal*, **11**, 215–227.

Cox, A., Holbrook, D. and Rutter, M. (1981). 'Psychiatric interviewing techniques VI. Experimental study: eliciting feelings'. *British Journal of Psychiatry*, **139**, 144–152.

Cox, A., Hopkinson, K. and Rutter, M. (1981). 'Psychiatric interviewing techniques II. Naturalistic study: eliciting factual information'. *British Journal of Psychiatry*, **138**, 283–291.

Cox, A., Rutter, M. and Holbrook, D. (1981). 'Psychiatric interviewing techniques V. Experimental study: eliciting factual information'. *British Journal of Psychiatry*, **139**, 29–37.

Creak, M. (1963). 'Childhood psychosis: a review of 100 cases'. *British Journal of Psychiatry*, **109**, 84–89.

Crisp, A. (1977). 'Diagnosis and outcome of anorexia nervosa'. *Proceedings of the Royal Society of Medicine*, **70**, 464–470.

Crome, L. (1960). 'The brain and mental retardation'. *British Medical Association*, **2**, 897–904.

Currie, K.H. and Brannigan, C. (1970). 'Behaviour analysis and modification with an austistic child'. In *Behaviour Studies in Psychiatry*, eds C. and S.J. Hutt. Oxford: Pergamon.

Dale, P.S. (1976). *Language Development: Structure and Function*. Hindsdale, Ill.: Dryden Press.

Davenport, C.W., Zoule, J.P., Kuhn, C.C. and Harrison, S.T. (1972). 'Cyclic vomiting'. *Journal of the American Academy of Child Psychiatry*, **11**, 66–87.

Davie, R., Butler, N. and Goldstein, H. (1972). *From Birth to Seven*. London: Longman.

Department of Health and Social Security (1971). *Youth Treatment Centres*. London: HMSO.

Dische, S. (1971). 'Management of enuresis'. *British Medical Journal*, **2**, 33–36.

Dockar-Drysdale, B. (1968). *Therapy in Child Care* (collected papers). London: Longman Green.

Dockar-Drysdale, B. (1973). *Consultation in Child Care*. London: Longman.

Drillien, C.M. (1969). 'School disposal and performance for children of different birth weight, 1953–1960'. *Archives of Disease in Childhood*, **44**, 562–570.

Driscoll, J.M. *et al.* (1982). 'Mortality and morbidity in infants less than 1,001 grams birth weight'. *Pediatrics*, **69**, 21–26.

Duvall, E.M. (1977). *Marriage and Family Development*, 5th edn. Philadelphia: Lippincott.

Earls, F. *et al.* (1982). 'Concurrent validation of a behavior problems scale to use with 3-year-olds'. *Journal of the American Academy of Child Psychiatry*, **21**, 47–57.

Earls, F. and Richman, N. (1980a). 'The prevalence of behavior problems in three-year-old children of West-Indian born parents'. *Journal of Child Psychology and Psychiatry*, **21**, 99–106.

Earls, F. and Richman, N. (1980b). 'Behavior problems in pre-school children of West Indian-born parents: a re-examination of family and social factors'. *Journal of Child Psychology and Psychiatry*, **21**, 107–117.

Eisenberg, L. (1966). 'Reading retardation: psychiatric and sociological aspects'. *Pediatrics*, **37**, 352–365.

Ekstein, R. and Wallerstein, J. (1956). 'Observations on the psychotherapy of borderline and psychotic children'. *Psychoanalytic Study of the Child*, **11**, 303–311.

Elkins, R., Rapoport, J.L. and Lipsky, A. (1980). 'Obsessive–compulsive disorders of childhood and adolescence – a neurobiological viewpoint'. *Journal of the American Academy of Child Psychiatry*, **19**, 511–524.

Ellis, R. (1980). *Inborn Errors of Metabolism*. London: Croom Helm.

Epstein, N.B., Bishop, D.S. and Levin, S. (1978). 'The McMaster model of family functioning'. *Journal of Marriage and Family Counselling*, **4**, 19–31.

Erikson, E.H. (1965). *Childhood and Society*. London: Penguin.

Erikson, E.H. (1968). *Identity and the Life Cycle*. London: Faber.

Eyman, R.K., Moore, B.C., Capes, L. and Zachofsky, T. (1970). 'Maladaptive behaviour of institutionalised retardates with seizures'. *American Journal of Mental Deficiency*, **74**, 651–659.

Eysenck, H.J. (1959). 'Learning theory and behaviour therapy'. *Journal of Mental Science*, **105**, 61–95.

Farrington, D.P. (1978). 'The family background of aggressive youths'. In *Aggression and Anti-social Behaviour in Childhood and Adolescence*, pages 73–94, eds L. Hersov, M. Berger and D. Shaffer. Oxford: Pergamon.

Fish, B. (1977). 'Neurobiologic antecedents of schizophrenia in children'. *Archives of General Psychiatry*, **34**, 1297–1313. (Reprinted in *Annual Progress in Child Psychiatry and Child Development*, 1978, eds S. Chess and A. Thomas. New York: Brunner/Mazel.)

Fisher, C. et al. (1974). 'A psychophysiological study of nightmares and night terrors'. *Journal of Nervous and Mental Diseases*, **158**, 174–188.

Flavell, J.H. (1963). *The Developmental Psychology of Jean Piaget*. Princeton: van Nostrand.

Fleck, S. (1976). 'A general systems approach to severe family pathology'. *American Journal of Psychiatry*, **133**, 669–673.

Folstein, S. and Rutter, M. (1977). 'Genetic influences and infantile autism'. *Nature*, **265**, 726–728 (Reprinted in *Annual Progress in Child Psychiatry and Child Development*, 1987, eds S. Chess and A. Thomas. New York: Brunner/Mazel.)

Forgays, D.G. (ed.) (1978). *Primary Prevention of Psychopathology. Volume 2: Environmental Issues*. Hanover, New Hampshire: University Press of New England.

Frankl, V.E. (1960). 'Paradoxical intention: a logotherapeutic technique'. *American Journal of Psychotherapy*, **14**, 520–535.

French, A. (1977). *Disturbed Children and Their Families*, New York: Human Sciences Press.

Freud, A. (1966). *Normality and Pathology in Childhood*. New York: International Universities Press and London: Hogarth.

Freud, A. (1972). *A Short History of Child Analysis*. London: Hogarth Press.

Freud, S. (1905). 'Three essays on the theory of sexuality'. *Standard Edition*, 7. London: Hogarth (1953).

Freud, S. (1923). 'Inhibitions, symptoms and anxiety'. *Standard Edition*, 7. London: Hogarth (1953).

Frith, V. (1978). 'Spelling difficulties'. *Journal of Child Psychology and Psychiatry*, **19**, 279–285.

Fundudis, T., Kolvin, I. and Garside, R.F. (1979). *Speech Retarded and Deaf Children: Their Psychological Development*. London: Academic Press.

Gaensbauer, T.J. and Harmon, R.J. (1981). 'Clinical assessment in infancy utilizing structured playroom situations'. *Journal of the American Academy of Child Psychiatry*, **20**, 264–280.

Garfinkel, B. and Golombek, H. (1977). 'Suicide and depression in childhood and adolescence'. In *Psychological Problems of the Child and his Family*, eds P. Steinhauer and Q. Rae-Grant. Toronto: Macmillan.

Garside, R.F. *et al.* (1975). 'Dimensions of temperament in infant school children'. *Journal of Child Psychology and Psychiatry*, **16**, 219–231.

Geleerd, E.R. (1958). 'Borderline states in childhood and adolescence'. *Psychoanalytic Study of the Child*, **13**, 279–295.

Gibbens, T.C.N. (1974). 'Preparing psychiatric court reports'. *British Journal of Hospital Medicine*, **12**, 278–284.

Gibbs, J.T. (1982). 'Psychosocial factors related to substance abuse among delinquent females: implications for prevention and treatment'. *American Journal of Orthopsychiatry*, **52**, 261–271.

Gil, D.G. (1975). 'Unravelling child abuse'. *American Journal of Orthopsychiatry*, **45**, 346–356.

Ginott, H.G. (1961). *Group Psychotherapy with Children*. New York: McGraw-Hill.

Gittelman-Klein, R. and Klein, D.F. (1971). 'Controlled imipramine treatment of school phobia'. *Archives of General Psychiatry*, **25**, 204–207.

Goetz, P.C., Succop, R.A. Reinhart, J.B. and Miller, A. (1977). 'Anorexia nervosa in children: a follow-up study'. *American Journal of Orthopsychiatry*, **47**, 597–603.

Gold, J. and Reisman, J. (1970). 'An outcome study of a day treatment unit school in a community mental health centre'. *American Journal of Orthopsychiatry*, **40**, 286–287.

Goldsmith, E. (1977). 'The future of an affluent society: the case of Canada'. *Ecologist*, **7**, 160–194.

Goldsmith, E. *et al.* (1972). 'A blueprint for survival'. *Ecologist*, **2**, 143.

Goodman, J.D. and Sours, J.A. (1967). *The Child Mental Status Examination*. New York: Basic Books.

Gordon, D. (1978). *Therapeutic Metaphors: Helping Others Through the Looking Glass*. Cupertino, CA: Meta Publications.

Gordon, S. and Davidson, N. (1981). 'Behavioral parent training'. In *Handbook of Family Therapy*, eds A. Gurman and D. Kniskern. New York: Brunner/Mazel.

Graham, P. (1974). 'Depression in pre-pubertal children'. *Developmental Medicine and Child Neurology*, **14**, 340–349.

Graham, P.J. (1981). 'Depressive disorders in children – a reconsideration'. *Acta Paedopsychiatrica*, **46**, 285–296.

Graham, P., Rutter, M. and George, S. (1973). 'Temperamental characteristics as predictors of behaviour disorders in children'. *American Journal of Orthopsychiatry*, **43**, 328–339.

Greenberg, L.M. and Stephans, J.H. (1977). 'Use of drugs in special syndromes'. In *Psychopharmacology in Childhood and Adolescence*, ed. J.M. Wiener. New York: Basic Books.

Grinder, J. and Bandler, R. (1981). *Trance-Formations*. Moab. Utah: Real People Press.

Grinker, J.A. (1981). 'Behavioral and metabolic factors in childhood obesity'. In *The Uncommon Child*, eds M. Lewis and L.A. Rosenblem. New York: Plenum.

Group for the Advancement of Psychiatry (1966). *Psychopathological Disorders in Childhood. Report No. 62*. New York.

Group for the Advancement of Psychiatry (1968). *Normal Adolescence: Its Dynamics and Impact*. New York: GAP. (Also London: Crosby Lockwood Staples, 1974.)

Gruber, A.R., Heck, E.T. and Mintzer, E. (1981). 'Children who set fires: some background and behavioural characteristics'. *American Journal of Orthopsychiatry*, **51**, 484–488.

Gualtieri, C.T. *et al.* (1982). 'Clinical studies of methylphenidate serum levels in children and adults'. *Journal of the American Academy of Child Psychiatry*, **21**, 19–26.

Gubbay, S.S. (1975). *The Clumsy Child*. London: Saunders.

Guilleminault, C., Eldridge, F.L., Simmons, F.B. and Dement, W.C. (1976). 'Sleep apnoea in eight children'. *Pediatrics*, **58**, 23–30.

Hack, M., Fanaroff, A.A. and Merkatz, I.R. (1979). 'The low birth-weight infant: evolution of a changing outlook'. *New England Journal of Medicine*, **301**, 1162–1165.

Haley, J. (1973). *Uncommon Therapy: The Psychiatric Techniques of Milton J. Erickson*. New York: Norton.

Haley, J. (1977). *Problem Solving Therapy*. San Francisco: Jossey-Bass.

Haley, J. (1980). *Leaving Home*. New York: McGraw-Hill.

Hamburg, B.A., Kraemer, H.C. and Jahnke, W.A. (1975). 'A hierarchy of drug use in adolescence'. *American Journal of Psychiatry*, **132**, 1155–1162.

Harlow, H.F. (1958). 'The nature of love'. *American Journal of Psychology*, **13**, 673–685.

Hartsough, C.S. and Lambert, N.H. (1982). 'Some environmental and familial correlates and antecedents of hyperactivity'. *American Journal of Orthopsychiatry*, **52**, 272–287.

Hassanyeh, F. and Davison, K. (1980). 'Bipolar affective psychosis with onset before age 16 years: Report of 10 Cases'. *British Journal of Psychiatry*, **137**, 530–537.

Hawton, K., O'Grady, J., Osborn, M. and Cole, D. (1982). 'Adolescents who take overdoses: their characteristics, problems and contacts with helping agencies'. *British Journal of Psychiatry*, **140**, 118–123.

Hazel, N. (1977). 'How family placements can combat delinquency'. *Social Work Today*, **8**, 6–7.

Hechtman, L. *et al.* (1976). 'Hyperactives as young adults'. *Canadian Medical Association Journal*, **115**, 625–630.

Helfer, R.E. and Kempe, C.H. (1968). *The Battered Child*. Chicago: University of Chicago Press.

Heller, T. (1954). 'About dementia infantilis' (translation). *Journal of Nervous and Mental Disease*, **119**, 471–477.

Henderson, A.S. (1971). In *Modern Perspectives in Adolescent Psychiatry*, ed. J.G. Howells. Edinburgh: Oliver and Boyd.

Hermelin, B. and O'Connor, N. (1970). *Psychological Experiments with Austistic Children*. Oxford: Pergamon.

Hersov, L. (1976a). 'Emotional disorders'. In *Child Psychiatry: Modern Approaches*, eds M. Rutter and L. Hersov. Oxford: Blackwell.

Hersov, L. (1976b). 'School refusal'. In *Child Psychiatry: Modern Approaches*, eds M. Rutter and L. Hersov. Oxford: Blackwell.

Hoag, J.M., Norriss, N.G., Himeno, E.J. and Jacobs, J. (1971). 'The encopretic child and his family'. *Journal of the American Academy of Child Psychiatry*, **10**, 242–256.

Hoefler, S.A. and Bornstein, P.H. (1975). 'Achievement place: an evaluative review'. *Criminal Justice and Behaviour*, **2**, 146–168.

Hong, K. (1978). 'The transitional phenomena'. *Psychoanalytic Study of the Child*, **3**, 47–49.

Hood, R. and Sparks, R. (1970). *Key Issues in Criminology*. London: Weidenfeld and Nicolson.

Hopkinson, K., Cox, A. and Rutter, M. (1981). 'Psychiatric interviewing techniques III. Naturalistic study: eliciting feelings'. *British Journal of Psychiatry*, **138**, 406–415.

Howells, J.G., ed. (1979). *Modern Perspectives in the Psychiatry of Infants*. New York: Brunner/Mazel.

Humphries, T., Kinsbourne, M. and Swanson, J. (1978). 'Stimulant effects on co-operation and social interaction between hyperactive children and their mothers'. *Journal of Child Psychology and Psychiatry*, **19**, 13–22.

Hundelby, J.D., Carpenter, R.A., Ross, R.A.J. and Mercer, G.W. (1982). 'Adolescent drug use and other behaviours'. *Journal of Child Psychology and Psychiatry*, **23**, 61–68.

Ingram, T.T.S. (1974). 'Psychomotor development and its disorders'. In *A*

Companion to Medical Studies, Vol. 3, Part 2, eds R. Passmore and J.S. Robson. Oxford: Blackwell.

Irving, H. (1981). 'Family mediation: a method for helping families resolve legal disputes'. In *Treating Families with Special Needs*, eds D.S. Freeman and B. Toute. Ottawa: Canadian Association of Social Workers.

Jalali, B., Jalali, M.D., Crocetti, G. and Turner, F. (1981). 'Adolescent and drug use: toward a more comprehensive approach'. *American Journal of Orthopsychiatry*, **51**, 120–130.

Jeavons, P. and Bower, B.D. (1964). *Infantile Spasms. A Review of the Literature and Study of 112 Cases*. London: Heinemann.

Jeavons, P., Harber, J.R. and Bower, B.D. (1970). 'Long-term prognosis in infantile spasms'. *Developmental Medicine and Child Neurology*, **12**, 413–421.

Jenkins, R.L. (1969). 'Classification of behaviour problems of children'. *American Journal of Psychiatry*, **125**, 1032–1039.

Johnson, O.G. and Bommarito, J.W. (1971). *Tests and Measurement in Child Development: Handbook 1*. San Francisco: Jossey-Bass.

Justice, B. and Duncan, D.P. (1976). 'Running away: an epidemic problem of adolescence'. *Adolescence*, **11**, 365–371.

Kandel, D. and Faust, R. (1975). 'Sequence and stages in patterns of adolescent drug use'. *Archives of General Psychiatry*, **32**, 923–932.

Kanner, L. (1943) 'Autistic disturbance of affective contact'. *Nervous Child*, **2**, 217–250.

Kanner, L. (1944). 'Early infantile autism'. *Journal of Pediatrics*, **25**, 211–217.

Keith, P.R. (1975). 'Night terrors'. *Journal of the American Academy of Child Psychiatry*, **14**, 477–489.

Kempe, C.H. (1971). 'Pediatric implications of the battered baby syndrome'. *Archives of Disease in Childhood*, **46**, 28–37.

Kempe, C.H. *et al.* (1962). 'The battered child syndrome'. *Journal of the American Medical Association*, **191**, 17–23.

Kendall, R.E. (1972). 'Schizophrenia: the remedy for diagnostic confusion'. *British Journal of Hospital Medicine*, **8**, 383–390.

Kennedy, W.A. (1965). 'School phobia: rapid treatment of fifty cases'. *Journal of Abnormal Psychology*, **70**, 285–289.

Kent, M.W. and Rolfe, J.E. (eds) (1978). *Primary Prevention of Psychopathology, Vol 3: Social Competence in Children*. New Hampshire: University Press of New England.

Kessler, M. and Albee C.W. (1977). 'An overview of the literature of primary prevention'. In *Primary Prevention of Psychopathology*, Vol. 1, eds W. Albee and J.M. Jolle. Hanover, New Hampshire: University Press of New England.

Kinard, E.M. (1982). 'Experiencing child abuse: effects on emotional adjustment'. *American Journal of Orthopsychiatry*, **52**, 82–91.

King, R.D., Raynes, N.V. and Tizard, J. (1971). *Patterns of Residential Care*. London: Routledge and Kegan Paul.

Kirman, B.H. and Bicknell, J. (1975). *Mental Handicap*. Edinburgh; Churchill-Livingstone.

Klein, M. (1932). *The Psychoanalysis of Children*. London: Hogarth.

Klein, M., (1948). *Contributions to Psycho-Analysis 1921–1945*. London: Hogarth.

Kolvin, I. *et al.* (1971). 'Studies in the childhood psychoses'. *British Journal of Psychiatry*, 118, 381–419.

Kolvin, I. and Fundudis, T. (1981). 'Electively mute children: psychological development and background factors'. *Journal of Child Psychology and Psychiatry*, 22, 219–232.

Kolvin, I., MacKeith, R.C. and Meadows, S.R. (eds) (1973). *Bladder Control and Enuresis*. London: Heinemann.

Kraus, J. (1981). 'Juvenile drug abuse and delinquency: some differential associations'. *British Journal of Psychiatry*, 139, 422–430.

Krupinski, J. *et al.* (1967). 'A community mental health survey of Heyfield, Victoria'. *Medical Journal of Australia*, 1, 1204–1211.

Kushlick, A. (1975). 'The need for residential care of the mentally handicapped'. *British Journal of Hospital Medicine*, 8, 161–167, (Reprinted in *Contemporary Psychiatry*, eds J. Silverstone and B. Barraclough. Ashford, Kent: Headley Bros.)

Lahey, M. and Bloom, L. (1977). 'Planning a first lexicon: which words to teach first'. *Journal of Speech and Hearing Disorders*, 42, 340–369.

Lansdown, R. (1978). 'Retardation in mathematics; a consideration of multifactorial determination'. *Journal of Child Psychology and Psychiatry*, 19, 181–185.

Larson, G., Allison, J. and Johnston, E. (1978). 'Alberta Parent Counsellors: a community treatment programme for disturbed youths'. *Child Welfare*, 57, 47–52.

Laslett, R. (1977). *Educating Maladjusted Children*. London: Crosby Lockwood Staples.

Latvik, N.J. (1977). 'Urban–rural differences in rates of disorder. A comparative psychiatric population study of Norwegian adolescents'. In *Epidemiological Approaches in Child Psychiatry*, pages 223–251, ed. P.J. Graham. London: Academic Press.

Leighton, A. (1965). 'Poverty and social change'. *Scientific American*, 212, No 5, 21–27.

Leissner, A., Powley, T. and Evans, D. (1977). *Intermediate Treatment*. London: National Childrens Bureau (8 Wakley Street, London, EC1V 7QE).

Leslie, S.A. (1974). 'Psychiatric disorders in the young adolescents of an industrial town'. *British Journal of Psychiatry*, 125, 113–124.

Levin, S., Rubenstein, J.S. and Streiner, D.C. (1976). 'The parent–therapist programme: an innovative approach to treating emotionally disturbed children'. *Hospital and Community Psychiatry*, 27, 407–410.

Liebman, R., Minuchin, S. and Baker, L. (1974). 'An integrated treatment program for anorexia nervosa'. *American Journal of Psychiatry*, 131, 432–436.

Linnihan, P.C. (1977). 'Adolescent day treatment'. *American Journal of Orthopsychiatry*, 47, 679–688.

Litt, C.J. (1981). 'Children's attachment to transitional objects'. *American Journal of Orthopsychiatry*, 51, 131–139.

Little, R.E. and Streissgath, A.P. (1981). 'Effects of alcohol on the foetus'. *Canadian Medical Association Journal*, **125**, 159–163.

Livingstone, S. (1972). 'Epilepsy in infancy, childhood and adolescence. In *Manual of Child Psychopathology*, ed. B.J. Wolman. New York: McGraw-Hill.

Lotter, V. (1966). 'Epidemiology of autistic conditions in young children. I Prevalence'. *Social Psychiatry*, **1**, 124–137.

Lotter, V. (1978). 'Childhood autism in Africa'. *Journal of Child Psychology and Psychiatry*, **19**, 231–244.

Lovaas, O.I., Koegel, R., Simmons, J.Q. and Long J.S. (1973). 'Some generalisations and follow-up measures on autistic children in behaviour therapy'. *Journal of Applied Behavioural Analysis*, **6**, 131–166.

Lynch, M.A. (1978). 'The prognosis of child abuse'. *Journal of Child Psychology and Psychiatry*, **19**, 175–180.

McFarlane, L.W., Allen, L. and Honzik, M.P. (1954). *A Development Study of the Behavior Problems of Normal Children between 21 Months and 14 Years*. Berkeley: University of California Press.

MacKeith, R. (1968). 'A frequent factor in the origin of primary enuresis: anxiety in the third year of life'. *Developmental Medicine and Child Neurology*, **10**, 465–470.

Marchant, R., Howlin, P., Yale, W. and Rutter, M. (1974). 'Graded change in the treatment of the behaviour of autistic children'. *Journal of Child Psychology and Psychiatry*, **15**, 221–227.

Martin, H.P. and Beezley, P. (1977). 'The emotional development of abused children'. *Developmental Medicine and Child Neurology*, **19**, 373–387.

Martin, J.A.M. (1980). 'Syndrome delineation in communication disorders'. In *Language and Language Disorders in Children*, eds L.A. Hersov, M. Berger and A.R. Nicol. Oxford and New York: Pergamon.

Martin, P.R. and Lefebvre, A.M. (1981). 'Surgical treatment of sleep-apnoea-associated psychosis'. *Canadian Medical Association Journal*, **124**, 978–980.

Masterson, J.S. (1972). *Treatment of the Borderline Adolescent: Developmental Approach*. New York: Wiley-Inter-Science.

Meiselman, K.C. (1978). *Incest*. San Francisco: Jossey/Bass.

Mendelson, W., Johnson, N. and Stewart, M. (1971). 'Hyperactive children as teenagers'. *Journal of Nervous and Mental Disease*, **153**, 273–279.

Miller, F.J.W., Court, S.D.M., Walton, W.S. and Knox, E.K. (1960). *Growing up in Newcastle-on-Tyne*. Oxford University Press.

Miller, L.C., Barrett, C.C. and Hampe, E. (1974). 'Phobias of childhood in a pre-scientific era'. In *Child Personality and Psychopathology: Current Topics*, ed. A. Davids. New York: Wiley.

Minde, K. and Minde, R. (1981). 'Psychiatric intervention in infancy'. *Journal of the American Academy of Child Psychiatry*, **20**, 217–238.

Minde, K. *et al.* (1980). 'Self-help groups in a premature nursery'. *Journal of Pediatrics*, **96**, 933–940.

Minde, K., Weiss, G. and Mendelson, N. (1972), 'A five-year follow-up study of

91 hyperactive school children'. *Journal of the American Academy of Child Psychiatry*, **11**, 595–610.

Minuchin, S. (1974). *Families and Family Therapy*. Cambridge, Mass: Harvard University Press.

Minuchin, S., Baker, L., Rosman, B.L., Liebman, R., Millman, L. and Todd, T.C. (1975). 'A conceptual model of psychosomatic illness in children'. *Archives of General Psychiatry*, **32**, 1031–1038.

Minuchin, S. and Fishman, H.C. (1981). *Family Therapy Techniques*. Cambridge, Mass: Harvard University Press.

Minuchin, S., Rosman, B.L. and Baker, L. (1978). *Psychosomatic Families: Anorexia Nervosa in Context*. Cambridge, Mass: Harvard University Press.

Morrison, J. and Stewart, M. (1976). 'Bilateral inheritance as evidence for polygenicity in the hyperactive child syndrome'. *Journal of Nervous and Mental Disease*, **158**, 226–228.

New English Bible (1970). Leviticus, Chap. 22, verses 20–22.

Newson, J. and Newson, E. (1968). *Four Years Old in an Urban Community*. London: Allen and Unwin.

Newson, J. and Newson, E. (1976). *Seven Years Old in the Home Environment*. London: Allen and Unwin.

Nielson, J. and Christenson, A.L. (1974). Thirty-five males with double Y chromosome'. *Psychological Medicine*, **4**, 28–37.

Norouha, M.J. (1974). 'Cerebral degenerative disorders of infancy and childhood'. *Developmental Medicine and Child Neurology*, **16**, 228–241.

O'Connor, D.J. (1977). 'Normal and problem drinking among children'. *Journal of Psychology and Psychiatry*, **18**, 279–284.

O'Connor, D.J. (1979). 'A profile of solvent abuse in school children'. *Journal of Child Psychology and Psychiatry*, **20**, 365–368.

O'Leary, K.D. and O'Leary, S.G. (1977). *Classroom Management: The Successful Use of Behaviour Modification*. Elmsford, NY: Pergamon.

Orvaschel, H., Weissman, M.M. and Kidd, K.K. (1980). 'Children and depression'. *Journal of Affective Disorders*, **2**, 1–16.

Osofsky, J.D. (ed.) (1979). *Handbook of Infant Development*. New York: Wiley.

Patterson, G.R. (1975). *Families: Application of Social Learning to Family Life*. Champaign, Ill.: Research Press.

Patterson, G.R. (1976). 'The aggressive child: victim or architect of a coercive system'. In *Behaviour Modification and Families*, eds E.J. Mash, L.A. Hamerlynck and L.C. Handy, New York: Brunner/Mazel.

Penrose, L.S. (1972). *The Biology of Mental Defect*. London: Sidgewick and Jackson.

Philipp, R. (1979). 'Conducting parent training groups: approaches and strategies'. In *New Directions in Children's Mental Health*, ed. S.J. Shamsie, New York: Sp. Medical and Scientific Books.

Pinkerton, P. (1958). 'Psychogenic megacolon in children; the implications of bowel negativism'. *Archives of Disease in Childhood*, **33**, 371–380.

Pinkerton, P. (1974). 'Inpatient treatment of children with psychosomatic disorders'. In *The Residential Psychiatric Treatment of Children*, ed. P. Barker, London: Crosby Lockwood Staples.

Pond, D. (1974). 'Residential psychiatric treatment of children with epilepsy and brain damage'. In *The Residential Psychiatric Treatment of Children*, ed. P. Barker. London: Crosby Lockwood Staples.

Power, M.J., Benn, R.T. and Morri, J.N. (1972). 'Neighbourhood, school and juveniles before the courts'. *British Journal of Criminology*, **12**, 111–132.

Poznanski, E.O. (1982). 'The clinical phenomenology of childhood depression'. *American Journal of Orthopsychiatry*, **52**, 308–313.

Provence, S. and Lipton, R. (1962). *Infants in Institutions*, New York: International Universities Press.

Puig-Antich, J. (1980). 'Affective disorders in childhood'. *Psychiatric Clinics of North America*, **3**, 403–424.

Puig-Antich, J. (1981). 'Antidepressant treatment in children: current state of the evidence'. In *Depression and Antidepressants*, eds E. Friedman and S. Gershon. New York: Raven.

Ramsey, C.V. (1943). 'The sexual development of boys'. *American Journal of Psychology*, **56**, 217–233.

Rantala, S.L. and Petri-Larmi, M. (1976). 'Haloperidol in the treatment of stuttering'. *Folia Phoniatrica*, **28**, 354–361.

Rapoport, J. *et al.* (1978). 'Dextroamphetamine: cognitive and behavioural effects in normal prepubertal boys'. *Science*, **199**, 560–562.

Reed, G.F. (1963). 'Elective mutism in children: a re-appraisal'. *Journal of Child Psychology and Psychiatry*, **4**, 99–107.

Rees, H.M.N. (1974). 'Assessment and treatment of language disordered children'. In *The Residential Psychiatric Treatment of Children*, ed. P. Barker, London: Crosby Lockwood Staples.

Ricciuti, H.N. (1981). 'Developmental consequences of malnutrition in early childhood'. In *The Uncommon Child*, eds M. Lewis and L.A. Rosenblum. New York: Plenum.

Richman, N. (1981a). 'A community survey of characteristics of one to two year olds with sleep disruptions'. *Journal of the American Academy of Child Psychiatry*, **20**, 281–291.

Richman, N. (1981b). 'Sleep problems in young children'. *Archives of Disease in Childhood*, **56**, 491–493.

Richman, N., Stevenson, J.E. and Graham, P.J. (1975). 'Prevalence of behaviour problems in 3-year-old children: an epidemiological study in a London borough'. *Journal of Child Psychology and Psychiatry*, **16**, 277–287.

Rist, K. (1979). 'Incest: theoretical and clinical views'. *American Journal of Orthopsychiatry*, **49**, 680–691.

Rivinus, T.M., Jamison, D.L. and Graham, P.J. (1975). 'Childhood organic neurological disease presenting as psychiatric disorder'. *Archives of Disease in Childhood*, **50**, 115–119.

Robins, L.N. (1966). *Deviant Children Grown Up*. Baltimore: Williams and Wilkins.

Robins, L. (1978). 'Sturdy childhood predictors of adult antisocial behaviour: replications from longitudinal studies'. *Psychological Medicine*, 8, 611–622.

Robinson, H.B. (1981). 'The uncommonly bright child'. In *The Uncommon Child*, eds M. Lewis and L.A. Rosenblum. New York: Plenum.

Rollins, N. and Piazza, E. (1981). 'Anorexia nervosa: a quantitive approach to followup'. *Journal of the American Academy of Child Psychiatry*, 20, 167–183.

Rosenthal, M.J. (1981). 'Sexual differences in the suicidal behaviour of young people'. In *Adolescent Psychiatry*, Vol. 9, eds S.C. Feinstein *et al.* University of Chicago Press.

Rubinstein, J.S. (1977). 'Institutions without walls for emotionally disturbed children'. *Hospital and Community Psychiatry*, 28, 849–851.

Russell, G.F.M. (1977). 'General management of anorexia nervosa and difficulties in assessing the efficacy of treatment'. In *Anorexia Nervosa*, ed. R. Vigersky. New York: Raven.

Russell, G.F.M. (1979). 'Bulimia nervosa: an ominous variety of anorexia nervosa'. *Psychological Medicine*, 9, 429–448.

Rutter, M. (1967a). 'The concept of "dyslexia" '. In *Planning for Better Learning* eds P. Wolff and R.C. MacKeith. London: Heinemann.

Rutter, M. (1967b). 'A children's behaviour questionnaire for completion by teachers: preliminary findings'. *Journal of Child Psychology and Psychiatry*, 8, 1–11.

Rutter, M. (1970a). 'Autistic children: infancy to adulthood'. *Seminars on Psychiatry*, 2, 435–450.

Rutter, M. (1970b). 'A children's behaviour questionnaire for completion by parents'. Appendix 6. In *Education Health and Behaviour*, eds M. Rutter, J. Tizard and M. Whitmore. London: Longman.

Rutter, M. (1971a). 'Psychiatry'. In *Mental Retardation*, Vol 3. New York: Grune and Stratton.

Rutter, M. (1971b). 'Normal psychosexual development'. *Journal of Child Psychology and Psychiatry*, 11, 359–383.

Rutter, M. (1972). *Maternal Deprivation Reassessed*. Harmondsworth: Penguin.

Rutter, M. (1973). 'Why are London children so disturbed?' *Proceedings of the Royal Society of Medicine*, 66, 1221–1225.

Rutter, M. (1976). 'Infantile autism and other child psychoses'. In *Child Psychiatry: Modern Approaches*, eds M. Rutter and L. Hersov. Oxford: Blackwell.

Rutter, M. (1979). 'Invulnerability or why some children are not damaged by stress'. In *New Directions in Children's Mental Health*, ed. S.J. Shamsie. New York: SP. Medical and Scientific Books.

Rutter, M. (1980a). 'School influences on children's behaviour and development'. *Pediatrics*, 65, 208–220.

Rutter, M. (1980b). *Changing Youth in a Changing Society*. Cambridge, Mass.: Harvard University Press.

Rutter, M. (1981). 'The city and the child'. *American Journal of Orthopsychiatry*, 51, 610–625.

Rutter, M. Bartak, L. and Lewman, S.L. (1971). 'Autism a central disorder of cognition and language?' In *Infantile Autism: Concepts, Characteristics and Treatment*, ed. M. Rutter. London: Whitefriars Press.

Rutter, M. and Cox, A. (1981). 'Psychiatric interviewing techniques: 1. Methods and measures'. *British Journal of Psychiatry*, 138, 273–282.

Rutter, M. and Cox, A. *et al.* (1981). 'Psychiatric interviewing techniques IV. Experimental study: four contrasting styles'. *British Journal of Psychiatry*, 138, 456–465.

Rutter, M. and Graham, P. (1968). 'The reliability and validity of the psychiatric assessment of the child: 1. Interview with the child'. *British Journal of Psychiatry*, 114, 563–579.

Rutter, M., Graham, P., Chadwick, O. and Yule, W. (1976). 'Adolescent turmoil; fact or fiction?'. *Journal of Child Psychology and Psychiatry*, 17, 35–56.

Rutter, M., Graham, P. and Yule, W.A. (1970). *A Neuropsychiatric Study in Childhood*. London: Heinemann.

Rutter, M. and Lockyer, L. (1967). 'A 5- to 15-year follow-up of infantile autism and specific developmental receptive language disorder'. *British Journal of Psychiatry*, 126, 127–145.

Rutter, M., Maughan, N., Mortimore, P. and Ouston, J. (1979). *Fifteen Thousand Hours*. London: Open Books.

Rutter, M. and Shaffer, D. (1980). 'DSM–III A step forward or back in terms of the classification of child psychiatric disorders'. *Journal of the American Academy of Child Psychiatry*, 19, 371–394.

Rutter, M., Shaffer, D. and Sturge, C. *A Guide to a Multi-Axial Classification Scheme for Psychiatric Disorders in Childhood and Adolescence*. Dept of Child and Adolescent Psychiatry, Institute of Psychiatry, London, SE8 8AF.

Rutter, M., Tizard, J. and Whitmore, K. (1970). *Education, Health and Behaviour*. London: Longman.

Rutter, M. and Yule, W. (1975). 'The concept of specific reading retardation'. *Journal of Child Psychology and Psychiatry*, 16, 181–197.

Safer, D.J. and Allen, R.P. (1976). *Hyperactive Children: Diagnosis and Management*. Baltimore: University Park Press.

Sallade, J. (1973). 'A comparison of the psychological adjustment of obese *vs.* non-obese children'. *Journal of Psychosomatic Research*, 17, 89–96.

Sarafino, E.P. (1979). 'An estimate of nationwide incidence of sexual offences against children'. *Child Welfare*, 58, 127–134.

Savicki, V. and Brown, R. (1981). *Working With Troubled Children*. New York: Human Sciences Press.

Schinke, S.P., Gilchrist, L.D. and Small, R.W. (1979). 'Preventing unwanted teenage pregnancy'. *American Journal of Orthopsychiatry*, 49, 81–88.

Schmitt, B.D. (1975). 'The minimal brain dysfunction myth'. *American Journal of Diseases of Children*, 129, 1313–1319.

Schofield, M. (1965). *The Sexual Behaviour of Young People*. London: Longmans.

Scott, P.D. (1977). 'Non-accidental injury in children'. *British Journal of Psychiatry*, 131, 366–380.

Sgroi, S.M. (1975). 'Sexual molestation of children'. *Children Today*, **4**, 18–21, May/June. (Reprinted in *Annual Progress in Child Psychiatry and Child Development*, 1976, eds S. Chess and A. Thomas. New York: Brunner/Mazel.)

Shaffer, D. (1974). 'Suicide in childhood and adolescence'. *Journal of Child Psychology and Psychiatry*, **15**, 275–291.

Shaffer, D. (1976). 'Enuresis'. In *Child Psychiatry: Modern Approaches*, eds M. Rutter and L. Hersov. Oxford: Blackwell.

Shaffer, D. and Fisher, P. (1981). 'The epidemiology of suicide in children and adolescents'. *Journal of the American Academy of Child Psychiatry*, **20**, 513–565.

Shaffer, D. and Greenhill, L. (1979). 'A critical note on the predictive validity of "the hyperkinetic syndrome"'. *Journal of Child Psychology and Psychiatry*, **18**, 61–72.

Shepherd, M., Oppenhein, B. and Mitchell, S. (1971). *Child Behaviour and Mental Health*. University of London Press.

Shields, J. (1976). 'Polygenic influences'. In *Child Psychiatry: Modern Approaches*, eds M. Rutter and L. Hersov. Oxford: Blackwell.

Silver, H.K. and Finkelstein, M. (1967). 'Deprivation dwarfism'. *Journal of Paediatrics*, **70**, 317–324.

Simmons, J.E. (1981). *Psychiatric Examination of Children*, 3rd edn. Philadelphia: Lea and Febiger.

Skynner, A.C.R. (1976). *One Flesh: Separate Persons*. London: Constable. (Published in USA as *Systems of Family and Marital Psychotherapy*. New York: Brunner/Mazel.)

Slade, P.D. and Russell, G.F.R. (1971). 'Developmental dyscalculia: a brief report on four cases'. *Psychological Medicine*, **1**, 292–298.

Sluckin, A. (1975). 'Encopresis: a behavioural approach described'. *Social Work Today*, **5**, 643–646.

Spitz, R.A. (1946). 'Anaclitic depression'. *Psychoanalytic Study of the Child*, **2**, 113–117.

Stanley, L. (1980). 'Treatment of ritualistic behaviour in an eight year old girl by response prevention'. *Journal of Child Psychology and Psychiatry*, **21**, 85–90.

Stewart, M.A., de Blois, C.S. and Cummings, C. (1980). 'Psychiatric disorder in the parents of hyperactive boys and those with conduct disorder'. *Journal of Child Psychology and Psychiatry*, **21**, 283–292.

Stott, D.H. (1960). 'The prediction of delinquency from non-delinquent behaviour'. *The Journal of Delinquency*, **10**, 195–210.

Strachan, J.G. (1981). 'Conspicuous firesetting in children'. *British Journal of Psychiatry*, **138**, 26–29.

Sturge, C. (1982). 'Reading retardation and antisocial behaviour'. *Journal of Child Psychology and Psychiatry*, **23**, 21–31.

Sussenwein, F. (1976). 'Psychiatric social work'. In *Child Psychiatry: Modern Approaches*, eds M. Rutter and L. Hersov. Oxford: Blackwell.

Szurek, S.A. and Berlin, I.N. (eds) (1973). *Clinical Studies in Childhood Psychosis*. New York: Brunner/Mazel.

Thomas, A. and Chess, S. (1977). *Temperament and Development*. New York: Brunner/Mazel.

Thomas, A., Chess, S. and Birch, H.G. (1968). *Temperament and Behaviour Disorders in Children*. New York University Press.

Thomlinson, R.J. (1981). 'Behavioural family intervention with the family of a mentally handicapped child'. In *Treating Families with Special Needs*, eds D.S. Freeman and B. Trute. Ottawa: Canadian Association of Social Workers.

Thompson, L.J. (1973). 'Learning disabilities; an overview'. *American Journal of Psychiatry*, **130**, 393–399.

Tizard, J. (1976). 'Nutrition, growth and development'. *Psychological Medicine*, **6**, 1–5.

Torgersen, A.M. (1981). 'Genetic factors in temperamental individuality'. *Journal of the American Academy of Child Psychiatry*, **20**, 702–711.

Torgersen, A.M. and Kringlen, E. (1978). 'Genetic aspects of temperamental differences in infants'. *Journal of the American Academy of Child Psychiatry*, **17**, 433–444.

Turgay, A. (1980). 'Conversion reactions in children'. *Psychiatric Journal of the University of Ottawa*, **5**, 287–294.

Van Buskirk, S.S. (1977). 'A two-phase perspective on the treatment of anorexia nervosa'. *Psychological Bulletin*, **84**, 529–538.

Vandersall, A. and Wiener, J.M. (1970). 'Children who set fires'. *Archives of General Psychiatry*, **22**, 63–71.

von Bertalanffy, L. (1948). *General Systems Theory*. New York: Braziller.

Vorrath, H.H. and Brendthro, L.K. (1976). *Positive Peer Culture*. Chicago: Aldine.

Vrono, M. (1974). 'Schizophrenia in childhood and adolescence'. *International Journal of Mental Health*, **2**, 1–116.

Wagner, B.R. and Breitmeyer, R.G. (1975). 'PACE: a residential, community oriented behaviour modification programme for adolescents'. *Adolescence*, **10**, 277–286.

Walton, J.N., Ellis, E. and Court, S.D.M. (1962). 'Clumsy children: developmental apraxia and agnosia'. *Brain*, **85**, 603–612.

Wardle, C.J. (1961). 'Two generations of broken homes in the genesis of conduct and behaviour disorders in children'. *British Medical Journal*, **2**, 349–354.

Wardle, C.J. (1974). 'Residential care of children with conduct disorders'. In *The Residential Psychiatric Treatment of Children*, ed. P. Barker, London: Crosby Lockwood Staples.

Weiss, G. (1981). 'Controversial issues of the pharmacotherapy of the hyperactive child'. *Candian Journal of Psychiatry*, **26**, 385–392.

Wender, P. (1971). *Minimal Brain Dysfunction in Children*. New York: Wiley.

Werry, J.S. (1972). 'Organic factors in childhood psychopathology.' In *Psychopathological Disorders in Childhood*, eds H.C. Quay and J.S. Werry. New York: Wiley.

Werry, J.S. (1982). 'An overview of pediatric psychopharmacology'. *Journal of the American Academy of Child Psychiatry*, **21**, 3–9.

Werry, J.S., Dowrick, P.W., Lampen, E.L. and Vamos, M.J. (1975). 'Imipramine in enuresis: psychological and physiological effects'. *Journal of Child Psychology and Psychiatry*, **16**, 289–299.

West, D.J. and Farrington, D.P. (1973). *Who Becomes Delinquent?* London: Heinemann.

Whittaker, J.K. (1979). *Caring for Troubled Children*. San Francisco: Jossey-Bass.

Whitten, C.F., Pettit, M.G. and Fischoff, J. (1969). 'Evidence that growth failure from maternal deprivation is secondary to undereating'. *Journal of the American Medical Association*, **209**, 1675–1682.

WHO (1977). *See* World Health Organisation.

Wieder, H. and Kaplan, E.H. (1969). 'Drug use in adolescence: psychodynamic meaning and pharmacogenic effect'. *Psychoanalytic Study of the Child*, **24**, 399–431.

Wiener, J.M. (ed) (1977). *Psychopharmacology in Childhood and Adolescence*. New York: Basic Books.

Wilson, J. (1974) 'Investigation of degenerative disease of the central nervous system'. *Archives of Disease in Childhood*, **47**, 136–170.

Wing, L. (1980). 'Childhood autism and social class; a question of selection?' *British Journal of Psychiatry*, **137**, 410–417.

Wingate, M.E. (1976). *Stuttering: Theory and Treatment*. New York: Irvington.

Winnicott, D. (1960). *The Maturational Process and the Facilitating Environment*. London: Hogarth.

Winnicott, D.W. (1965). *The Family and Individual Development*. London: Tavistock.

Wolff, S. and Barlow, A. (1979). 'Schizoid personality in childhood: a comparative study of schizoid, autistic and normal children'. *Journal of Child Psychology and Psychiatry*, **20**, 29–46.

Wolkind, S.N. (1974). 'Sex differences in the aetiology of antisocial disorder in children'. *British Journal of Psychiatry*, **125**, 125–130.

Wolkind, S. (1981). 'Depression in mothers of young children'. *Archives of Disease in Childhood*, **56**, 1–3.

Wolkind, S. and Rutter, M. (1973). 'Children who have been "in care" – an epidemiological study'. *Journal of Child Psychology and Psychiatry*, **14**, 97–105.

Woodward, J. and Jackson, D. (1961). 'Emotional reactions in burned children and their mothers'. *British Journal of Plastic Surgery*, **13**, 316–324.

World Health Organisation. (1977a). *International Classification of Diseases*. 1975 Revision. Geneva: WHO.

World Health Organisation. (1977b). *Child Mental Health and Psychosocial Development*. Geneva: WHO.

Wynn, A. (1974). 'Health care systems for pre-school children'. *Proceedings of the Royal Society of Medicine*, **67**, 340–343.

Yalom, I. (1975). *The Theory and Practice of Group Psychotherapy*, 2nd edn. New York: Basic Books.

York, P. and York, D. (1980). *Toughlove: A Self Help Manual for Parents Troubled by Teenage Behaviour.* Sellersville, Pennsylvania: Community Service Foundation.

Youngerman, J. and Canino, I. (1978). 'Lithium carbonate use in children and adolescents'. *Archives of General Psychiatry,* **35,** 216–224.

Yule, W. (1967). 'Predicting reading ages on Neal's analysis of reading disability'. *British Journal of Educational Psychology,* **37,** 252–255.

Yule, W. and Carr, J. (eds) (1980). *Behaviour Modification for the Mentally Handicapped.* London: Croom Helm.

Zax, M., Samcroff, A.J. and Babigian, H.M. (1977). 'Birth outcomes in the offspring of mentally disordered women'. *American Journal of Orthopsychiatry,* **47,** 218–230.

Glossary

This glossary is intended primarily for readers who may not have a medical or psychological background. Certain terms which are adequately explained where they occur in the text have been omitted.

Affect Mood. Thus an *affective psychosis* is one in which the primary feature is deviation from normal of the mood (e.g. towards depression).

Agenesis Failure to grow normally.

Amino acid An organic nitrogen-containing compound made up of amino and acidic groups. Proteins are more complex compounds composed of amino acids arranged in various patterns.

Amniotic fluid The liquid surrounding the foetus in the uterus. It is enclosed by a membrane, the *amnion.*

Anal fissure A longitudinal ulcer in the wall of the anal canal. Often causes severe pain on defecation.

Anorexia Loss of appetite.

Antibiotic A drug which controls infections by acting against the causative organisms. An example is penicillin.

Anticonvulsant Acting against or preventing fits, that is any of the varieties of epilepsy.

Anti-Parkinsonian drug A drug which controls the symptoms of Parkinsonism (see below).

Aphonia Inability to phonate normally despite normal articulation, with the result that subject talks in a whisper. Often a hysterical symptom (see Chapter 5).

Apraxia The inability to carry out a purposeful action despite possession of the ability to perform all the individual movements required for the action. The subject cannot synthesise movements to produce the desired result.

Autistic Behaviour controlled by factors within the individual, rather than by the reality situation in which he is living.

Autonomic nervous system A system of nerves supplying heart muscle, blood vessels and certain glands. Affects heart rate, blood pressure and action of glands.

Autosomal To do with those chromosomes not involved in sex determination. An autosomal gene is one carried on any chromosome but a sex chromosome.

Barium enema A special type of X-ray in which a barium compound is given as an enema to show up the rectum (the terminal part of the intestinal canal) and the colon (the part above it) radiographically.

Basophilic stippling The stippling of the red blood cells, shown up on microscopic examination of the cells, suitably stained.

Benzodiazepine The chemical name of a group of substances some of which (e.g. chlordiazepoxide) are thought to have a tranquillising, anxiety-reducing action.

Body-image The view which an individual has of the size, shape and nature of his body. In part this is made up of feelings and ideas of which the subject is not fully consciously aware.

Carbohydrate A group of organic chemical compounds made up of carbon, hydrogen and oxygen atoms arranged in a particular way. An example is glucose. Carbohydrates are very important constituents of the body and of the diet.

Centile Centile ranking puts a series of scores or values in order according to the percentage which occurs at or below each figure. Thus if the heights of a group of children of a certain age are so arranged, the 50th centile will be that height at or below which half of the children's heights fall. Similarly one in ten will fall at or below the 10th centile, and 97 in 100 will be at or below the 97th centile.

Cerebral cortex The outer, surface, layer of the brain. Also known as the grey matter, it is infolded to increase its area. It is vital for many associative mental processes notably those concerned with thought. Incoming neurological messages are also received in the cortex, and outgoing ones (for example those leading to voluntary movements of limbs) originate in it.

Cerebral dominance One or other lateral half of the higher part of the brain (the cerebral cortex) is normally dominant. In right-handed individuals the left cerebral hemisphere (which controls the right side) is thus the dominant one.

Cerebral palsy Weakness of various muscle groups, sometimes widespread and usually present from early in life, due to damage or maldevelopment of the brain. Many forms exist. The muscles are often abnormally stiff and rigid (or 'spastic'), though this is not so in all forms. Cerebral palsied patients are often referred to as *spastics.*

Chelating agent A chemical substance which combines with, and thus inactivates, metallic ions. Such agents are therefore useful in treatment of lead poisoning and also in removing excess copper from the body in hepato-lenticular degeneration.

Chorea A group of conditions in which there are involuntary movements (of face, tongue, limbs, etc.) which consist of parts of normal organised movements. They are not under voluntary control however, and are fragmented, irregular and purposeless. The movements themselves are called *choreiform* movements.

Chromosomes Very small bodies contained in the nuclei of cells. The normal human complement is twenty-three pairs of chromosomes. The chromosomes carry the genetic material responsible for controlling the development of cells and thus of the whole organism.

Cluster analysis A statistical technique which groups together variables which have more in common with each other than with variables in other groups.

Colon The part of the intestine immediately before the rectum. Shorter and of larger diameter than the small intestine which precedes it.

Conditioning A term derived from learning theory. It describes various ways in which human beings and animals can be systematically taught to respond in particular ways to stimuli of one sort or another. In Pavlov's classical experiment a dog was conditioned to salivate by giving food at the same time as a bell was rung; then when the bell only was rung it still salivated — a *conditioned response*. In *operant conditioning* the dog might be put in a position in which it could obtain food by pressing a lever. Doing this at first by chance (or by coaxing) it would learn how the action was rewarded and would thus be conditioned to perform it repeatedly.

Conflict A clash between the demands of reality and those of unconscious drives and feelings. This can lead to anxiety and other
forms of emotional disorder, the cause not being consciously
understood by the subject.

Contingency This refers to the consequences which follow particular
behaviours. In behaviour therapy these are planned so as to bring
about changes in behaviour.

Control group A group of subjects in an experiment, or the investigation of a treatment method, who do not receive the procedure
or treatment under investigation. Normally the control group
should be matched as closely as possible to the *experimental*
group.

Convulsions An alternative term for major epileptic fits, and often
used to describe such fits when they occur in babies and young
children.

Coproporphyrin A breakdown product of haemoglobin, the red
oxygen-carrying substance in the red blood cells.

Cystic fibrosis A disorder affecting various glands in the body. It
causes the mucus secreted by the glands to be abnormally thick so
that, for example, the secretions of the pancreas are abnormal,
causing intestinal symptoms and sometimes death, especially in
babies. Also affects the lungs and other parts of the body.

Defence The process of dealing with feelings such as anxiety or guilt
by means of mental mechanisms such as those described in Chapter 1.

Delirium A state of clouded consciousness with confusion and disorientation, often due to an acute febrile illness or to excessive
doses of drugs acting on the brain. Can also occur in various forms
of acute brain disease.

Dementia The deterioration of intellectual function, usually due to
degeneration of or damage to areas of the brain.

Depression A state of morbid sadness or lowering of mood.

Desensitisation Treating undue sensitivity to a stimulus by carefully
graduated, controlled and increasing exposure to the stimulus.
The latter may be a physical allergen (like pollen in hay fever or
asthma) or an object or situation which causes fear or anxiety (as
in phobic states, see Chapter 5).

Developmental Used in a special sense to describe certain disorders
which are considered to be primarily anomalies of the development of normal function, e.g. speech.

Diabetes In the commonest of this group of diseases, diabetes melli-
tus, the blood sugar level is raised and there are thirst, production
of excess amounts of urine and other serious symptoms. Can be
fatal, but responds to insulin, other drugs and diet.

Dominant In genetics, a dominant trait is one which is manifested
when the factor (or *gene*) concerned is carried on only one of a
pair of chromosomes.
By comparison a *recessive* trait is only manifested when the trait
is carried on both members of a pair of chromosomes.

Echolalia The repetition, inappropriately, of words or phrases
spoken to the subject. In *delayed echolalia*, the repetition occurs
later, perhaps by hours or even days.

Electroencephalograph Often known as an EEG, this is a record of
the variations in electrical potential between different parts of the
brain. Normally a number of channels are recorded simultaneously
using electrodes placed at different points on the skull.

Encephalitis Inflammation of the brain, having a variety of causes.

Encephalopathy Disease of, or affecting the brain.

Endocrine Endocrine glands are those which produce hormones
which circulate in the blood stream to produce various general
effects on the function of the body. Endocrine disorders are those
in which the functioning of these glands, or of the hormones they
produce, is abnormal.

Enema The introduction of a liquid into the rectum, usually to
promote the evacuation of faeces.

Enzyme Enzymes are complex chemical substances with the role of
enabling particular chemical reactions to take place in the body.
Numerous enzymes are known to exist, facilitating a vast number of
chemical processes needed for the normal functioning of the body.

Fantasy The production of mental images to provide gratification or
satisfaction often not obtainable in reality. The term *fantasy* is
also often used for the images themselves.

Gene penetrance Refers to the proportion of individuals in whom a
gene has an effect. If a dominant gene has an effect in every
individual carrying it, penetrance is 100 per cent. If only a proportion of the individuals are affected the penetrance is less and is
expressed as the percentage of individuals who are affected.

Hallucination The subjective experience of a sensory perception not
arising in the external world. Thus auditory hallucinations may
take the form of hearing voices when no one is actually speaking;

and visual hallucinations of seeing things which in reality are not there.

Hemiplegia Paralysis, often with stiffness and increased tone, of the muscles, affecting one half (left or right) of the body. Due to a neurological disorder involving the opposite side of the brain, or spinal cord.

Hormone Substance produced by an endocrine gland (see above), to circulate in the blood stream and carry out its particular function.

Hyperkinesis Excessive motor activity, with little apparent purpose.

Hypochondriasis Excessive preoccupation with physical symptoms, often seen in unduly anxious individuals.

Hypomania A milder form of mania (see below).

Ideas of reference An idea of reference is the belief that something in the subject's environment or experience refers to the subject when in fact it does not. Chance remarks, glances, gestures, advertisements, statements on radio or television and almost anything else may be regarded in this way.

Identification The acquisition of the views and attitudes of another person as a result of a close, usually loving or admiring, relationship with that person.

Illusion A false perception of reality, as when sensory data are misinterpreted. By contrast a *delusion* is a false belief held in spite of evidence to the contrary.

Infection A disease caused by the establishment and multiplication in the body of organisms such as bacteria or viruses.

Institutionalisation The effects upon individuals of a prolonged period of living in the impersonal atmosphere of an institution. Characterised by overdependence on the staff, loss of initiative and a progressive inability to cope with life in the outside world.

IQ Intelligence quotient. See Chapter 14.

Maladjusted Primarily an administrative, educational term used to describe a group of children requiring a certain special type of educational provision. Also sometimes used, loosely, to describe any child who is emotionally disturbed in one way or another.

Malocclusion The condition that exists when the teeth do not meet in the most efficient way.

Mania A state of excitement, euphoria, excessive activity and impaired judgement. The opposite of depression.

Meningitis Inflammation of the meninges, the membranes covering the brain and spinal cord.

Metabolic Metabolism is the process whereby substances entering the body are processed, used in various ways, and their breakdown products excreted from the body. Metabolic processes are those concerned with this, and metabolic disorders are those in which some of the processes are not functioning normally.

Micturition The passage of urine.

Mutism Emotionally determined refusal to speak despite the physical capacity to do so.

Myelin A substance forming the sheaths of nerves. Loss of their myelin sheaths causes failure of the function of nerves, as in *demyelinating diseases.*

Neurological To do with the nervous system, that is the brain and spinal cord, and the nerves connected with them.

Nystagmus Repeated, quick to-and-fro movements of the eyes.

Organic To do with the physical structures of the body. Thus an *organic disease* is one in which there is demonstrable physical abnormality of the parts or organs involved.

Otologist A specialist in disorders of the ear and of hearing.

Palpitation The sensation of rapid beating of the heart.

Parkinsonism A condition in which there is muscular rigidity, tremor which is worse on voluntary movement and weakness of voluntary movements. The muscles of the face and also those responsible for speech may be affected as well as the limb muscles. Usually due to damage to or disease of certain structures in the base of the brain. Can also be caused as a side-effect of various drugs used in psychiatry.

Peptic ulcer A form of ulceration of the inside of the wall of the stomach or the duodenum (the part of the alimentary tract into which the stomach leads).

Phenothiazine The generic name of a group of drugs used to control some form of psychotic behaviour (notably schizophrenia). They are also used as tranquillisers for other conditions, and have other medical uses. The first one brought into clinical use was chlorpromazine, but many others are now available.

Phobia An irrational fear.

Photophobia A dislike, and often active avoidance, of light. Occurs in certain brain diseases, e.g. encephalitis and meningitis.

Plasma The clear yellowish liquid in which the blood cells are suspended.

Projection A term used in psychology for ideas arising from within an individual which are attributed to some other person or object. (See also Chapter 1).

Psychiatrist A medically qualified practitioner who has specialised in the study and treatment of patients with disorders affecting the mind.

Psychologist A person with training and expertise in the scientific study of behaviour. Psychologist are non-medical graduates who, after their university course, often do further training in their special branch of psychology. Clinical and educational psychologists are those mainly concerned in child psychiatry.

Psychopathology The abnormalities of the mind, often mainly unconscious, responsible for or associated with mental and emotional disorders.

Pyloric stenosis Obstruction at the lower end of the stomach, where it joins the duodenum. Can be a congenital disorder requiring operative treatment in the early days or weeks of life.

Recessive See under *Dominant.*

Reference See *Ideas of reference.*

Regression The reversion to a mode of behaviour and/or an emotional state appropriate to a younger age.

Rubella German measles.

Spastic Showing increased muscle tone. People suffering from cerebral palsy are sometimes referred to as 'spastics' because of the increased tone which is a feature of many forms of the condition.

Spina bifida In this condition there is a defect in the vertebral column, and often also in the underlying spinal cord. May be symptomless in mild cases, or may cause mild or severe neurological disorders.

Standard deviation A measure of the scatter of a series of values round the mean. The amounts by which each of the values differs from the mean are taken and each is squared. The square root of the mean of these squares is the standard deviation. In practice the following formula is used.

$$SD = \sqrt{\frac{\Sigma \, (\Upsilon - \bar{\Upsilon})^2}{n - 1}}$$

where *n* is the number of values of the measurement, Υ; $\bar{\Upsilon}$ is the mean of all the values of Υ and Σ signifies 'the sum of'.

Subarachnoid haemorrhage Bleeding from one of the arteries lying beneath the arachnoid membrane, which covers the surface of the brain. Is often due to a congenital aneurysm (or saccular swelling) on the artery.

Subdural haematoma An accumulation of blood resulting from bleeding underneath the dura, a membrane covering the brain, superficial to the arachnoid. Subdural haemorrhage often develops slowly following a head injury.

Sublimation The expression through socially acceptable behaviour of drives, where the direct expression would be unacceptable.

Suppository A solid preparation of a drug for rectal administration.

Syphilis A venereal disease due to an organism, *Treponema pallidum*. In its later stages it can affect the central nervous system and cause dementia and other abnormalities.

Systemic infection An infection affecting the body as a whole.

Temporal lobe One of the areas of the cortex of the brain. The temporal lobes are situated in the lower, lateral parts of each cerebral hemisphere.

Toxaemia The presence in the circulating blood, and thus in the body tissues generally, of harmful substances (toxins) formed by infective agents like bacteria or viruses, or produced in the body cells as a result of a disease, injury or other disorder.

Toxoplasmosis A disease due to protozoal organisms (*Toxoplasma*) affecting muscle fibres and other cells.

Tranquilliser A drug with the primary action of reducing anxiety and tension or quietening disturbed, restless, aggressive or psychotic behaviour.

Tricyclic Tricyclic antidepressants are so called because of their chemical structure. The first of the modern antidepressant drugs to be brought into use was a tricyclic compound, imipramine, and several other related drugs are now also in use.

Truancy The wilful avoidance of school.

Urethra The passage leading from the bladder to the exterior, for the passage of urine and also, in the male, seminal fluid.

Index

Abused children, 186
Access disputes, 239–240
Accident prevention, 272
Accidents, 270
Accommodation, 248
Adams, P.L., 82, 244
Adaptive functioning, 36
Adjustment disorders/reactions, 85,
    122, 139–142, 171
Adolescence, disorders in, 200–216
Adolescent conduct disorders, 206–211
Adolescent development, 12–16
Adolescent drug taking, 207–211
Adolescent gangs, 64, 205
Adolescent groups, 205–206
Adolescent turmoil, 15, 204
Adolescent Psychiatry, 213
Adrenocorticotrophic hormone, 107
Affective disorders/psychoses, 95,
    114–119, 211, 212–213
  causes, 115
  description, 115–117
  outcome, 119
  treatment, 117
Affective involvement, 53, 63
Affective problems, 51
Affective responsiveness, 52–53
Aggressive behaviour, 62, 64, 65–66,
    144, 157, 160, 202, 254, 260
Agoraphobia, 74, 79, 80
Akinetic attacks, 157
Albee, G.W., 269, 176
Alberta Parent Counsellors, 263
Alcoholism, 270
Alcohol use/abuse, 117, 208–210

Allen, F.H., 244
Allen, R.P., 135, 136
Allergy, 176, 178, 180
Alternative families, 241, 263–264
Amaurotic family idiocy, 109
American Psychiatric Association, 35,
    58, 73, 95, 121, 134, 139, 161,
    181, *see also* DSM-III
Amini, F., 209
Amitriptyline, 124, 127, 256, 258
Amniocentesis, 270, 272
Amphetamine drugs, 120, 137, 207,
    209, 210, 255
Anaclitic depression, 116–117
Anaemia, 108, 190
Anastasi, A., 226
Anders, T.F., 189
Anderson, L.M., 238
Andrews, K., 153
Anorexia nervosa, 90, 173, 175,
    181–183, 190, 254, 260
Anthony, E.J., 129
Anticipatory anxiety, 153
Anticipatory guidance, 274
Anticonvulsant drugs, 160, 255, 256
Antidepressant drugs, 117, 215, 256
Anti-Parkinsonian drugs, 109
Antisocial behaviour, 118, 136, 137,
    138, 160, 163, *see also* Conduct
    disorders
Anxiety disorders/states, 73, 74,
    78–79, 211
Anxiolytics, 256
APA, *see* American Psychiatric
    Association

Aphonia, 84
Approved schools, 267
Apraxia, 171
Archipeligo children, 143
Arithmetic tests, 221—222
Articulation disorders, 169—171
Asperger, H., 143
Assessing children, 39
Asthma, 172, 173, 175, 175—178,
     180, 181, 195
Atropine, 120
Attachment behaviour, 2—3, 4, 10
Attainment tests, 221—222
Attention deficit disorder, 134—138
Atypical anxiety disorder, 74
Atypical developmental disorder, 161
Audiometry, 169
Audiophonic difficulties, 164
Australia, epidemiological studies in, 38
Autism, *see* Infantile autism
Autistic aloneness, 98—99
Autistic psychopathy of childhood, 143
Auto-immune reactions, 178
Autonomy versus shame, 4
Avoidant disorder, 73, 79
Awad, G., 239

Bagley, C., 157
Bakwin, H., 122
Balbernie, R., 61, 142, 143, 150
Baldwin, J.A., 233
Bandler, R., 245
Barbiturates, 207, 209, 210
Barium enema, 132
Barker, P., 16, 27, 35, 42, 48, 72, 92,
     107, 111, 114, 245, 247, 256,
     260, 262, 263, 274
Barlow, A., 143, 144
Barnhill, L.H., 18—19
Bartak, L., 99
Basic Family Therapy, 48, 114, 247,
     248
Basic trust, 2
Battered child syndrome, 233
Bayley Scales of Infant Development,
     186, 219—220
Beard, R.M., 1, 3, 12, 15
Bedwetting, *see* Enuresis
Beezley, P., 235
Behavioural adjustment, in pre-school
     children, 186
Behavioural styles, 2

Behaviour control (in families), 53—54
Behaviour, disorders, 194, 196, *see*
     also Conduct disorders
     drug treatment of, 256
Behaviour therapy, 241, 252—255
     for tics, 152
     in autism, 103—104
     in conduct disorders, 71
     in elective mutism, 156
     in encopresis, 133
     in enuresis, 124—127
     in hyperkinesis, 137
     with mentally retarded children,
          197—198
Belle indifférence, 84
Bellman, M., 128, 134
Bender Visual Motor Gestalt Test, 225
Bender, L., 82
Bene—Anthony Family Relations Test,
     223
Benzodiazepine drugs, 91
Benztropine, 109
Berecz, J.M., 80
Berg, I., 123
Berger, M., 162, 163
Berlin, I., 103
Berney, T., 90, 91
Berry Visual Motor Test, 225
Bever, T.G., 167
Bhanji, S., 182
Bicknell, J., 191, 195
Birch, H.G., 26
Bille, B., 178
Biller, H.B., 62
Binge eating, 182
Bipolar affective disorder, 114, 212,
     258
Birmingham, England, epidemiological
     study in, 154
Birth injury, 22
Birth trauma, 270
Blackburn, epidemiological studies in,
     38, 75
Bloom, L., 169
Blueprint for Survival, 277
Blumberg, H., 207
Boatman, B., 238
Bommarito, J.W., 226
Bonding, 1, 2—3, 60—61
Borderline states/personality, 144, 145
Bornstein, P.H., 254
Bower, D., 107

Bowlby, J., 1, 2, 4, 10, 30, 61
Bradley, S., 154
Brain damage/injury, 23, 97, 106—110, 119, 153, 158, 159, 173, 190, 191, 194, 195—196
  drug treatment in, 256
  in child abuse cases, 235, 237
Brain disorder, 225
Brannigan, C., 103
Breath-holding spells, 191
Breitmeyer, R.G., 254
Brendthro, L.K., 71, 261
Bridgland, M., 264
Bright children, 22
Bristol Social Adjustment Guide, 23, 223, 275
British Child Development Study, 23
British Medical Journal, 121
Broderick, C.B., 10
Broken homes, 62, 115
Bronchial asthma, *see* Asthma
Bronfenbrenner, V., 278
Brown, B., 154, 155, 156
Brown, G.W., 30
Brown, R., 47
Brown, S.L., 27
Brownies, 11
Bruch, H., 181
Bulimia, 182
Burquest, B., 214
Busch, F., 9
Buzzer ulcers, 127

Cade, B., 244
Caffey, J., 233
Cameron, J.R., 25
Canadian Tests of Basic Skills, 221
Canino, I., 259
Cannabis, 120
Cantwell, D., 255
Capes, M., 203
Caplan, G., 268, 269, 274, 275
Caplan, H.L., 83
Care Can Prevent, 274
Caretaker self/selves, 143
Caring for Troubled Children, 262
Carr, J., 198
Carter, E.A., 16
Castration fears, 6
Catell's Children's Personality Questionnaire, 224
  lipidosis, 102

Cerebral palsy, 170
Chamberlain, C., 239
Changing Youth in a Changing Society, 200
Character-disordered family, 238
Chazen, R., 262
Chelating agents, 108
Chess, S., 2, 22, 26, 61
Child abuse, 233—237
  assessment, 235
  causation, 233—234
  clinical features, 234—235
  epidemiology, 233
  outcome, 237
  prevention, 237
  treatment, 235—237
  welfare agencies, 227, 236, 262, 265—267, 271
  X-rays in, 233, 234, 235
Childhood Disorder: A Psychosomatic Approach, 174
Childhood schizophrenia, 95
Child Mental Health and Psychosocial Development, 271
Children's Aid Societies, 227
Children's Apperception Test, 222
Children's hearings, 227
Children's homes, 266
Chloral, 259
Chlordiazepoxide, 91, 257
Chlorpromazine, 114, 183, 255, 256, 257, 259
Christenson, A.L., 21
Chromosome abnormalities, 21
Cigarettes, 209, 210
Classification of disorders, 32—37
Cleveland, Ohio, 9
Clomipramine, 91
Clumsy children, 171, 225
Clutter, 153
Cocaine, 120, 207, 209, 211
Cohen, D.J., 97, 151
Cohen, I.L., 104
Communication (in families), 52, 63
Community homes, 267
Community workers, 247
Compensation, 7
Compulsions, 8, 80—82
Concrete operations, 5, 10, 12
Conditioning, 253
  in developmental language disorders, 169

in enuresis, 124–127
Conduct disorders, 22, 58–72, 157
  causes, 60–64
  definitions, 58
  description, 64–69
  in adolescence, 202–203, 204
  outcome, 72
  prevelance, 60
  treatment, 69–72, 261–262
  types, 58–59
Conflict avoidance, 174, 175
Conflict resolution, 174, 182
Confusion states, 95, 119–120
Congenital auditory imperception, 169
Congenital heart conditions, 173
Congenital syphilis, 270
Connell, P., 119
Conscience formation, 5, 6–7, 11–12,
  206
Constipation, *see* Encopresis
Constitutional factors, 20–23, 61
Conversion disorder/hysteria, 74, 83
Convulsions, 120
Coolidge, J.C., 202
Co-operative play, 12
Coping skills, 271, 275
Coprolalia, 152
Coproporphyrin, 108
Corbett, J., 151
Cordoza, V.G., 273
Correctional schools, 266
Cortical blindness, 109
Cotswold Community, 150
Court reports, 228–232
Cox, A., 42
Creak, M., 109
Credit counsellors, 247
Crime, 31, 277
Crisp, A., 181
Crome, L., 195
Cub scouts, 11
Cultural deprivation, 270, 272–273
Custody disputes, 239–240
Cystic fibrosis, 173

Dale, P.S., 167
Davison, K., 212, 215, 259
Day care, 192, 247
Daypatient treatment, 241, 262–263
Deafness, 102, 168
Defence mechanisms, 7–9, 11–12, 77

Delinquency, 22, 31, 64, 65, 66, 68,
  116, 202, 208, 209, 266, 277
Delinquent behaviour, 254
Delinquent neighbourhoods, 62
Delirium, 119–120
Delusional perception, 113
Delusions, 112
Dementia, 95
Dementia infantilis, 110
Demyelination, 109
Department of Health and Social
  Security, 150
Dependence/independence conflict,
  204
Depersonalisation/depersonalisation
  disorder, 74, 85
Depression, 31, 70, 72, 89, 114–119,
  178, 181, 189
  drug treatment of, 256–258
  in adolescence, 201, 209, 211,
  212–214, 215
  neurotic, 85–87
Depressive equivalents, 116
Deprivation
  cultural, 179, 272–273
  emotional, 194, 215
  physical, 194
  sensory, 168
Deprivation dwarfism, 179
Deprived children, 72
Derealisation, 85
Desmethylimipramine, 258
De-urbanisation, 277
Developmental apraxia, 171
Developmental arithmetic disorder,
  161
Development articulation disorder,
  161
Developmental dyslexia, 164
Developmental history, 42
Developmental language disorders,
  102, 103, 161, 165–169, 265
Developmental reading disorder, 161,
  162–164, 171
Dextroamphetamine/dexampheta-
  mine, 137, 257
Diabetes, 122, 173, 175, 195
Diagnostic and Statistical Manual,
  see DSM-III
Diarrhoea, 130, 178
Diazepam, 91, 188, 257
Dichloralphenazone, 259

Difficult children, 25
Diffuse cerebral sclerosis, 109
Dische, S., 124
Disengagement, 28, 50
Disintegrative psychosis, 95, 97,
    105–111
    causes, 106
    descriptions, 106–110
    outcome, 111
    treatment, 110–111
Disobedience, 64
Displacement, 7, 79
Dissociative disorders/states, 74, 83,
    85
Dockar-Drysdale, B., 61, 142, 150
Dopamine, 51
Down's syndrome, 21
Draw-a-Person Test, 222–223
Drillien, C.M., 22
Driscoll, J.M., 22
Drop attacks, 157
Drug abuse, 65, 117, 120, 207–211
Drug treatment, 72, 104, 241,
    255–260
    for mentally retarded children, 198
DSM-III. 35–37, 56–57, 58–59, 64,
    68, 73–74, 78, 79, 80, 83, 85,
    87, 90, 95, 98, 100, 102, 103,
    106, 114, 115, 116, 117, 121,
    134, 135, 138, 139, 140, 144,
    146, 148, 149, 161, 167, 169,
    182
Duncan, D.P., 207
Duration of disorders, 269
Duvall, E.M., 16, 17–18
Dwarfism, 179
Dysarthria, 170, *see also* Articulation
    disorders
Dysfunctional families, 28–30, 63,
    234
Dyslexia, 164
Dysthymic disorder, 87

Earls, F., 185, 186
Early infantile autism, *see* Infantile
    autism
Early intervention programmes, 192
Easy children, 25
Echolalia, 99, 103
Eczema, 173, 174, 176
Edinburgh children, 22

Educational attainment tests, 217,
    221–222
Educational measures, 241, 264–265
Ego integrity versus despair, 16
Eisenberg, L., 162
Ekstein, R., 144
Elective mutism, 90, 144, 147,
    154–156
Elkins, R., 82
Emergency feelings, 53
Emotional disorders, 73, *see also*
    Neurotic disorders
Emotional maturity, 75
Encephalitis, 107
Encopresis, 127–134, 155, 161, 194
Enmeshment, 28, 50, 175, 182
Enuresis, 121–127, 155, 161, 184,
    185
    causes, 122
    investigation, 123–124
    outcome, 127
    prevalence, 121–122
    treatment, 123–127, 254, 258
Environmental changes, 246–247
Environmental factors, 20, 26–32, 61,
    194
Epidemiology, 269
Epilepsy/epileptic children, 61, 72,
    119, 122, 157–160, 173, 188,
    190, 191
    in autistic children, 97
    in disintegrative psychoses, 110
    in mentally retarded children,
        195–196, 198
    treatment, 160, 255, 256
Epiloia, 108
Erickson, M., 245
Erikson, E.E., 1, 2, 4, 5, 11, 13, 16
Examining the child, 42–48
Eyman, R.K., 195
Eysenck, H.J., 76

False self/selves, 143, 148
Family
    break-up, 277
    care programme, 263
    development, 1, 16–19
    disharmony, 270, 272
    functions, 52
    homeostasis, 174
    mediation, 239–240
    Service Agencies, 227

service units, 276
structure, 50
systems, 17, 27–30, 48–54
therapy, 241, 247–251
   and child abuse, 236, 238
   for adolescent disorders,
     214, 215
   for young children's disorders,
     192
   in conduct disorders, 70
   in elective mutism, 156
   in food refusal, 190
   with mentally retarded
     children, 197
   transition points, 18–19
Fantasy/fantasies, 8, 120, 244
Farrington, D.P., 202, 274
Father absence, 62
Faust, R., 209
Fears, irrational, 77
Feeding problems, 189–190
Finger-sucking, 191
Finkelstein, M., 179
Fire-setting, 68–69
First year, 2–3
Fish, B., 112
Fisher, C., 188
Fisher, P., 118, 213
Fishman, C., 248
Fixation points, 76
Flavell, J.H., 1
Fleck, S., 17
Fluphenazine, 114, 256, 257
Focal epilepsy, 157
Foetal alcohol syndrome, 23
Folstein, S., 96
Food fads, 190
Food refusal, 189
Forgays, D.G., 269
Formal operations, 12, 15
Formulation, diagnostic, 54–56
Foster care workers, 263
Foster homes/parents, 262, 266
Four Years Old in an Urban Community, 186
Frankl, V.E., 245
French, A., 28
Freud, A., 1, 76, 243
Freud, S., 1
Frostig Test of Developmental
   Perception, 225
Frozen children, 143

Fugue, psychogenic/hysterical, 85
Fundudis, T., 154, 156

Gaensbauer, T.J., 186, 187
Garfinkel, B., 118
Garside, R., 11
Gates–MacGintie Reading Tests, 221
Gaze avoidance, 99
Geleerd, E.R., 144
Generalised anxiety disorder, 74, 79
General reading retardation, 162
General systems theory, 27
Generativity versus stagnation, 16
Genetic counselling, 272
Genetic factors in primary prevention,
   269–270
Genital stage, 5
Gesell Developmental Schedule, 220
Gibbens, T., 232
Gibbs, J.T., 208
Gifted children, 22
Gil, D.G., 234
Gilles de la Tourette's syndrome, 151,
   152
Ginott, H.G., 251
Gittelman-Klein, R., 91
Gliosos, 109
Glue sniffing, 210–211
Goetz, P.C., 183
Gold, J., 262
Goldsmith, E., 277
Golumbek, H., 118
Goodman, J.D., 48
Gordon, D., 245
Graham, P., 48, 85, 116, 194
Grand mal, 157
Greenberg, L.M., 152
Greenhill, L., 135
Griffiths Mental Development Scale,
   219
Grinder, J., 245
Grinker, J.A., 179
Group delinquent reaction, 64
Group for the Advancement of
   Psychiatry, 13, 15
Group homes, 266
Group tests, 225–226
Group therapy, 71, 134, 241,
   251–252
Gruber, A.R., 69
Gualtieri, C.T., 255

Gubbay, S.S., 172
Guilleminault, C., 189

Habit spasms, 151
Hack, M., 22
Haley, J., 28, 49, 214, 245
Hallucinations, 112, 113, 114, 120
Hallucinogens, 207, 210
Haloperidol, 104, 110, 114, 137,
    152, 154, 198, 255, 256, 257
Hamburg, B.A., 209
Harlow, H.F., 3
Harmon, R.J., 186, 187
Harris, M., 153
Hartsough, C.S., 136
Hashish, 210
Hassanyeh, F., 212, 215, 259
Hawton, K., 213
Hazel, N., 72, 263
Head-banging, 100, 198
Head injury, 173
Health visitors, 276
Hechtman, L., 138, 203
Heller's syndrome, 110
Help for Parents, 241, 246—247
Hemiplegia, 196
Hemispherectomy, 196
Henderson, A.S., 201
Hepatitis, 209
Hermelin, B., 102
Heroin, 120, 209
Hersov, L., 73, 88, 203
Hirschprung's disease, 129, 132
History taking, 39—42
Hoag, J.M., 129, 134
Hoefler, S.A., 254
Holbrook, D., 42
Home Office, 267
Homeostasis, 28, 249
Hopkinson, K., 42
Hostels, 266
Housebreaking, 64
House—Tree—Person Test, 223
Howells, J.G., 184
Humphries, T., 137
Hundleby, J.D., 209
Huntington's chorea, 109
Hyperactivity, 184, 195, *see also*
    Hyperkinetic syndrome
    in adolescence, 203
Hyperkinetic syndrome/behaviour,
    65, 72, 134—138, 161

drug treatment, 255—256
    in adolescence, 203
Hypervigilance, 235
Hypnagogic hallucinations, 189
Hypochondriacal disorder/neurosis,
    74
Hysterical aphonia, 84
Hysterical disorder/neurosis, 74, 78,
    181, 211
Hysterical-manipulative patients,
    183

ICD-9, 64, 69, 73, 78, 79, 85, 94—95,
    97, 105, 121, 134, 139, 144,
    145, 146, 149, 161
Identification, 5, 6
Identity versus role confusion, 13
Illinois Test of Psycholinguistic
    Abilities, 224
Imaginary playmates, 8
Imipramine, 91, 117—118, 124, 127,
    256—258, 258
    adverse effects, 258
Impulsions, 82
Impulsive behaviour, 256
Incest, 237—239
Incest, 239
Incidence of disorders, 269
Individual psychotherapy, 241—246
    in conduct disorders, 71
Industry versus inferiority, 11
Infantile autism, 95—105, 184
    and mental retardation, 195
    causes, 96—98
    description, 98—103
    drug treatment of, 259
    outcome, 105
    prevalence, 96
    residual state, 103, 105
    treatment of, 103—105
Infantile eczema, 173
Infantile myoclonic epilepsy, 107
Infantile psychosis, 95, 96
Infantile spasms, 107
Infant psychiatry, 184—192
Infectious diseases, 272
Ingram, T.T.S., 163
Inhalants, 207
Initiative versus guilt, 5
Inpatient treatment, 241, 260—262
Institute of Psychiatry, London, 33
Institutional care, 197

Institutionalisation, 196
Instrumental problems, 51
Insulin, 183
Intelligence in infantile autism, 105
Intelligence quotient, 162
Intelligence tests/testing, 217–221
Intermediate treatment, 274
Intermediate Treatment, 274
International Classification of Diseases, 33, 58, *see also* ICD-9
Interpretations, 243, 244
Intervening variables, 269
Interviewing parents, 39–42
Intimacy versus isolation, 16
Intuitive sub-stage, 10, 12
IQ, *see* Intelligence quotient
Irving, H., 239
Isle of Wight study, 14–15, 23–24, 38, 60, 66, 69, 75, 116, 128, 135, 162, 193, 194, 195, 196

Jalali, B., 207
Jeavons, P., 107
Jenkins, R.L., 64
Joffe, J.M., 269
Joining in family therapy, 248
Journal of the American Academy of Child Psychiatry, 184
Justice, B., 207

Kandel, D., 209
Kanner, L., 95, 97, 98
Kaplan, E.H., 215
Keith, P.R., 188
Kempe, C.H., 233
Kendall, R.E., 112
Kennedy, W.A., 92
Kent Family Placement Project, 263
Kent, M.W., 269
Kessler, M., 276
Kinard, E.M., 236
Kindergarten, 9
King, R.D., 196, 266
Kirman, B., 195
Klein, D.F., 91
Klein, M., 1, 243
Knight's move, 112
Kolvin, I., 96, 98, 121, 123, 154, 156
Kraus, J., 65
Kringlen, E., 22
Krupinski, J., 38, 201
Kushlick, A., 193

Lahey, M., 169
Lambert, N.H., 136
Language development, 165–167, 184
Language Development: Structure and Function, 167
Language disorder, 167–169, 170
in autism, 98, 99
Lansdown, R., 165
Large family size, 271
Larsen, G., 263
Latency period, 10
Late-onset psychosis, 111, 259
Latvik, N.J., 201
Laxatives, 133
Lead poisoning/encephalopathy, 108, 190–191, 270
Learning disorder(s)/problems, 32, 136, 138, 144
Learning theory, 246, 252
Lefebvre, A., 189
Leighton, A., 272, 273
Leissner, A., 274
Leslie, S., 38, 60, 75, 201
Levin, S., 263
Liedman, R., 181
Limit setting, 242
Lincoln–Oseretsky Motor Development Scale, 225
Linnihan, P.C., 262
Lipidoses, 109
Lipton, R., 9
Lithium carbonate, 215, 258–259
Litt, C.J., 9
Little, R.E., 23
Livingstone, S., 191
Lloyd, H., 154, 155
Lockyer, L., 98
London, epidemiological studies in, 38, 75, 96, 162, 185
Longo, D., 18–19
Lormier, B.M., 239
Lotter, V., 96
Lovaas, O.I., 103, 104
LSD, *see* Lysergic acid diethylamide
Lynch, M.A., 237
Lysergic acid diethylamide, 120, 207, 209, 210

MacKeith, R., 122
Maintenance, 248
Major depression/depressive disorder, 115–116, 257

Major epilepsy, 157
Malnutrition, 24, 194
Mania, 114, 212, 259
Manic-depressive disorder/psychosis,
    85, 114, 115, 212, 215
    treatment of, 159
Marchant, R., 100
Marijuana, 207, 208, 209, 210
Martin, H.P., 235
Martin, J.A.M., 167
Martin, P.R., 189
Masterson, J.S., 144
Masturbation, 6, 10, 14, 66, 191
Maternal depression, 30
Maternal deprivation, 30
Mathematical retardation, 165
Mattingly, D., 182
Maudsley Hospital, London, 42, 83,
    151, 152
MBD, *see* Minimal brain damage/
    dysfunction
McFarlane, L.W., 201
McGoldrick, M., 16
McMaster model of family functioning,
    51–54
Meiselman, K.C., 238
Mendelson, W., 203
Meningitis, 119
Mental handicap/retardation, 153,
    168, 172, 190, 193–199
    and autism, 94, 98, 102
    causes, 194–196
    prevalence of emotional disorders
        in, 193–194
    prevention of, 268, 270
    treatment of emotional disorders
        in, 196–199
Mental mechanisms, *see* Defence
    mechanisms
Merrill–Palmer Scale, 219
Metachromatic leukodystrophy, 109
Methylphenidate, 137, 198, 255–256,
    257
Middle childhood, 10–12
Middlesex, epidemiological study in,
    96
Migrane, 173, 174, 178, 179
Miller, F.J.W., 185
Miller, L.C., 80
Mimesis, 248
Minde, K., 184, 192, 203
Minde, R., 184, 192

Minimal brain damage/dysfunction,
    136
Minor epilepsy, 157
Minuchin, S., 18, 28, 49, 49–50, 174,
    175, 182, 183, 248
Mixed developmental disorder, 161,
    172
Mixed disturbance of conduct and
    emotions, 69
Mongolism, *see* Down's syndrome
Morrison, J., 135
Mulberry Bush School, 149–150
Multiaxial systems (of classification),
    32–33, 56
Multiple personality, 74, 85
Multiproblem family, 238

Nail-biting, 191–192, 195
National Children's Bureau, 277
Neale Analysis of Reading Ability, 221
Negative reinforcement, 254
Neurolinguistic programming,
    245–246
Neurotic–depressive disorders, 78,
    85–87
Neurotic disorders/symptoms, 73–93,
    153, 188
    causes, 73
    classification, 73–74
    definition, 73
    description, 77–90
    in adolescence, 201–202, 204
    prevalence, 75
Newcastle-on-Tyne, epidemiological
    study in, 154, 185
New Jersey schools, 207
Newson, J. and E., 62, 186
New York longitudinal study, 25
Nielson, G., 21
Nightmares, 188
Night terrors, 187–188
NLP, 245–246
Non-accidental injury, 233, *see also*
    Child abuse
Non-retentive soiling, 130–131
Norouha, M.J., 106
Nursery school, 9

Obesity, 173, 179–180
Obsessions/obsessional ideas, 8

Obsessive—compulsive disorder/
    neurosis, 74, 78, 80—82, 211,
    252
    treatment, 82, 254
O'Connor, D.J., 210, 211
O'Connor, N., 102
Oedipal stage, 6
O'Leary, K.D. and S.G., 255
Oliver, J.E., 233
Operant conditioning, 253, 254
Oral stage/conflict, 2, 76
Orphanages, 60, 168, 267
Orphenadrine, 109
Orvaschel, H., 85
Osofsky, J.D., 184
Overactivity, 185, *see also* Hyper-
    kinetic syndrome
Overanxious disorder, 73, 79
Overprotection, 90, 91, 171, 174,
    175, 182

Pad and buzzer, 124
Panic disorder, 74, 79
Paradox/paradoxical intention, 245
Paranoid ideas, 144
Paranoid schizophrenia, 113
Parental child, 30
Parental depression, 70, 86
Parental deprivation, 30
Parental mental illness, 271
Parent groups, 252
Patterson, G.R., 255
Peabody Picture Vocabulary Test,
    219
Peer group influences, 205
Penicillamine, 109
Penrose, L., 20
Peptic ulcer, 173, 174, 179
Periodic syndrome, 173, 178
Perphenazine, 114, 256, 257
Personality
    categories, 145, 146
    disorders, 35, 142—150
    tests, 217, 222—224
Pervasive developmental disorder, 95,
    102
Petit mal, 157—158
Petri-Larmi, M., 154
Phenobarbitone, 61, 157, 255
Phenothiazine drugs, 110, 114, 137,
    198, 215, 255—257, 259
Phenylketonuria, 20—21

Phenylpyruvic oligophrenia, 20—21
Philadelphia Child Guidance Clinic,
    183
Philipp, R., 252
Phobias/phobic disorders, 74, 77, 78,
    79—80, 211
    monosymptomatic/simple, 77, 80,
    253—254
Physical handicap, 173
Physical illness, 270
Piaget, J., 1, 3, 5, 10, 12, 15
Piazza, E., 183
Pica, 190—191
Pinkerton, P., 129, 133, 173
Playgroup(s), 9, 247
Pneumonia, 119
Poisons, 270
Polygenic influences, 21, 22, 135
Pond, D., 160
Positive peer culture, 71
Positive reinforcement, 254
Post-traumatic stress disorder, 74
Pot, 210
Power, M.J., 63
Poznanski, E.O., 116
Pragmatic abilities, 166
Pre-conceptual stage, 10
Pregnancy, 205
    risk factors, 270
Premature birth, 22
Premature infants, 22, 192
Prematurity, 270
Pre-operational period, 10, 12
Pre-school period, 5—10
Prevalence of disorders, 38, 268—269
Prevention of child psychiatric
    disorders, 268—278
Preventive intervention, 274
Preventive measures, 272—275
Primary experience, 143
Primary prevention, 268, 269—275
Principles of Primary Prevention, 269
Problem solving, 51
Projection, 7—8
Promethazine, 259
Promiscuity, 116
Pronominal reversal, 99, 103
Protective factors, 271—272
Provence, S., 9
Pseudosomatic disorders, 173
Psychoanalysis, 243
Psychogenic amnesia, 74

Psychogenic fugue, 74
Psychomotor retardation, 213
Psychosexual disorders, 149
Psychosis/psychotic disorders,
 94–120, 122
 classification, 94–95
 definition, 94
 in adolescence, 203
Psychosocial stressors, 35
Psychosomatic disorders, 173–183
Psychosomatic Families, 175
Puig-Antich, J., 114, 116, 117, 256

Rantala, S.L., 154
Rapoport, J., 137
Rationalisation, 7
Raven's Progressive Matrices, 219
Reaction formation, 7
Reading quotient, 162
Reading retardation, 66, *see also*
 Specific reading retardation
Reed, G.F., 156
Rees, H.M.R., 100, 168
Reframing, 245
Regression, 122, 130, 170
Reinforcement/reinforcing behaviour,
 61
Reisman, J., 262
Rejection/rejecting attitudes, 62, 115
Remedial education/teaching, 71, 137
 164
Removal from parental care, 241,
 265–267
Repression, 7
Residential treatment, 71, 104, *see
 also* Inpatient treatment
Resonance, 50
Respondent conditioning, 253
Response prevention, 82, 254
Retentive soiling, 129–130
Reversed caring, 235
Reynell Developmental Language
 Scales, 224
Richman, N., 185, 187
Rigidity, in families, 174, 175, 182
Risk factors in primary prevention,
 269–271
Ritalin, *see* Methylphenidate
Rituals, 81
Rivinus, T.M., 84
Robins, L., 72, 93, 216
Robinson, H.B., 22

Rocking, 100, 198
Roles (in families), 52, 63
Rolfe, J.E., 269
Rollins, N., 183
Rorschach Test, 222
Rosenthal, M.J., 213
Rowe, P., 10
Rubella, 22, 97, 270
Rubinstein, J.S., 72
Running away, 64, 86, 87, 116, 144,
 207, 212
Russell, G.F.M., 165, 182, 183
Rutter, M., 10, 14, 15, 23, 30, 31, 33,
 37, 38, 48, 60, 62, 63, 66, 69,
 72, 75, 96, 97, 98, 103, 111,
 128, 135, 161, 162, 163, 193,
 195, 196, 201, 203, 204, 216,
 272, 273, 274, 275

Safer, D.J., 135, 136
Sallade, J., 179
Sameness, desire for in autism, 100,
 102
Sarafino, E.P., 238
Savicki, V., 47
Scapegoat/scapegoating, 29–30,
 63, 115, 261
Schilder, P., 82
Schilder's disease, 109
Schinke, S.P., 205
Schizoid personality, 143–145, 146
Schizophrenia/schizophrenic
 psychosis, 98, 111–114, 181
 causes, 111
 description, 111–114
 in adolescence, 211
 outcome, 114
 prevalence, 111
 treatment, 114, 259
Schizophrenic syndrome of childhood,
 95
Schmitt, B.D., 136
Schneider, K., 112
Schofield, M., 14
School counsellors, 247
School environment/influences,
 30–31, 63
School failure, 64
School phobia, *see* School refusal
School refusal, 65, 77, 88–90, 144
 in adolescence, 202, 211
 treatment, 91–92

Schools for maladjusted children, 264
Scott, P., 233, 235, 237
Secondary prevention, 268, 275–276
Second year, 3–5
Self-esteem, 11
Self-help groups, 275
Senokot, 133
Sensori-motor period, 3
Separation anxiety/disorder, 2, 3, 73,
    79, 88, 90
Serotin, 151
Sex differences in susceptibility to
    stress, 271
Sex play, 6, 10
Sex role, 6, 205
Sexual abuse, 237–239
Sexual development, 6, 13–14, 200,
    205
Sexual misconduct, 64, 66
Sexual molestation, 235
Sgroi, S.M., 235
Shafer, G., 238
Shaffer, D., 37, 118, 123, 124, 135,
    212
Shepherd, M., 191
Shields, J., 21, 22
Silver, H.K., 179
Simmons, J.E., 48
Skynner, A.C.R., 30, 77, 90, 91
Slade, P.D., 165
Sleep apnoea, 189
Sleep disorder/difficulty, 46, 78, 86,
    116, 137, 173
    drug treatment, 259
Sleep problems, in young children,
    187–189, 191
Sleep-walking, 188
Sloman, L., 154
Sluckin, A., 133
Snake phobia, 253
Social environment, 31
Social learning theory, 252
Social phobia, 73, 80
Social service departments, 267
Social skills development, 252
Social work(ers), 246–247
Soiling, 173, *see also* Encopresis
Solvent inhalation, 210–211
Somatisation disorder, 74
Somatoform disorders, 74
Somatopsychic disorders, 173
Sours, J.A., 48

Sparks, R., 68
Specific arithmetical retardation, 161,
    164–165
Specific developmental disorders, 35,
    161–172
Specific motor retardation, 161,
    171–172
Specific reading retardation, 66,
    162–165, 204
Speech development, 4
Speech disorders, 167–169
Speech therapy, 156, 241, 265
Spelling difficulty, 163, 164
Sphingolipids, 109
Spitz, R., 116
Stammering, *see* Stuttering
Stanford–Binet Intelligence Scale,
    218–219
Stanley, L., 82
Stealing, 64, 65, 144
Stephans, J.H., 152
Stewart, M., 135
Stewart, M.A., 59
Stimulant drugs, 255
Stott, D.H., 275
Strachan, J.G., 69
Stranger anxiety, 3, 8
Strategic therapy, 244–246
Streissgarth, A.P., 23
Sturge, C., 163
Stuttering, 153–154, 195
Subacute sclerosing panencephalitis,
    110
Sublimation, 68, 88
Suicide/suicidal behaviour, 115,
    118–119, 144, 212, 213–214,
    215, 260
Supportive therapy, 243, 244
Sussenwein, F., 246
Swinson, R., 35
Syllabic speech, 154
Syntax, 165, 167
Syphilis, 22, 270
Systematic desensitisation, 253
Systems/systems theory, 17, 27–30
Systems therapy, 247
Szurek, S.A., 103

Tantrums, *see* Temper tantrums
Tay-Sachs disease, 109
Temperament/temperamental
    characteristics or styles, 2, 11,

20, 22, 25–26, 61, 136, 184, 187, 271
Temper tantrums, 4, 9, 64, 66, 136, 144, 157, 186–187, 198
  behaviour therapy for, 254
Temporal lobe epilepsy, 157, 159
Tertiary prevention, 268, 276
The Clumsy Child, 172
Thematic Apperception Test, 222
The Residential Psychiatric Treatment of Children, 262
Thioridazine, 256, 257
Thomas, A., 2, 25, 26, 61
Thompson, L.J., 163
Thought
  blocking, 112
  broadcasting, 113
  disorder, 112, 113
  insertion, 112, 113
  withdrawal, 113
Tics, 151–152
Tizard, J., 193, 195
Tobacco, 210
Token economy, 254
Torgersen, A.M., 22, 26
Toughlove, 275
Tourette's disorder/syndrome, 152
Toxaemia of pregnancy, 270
Toxoplasmosis, 22, 270
Tracking, 248
Training schools, 266–267
Tranquillisers, 72, 210
Transactional patterns, 51
Transitional objects, 8–9
Transitional phenomena, 9
Transition points, 18–19
Triclofos, 259
Tricyclic antidepressants, 91, 124, 257–258
Truancy, 65, 88, 116, 160, 164
  treatment, 71–72
Tuberous sclerosis, 108
Turgay, A., 84–85
Twin studies, 21, 26, 96, 122, 123

Ulcerative colitis, 173, 178, 181
Unintegrated children, 143

Van Buskirk, S.S., 183
Vandalism, 64, 68
Vandsersall, A., 69
Vineland Social Maturity Scale, 223

Visuo-spatial difficulties, 163
Von Bertalanffy, L., 27
Von Bogaert's disease, 110
Vorrath, H.H., 71, 261
Voyeurism, 149
Vrono, M., 111

Wagner, B.R., 254
Wallerstein, J., 144
Walton, J.N., 171
Wardle, C.J., 58, 62
Wechsler Intelligence Scale for Children, 171, 193, 217–218
Wechsler Pre-School and Primary School Intelligence Scale, 218
Weinstein, P., 189
Weiss, G., 137
Welfare feelings, 53
Wender, P., 136
Werry, J.S., 124, 136, 260
West, D.J., 274
Whitmore, K., 193, 195
Whittaker, J.K., 262
Whitten, C.F., 179
WHO, see World Health Organisation
Wide Range Achievement Test, 221
Wieder, H., 215
Wiener, J.M., 69, 260
Wilson, J., 106
Wilson's disease, 108
Wiltshire, England, study of child abuse in, 233
Wing, L., 96
Wingate, M.E., 154
Winnicott, D., 8, 61, 143, 148
Wolff, S., 143, 144
Wolkind, S., 30, 60, 62
World Health Organisation, 33, 58, 94, 134, 139, 161, 271
Writing disorder/difficulty, 163, 171
Wynn, A., 237

Yalom, I., 252
York, P. and D., 275
Young children's disorders, 184–192
  assessment, 186
  common problems, 186–192
  prevalence, 185–186
  treatment, 192
Youngerman, J., 259
Youth treatment centres, 150
Yule, W., 162, 163, 194, 198

Zax, M., 30